FIBRINOGEN

MEMOIRS

FIBRINOGEN MEMOIRS

Journeys of a Clot Doctor

Michael W. Mosesson

IPBooks Inc
New York• http://www.IPBooks.net

Fibrinogen Memoirs
Published by IPBooks, Queens, NY
Online at: www.IPBooks.net
Copyright © 2020 by Michael W. Mosesson

All right reserved. Printed in the United States of America. This book may not be reproduced, transmitted, or stored, in whole or in part by any means, including graphic, electronic, or mechanical without the express permission of the author and/or publisher, except in the case of brief quotations embodied in critical articles and reviews.

Cover Design original concept by Kathy Kovacic
Final Front and Back Cover Design by Lisa Roma Wacholder
Cover Micrographic Image courtesy of Michael W. Mosesson

ISBN 978-1-949093-65-0

Fibrinogen Memoirs: Journeys of a Clot Doctor / Michael W. Mosesson – 1st edition
Medicine – Science – Memoir – Blood
260 pp

DEDICATION

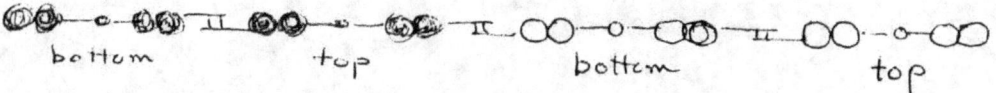

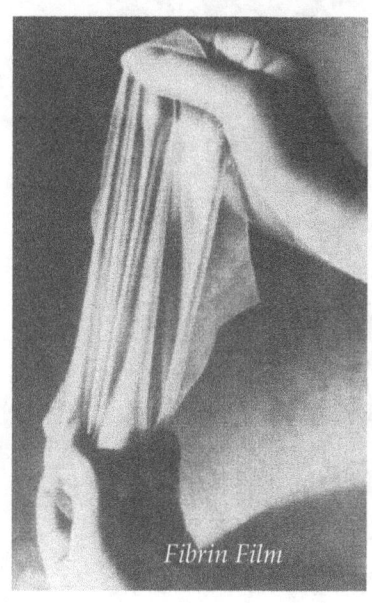
Fibrin Film

John Douglass Ferry (1912-2002) was a polymer chemist whose seminal contributions provided the framework for our present understanding of Fibrin assembly, structure, and elasticity. His published work and his insights are cited in several places in this book, most prominently in the chapter 'Fibrin, The Perfect Bioelastomer.' Ferry's prescient letter (*which contained the pencil drawing above*) led to a 'Eureka!' moment that clarified the ineluctable relationship between my proposed structure of an assembled fibrin polymer and its known elastic properties. I am grateful to have known him, befriended him, exchanged ideas, honored him, and profited from his remarkable abilities as a teacher and scientist.

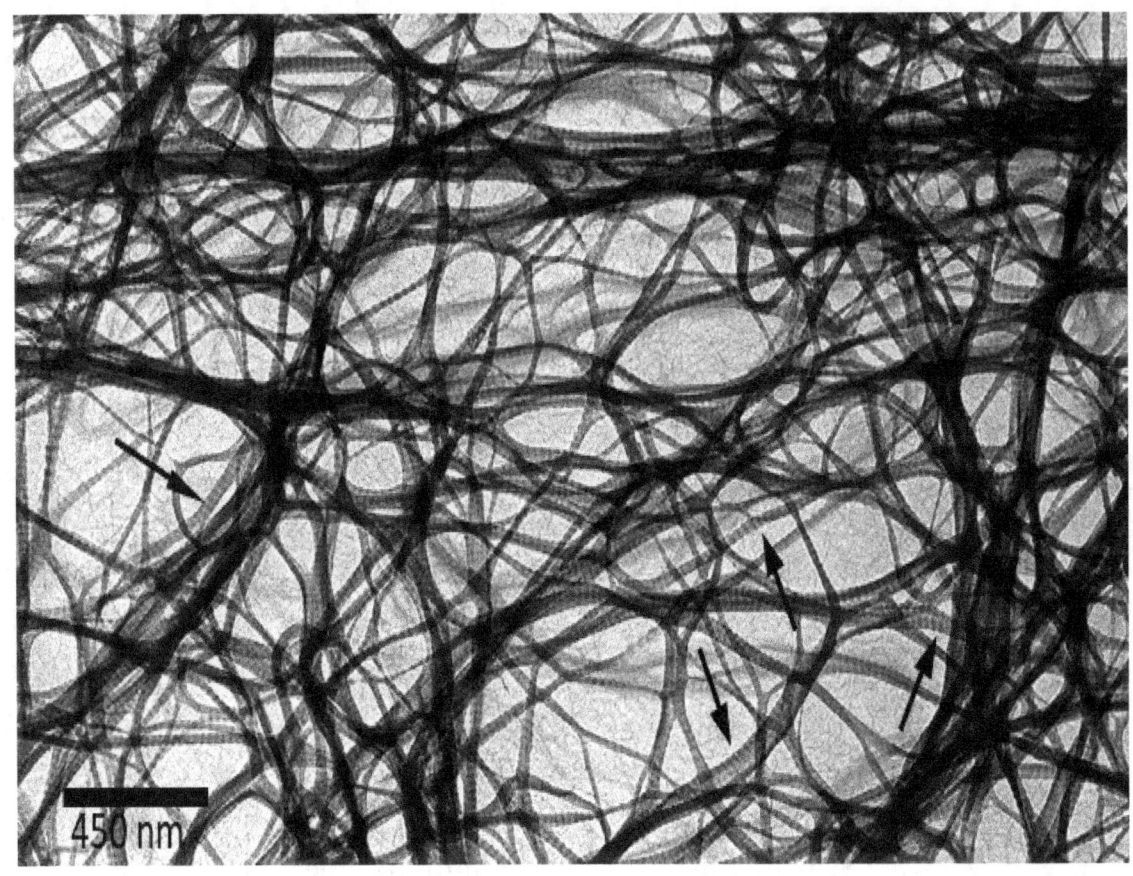

Cover Image: An electron micrographic image of the fibrin clot network shown on the cover. At this high magnification one can easily appreciate the cross-banding of network fibers (**arrows**). Spacing between bands is 22.5 nm [1 nm=10^{-9} meters], a length exactly one-half that of a fibrin molecule [ ]. The bar at the bottom left is 10 times the length of a fibrin molecule. The band spacing reflects a half-staggered arrangement of 45 nm fibrin molecules to form double-stranded 'thin' fibrils. These fibrils [ ] then associate side-to-side to form the branching thick fiber clot network shown above.

TABLE OF CONTENTS

COVER PAGE LEGEND		vii
ACKNOWLEDGEMENTS		x
PREFACE		xii
I.	THE TRANSITION TO A PHYSICIAN/SCIENTIST	1
II.	FIBRINOGEN 101	9
III.	PILOT IN COMMAND, 1961-2013	19
IV.	POTPOURRI OF DISCOVERIES AND REMEMBRANCES	33
V.	MY SEARCH FOR THE STRUCTURE OF FIBRINOGEN	61
VI.	FIBRIN, THE PERFECT BIOELASTOMER	77
VII.	MOLECULAR ARRANGEMENTS AT THE CORE OF FIBRIN BRANCHES	105
VIII.	ANTITHROMBIN I AND THE TRANSGENIC MOUSE THAT ROARED	111
IX.	THE FIBRINOLYTIC POTENTIAL OF BLOOD	125
X.	SWEET CLOVER DISEASE OF CATTLE AND THE PRODUCTION OF TRANSGENIC FIBRINOGEN IN COWS' MILK	151
XI.	ORIGINS OF THE INTERNATIONAL FIBRINOGEN RESEARCH SOCIETY *A Personal Account*	157
XII.	TRANSITIONS TO THE FOOD AND DRUG ADMINISTRATION *By John S. Finlayson*	161
ANNOTATED BIBLIOGRAPHY		213
THE AUTHOR		245

ACKNOWLEDGEMENTS

I began writing *Fibrinogen Memoirs* more than 11 years ago. After completing about ten chapters, I came to the belief that the subject matter might not appeal to a general audience. Accordingly, I printed out 25 copies and distributed them to some friends and scientific associates for review. Feedback was encouraging, but nevertheless I decided that was as far as I was going to go with publishing these stories. Some years later, I reconnected by chance with *Arnie Richards*, whom I knew as a fellow student from long gone days at Erasmus Hall High School, Brooklyn College, and SUNY-Downstate Medical Center. As our relationship rekindled, we spent profitable times together revisiting and recalling our lives and careers. This past March, shortly after COVID-19 had emerged in earnest in Florida, we met for lunch (outside) one day to continue our discussions. I knew that Arnie was a Psychoanalyst, but I did not know that he was also the Publisher of *IPBooks*. Our conversation turned to the Memoirs, and he agreed to review the manuscript. After he had read it, he enthusiastically encouraged me to pursue its publication with IPBooks. I am most grateful for that encouragement.

During my scientific career I have authored hundreds of peer-reviewed papers, review articles, book chapters, and compiled and edited books. 'Memoirs' is my first 'Storybook.' In that connection, I congratulate *Kathy Kovacic* for her skill in crafting the Book Cover design. Further, I was fortunate that *Lisa Roma Wacholder* undertook the task of editing the raw manuscript and turning it into Book form. Her contributions included not only expert formatting, layout and organization of text and figures, but she also helped perfect the final cover design, clarify much of the narrative by critiquing and by her abiding interest in gaining a 'non-technical' understanding of the contents. I am grateful for those efforts.

August 1, 2020

PREFACE

I began writing these chapters and sections more than 11 years ago while still a Senior Investigator at the Blood Research Institute. I hoped to convey how and why I undertook investigating Fibrinogen, Fibrin Network Assembly, Coagulation, Thrombosis, and Fibrinolysis, and identify the men and women who were my associates in those endeavors. During my long career I encountered many challenges and issues, most of which I was able to solve or resolve successfully. The narratives cover my successes and failures and include contextual descriptions of interactions with associates and co-workers. I hope in this manner to elucidate the personal circumstances that surrounded and influenced my work. I have also included a chapter on my flying career which began shortly after beginning my research career in 1961 and ended more than fifty years later near the end of that career. There is also a chapter containing a personal account of the founding of *The International Fibrinogen Research Society*.

I intend these chapters to be scientifically accurate representations of the problems and issues that I faced without excessive or confusing detail. Throughout I have flagged colleagues and associates who contributed to these works or to my activities. In one case [chapter IX) when I was unsuccessful in resolving an issue to my satisfaction, I appended a detailed roadmap for others to follow should they wish to. I tried to construct each chapter and frame each issue in a manner that would be understandable for readers without a formal background in blood coagulation, or protein chemistry. I also hope the book will serve as a valuable scientific and historical legacy for my colleagues, my children, and grandchildren, and for my many associates and friends.

I would be remiss if I did not thank John S. Finlayson for contributing a chapter concerned with the early days of the Division of Biologics Standards and its evolution as a part of the Food and Drug Administration (FDA). John played an important role in shaping my writing skills at the start of my career. He was a role model for his meticulous and unerring ability to clearly explain, discuss, and dissect scientific results. His influence on me has lasted for more than fifty years and we have never lost touch.

Finally, I am grateful that my wife Shirley graciously and lovingly put up with my many absences from home, my foibles, and enabled me to stay focused on what turned out to be my life's work.

Michael Mosesson   *April 27, 2020*

CHAPTER I

TRANSITION TO A PHYSICIAN / SCIENTIST

My Anna

I was born at The Beth Israel Hospital in Manhattan on the last day of 1934 and was named after my father's brother, Michael William, who had died in the 1918-1920 flu pandemic along with his sister, Anna Mosesson. When I was an infant, we moved to 420 Avenue "F" (Apartment 4E) in Flatbush, Brooklyn, a place that was to be home for the next 24 years. Difficult as those times were with America in the middle of The Great Depression', my folks had sufficient resources to hire a live-in Nanny, *Anna Stranzel*. Anna was 17 years of age at the time and came from a depressed coal-mining town in Pennsylvania called Scranton.

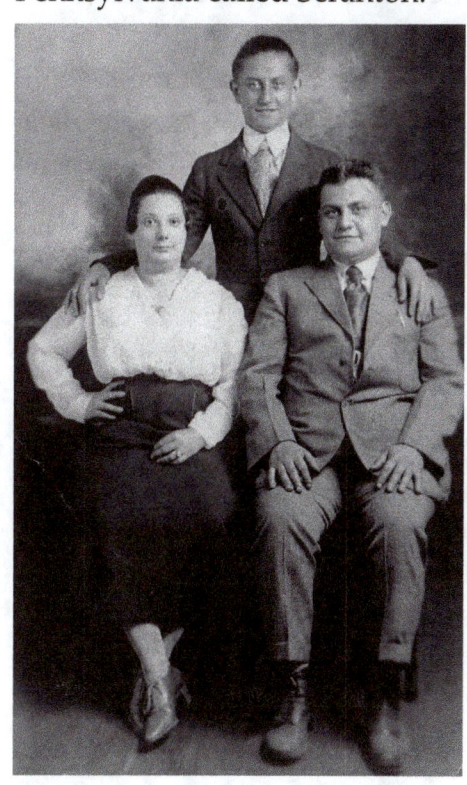

MWM-I is seated beside his wife, and my Dad, Benjamin, is standing.

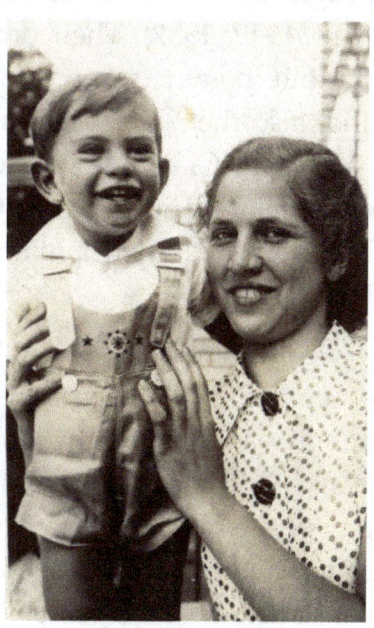

Me and my Anna.

My parents treated her like their own daughter, and for me she was always '*My Anna*.' I need no pictures to remember her face, her smile, and her love. Even at this end stage of my life, I sometimes still dream that Anna will 'show up' once again. Anna was my proxy mother for more than five years. Eventually, she returned to Scranton, and married, I was told. I know little more about her life away from us. She stayed in contact and for a few years came back to visit us. Those visits lasted until after grade school. Whenever she came to our apartment, I hugged her as I had often done before, and begged 'my Anna' not to leave me again. I am sure that at that time I resented her having left me without an explanation. I realize now how deeply I loved her and love her still. She fulfilled the role of *Mother* during an important phase of my life, and that memory remains with me.

The Brooklyn Dodgers

I lived at home until completing Medical School in 1959. It was relatively easy to support myself by working summers and holidays as a waiter/busboy in 'The Borscht Belt' (The Catskills) or in Atlantic City, New Jersey. One summer I ran an Arts and Crafts shop at a children's summer camp and doubled up as a Bunk Counselor. I had no prior experience in running an Arts and Crafts enterprise, but I easily mastered lanyard making, clay object casting and enameling, plus other sundry arts and crafts, and was able to meet The Camp Director's requirement that each camper bring home at least one completed project at summer's end.

I was a diehard fan of The Brooklyn Dodgers. It went without saying that if you rooted for The Dodgers you could not also be a New York Yankee or a New York Giants fan. The Yankees were important rivals of The Dodgers since they dominated American League baseball and tortured Dodger fans by beating them in four World Series (1941, 1947, 1949, 1952). Their domination ended in 1955 when Johnny Podres pitched a 2-0 shutout in game seven. It was the Brooklyn Dodgers' first World Series Championship, and, also their last, because after that season the franchise moved to Los Angeles. The New York Giants moved to San Francisco that same year, leaving The Yankees as the only major league baseball team in New York, a situation that remained until 1962 when The New York Metropolitans (The New York Mets) came to town with Casey Stengel as manager.

Although The New York Giants did not usually field good teams, there was one exception in 1951. By August of that year The Dodgers had a 13-game lead on The Giants, and I was confidently looking forward to another World Series encounter with the Yankees. That did not happen. The Dodgers and Giants wound up in a flat tie on the last day of the regular season, forcing a deciding playoff game that took place at the oblong shaped Polo Grounds, then The Giants' home field. The Polo Grounds had been constructed for the game of Polo, not for baseball. The centerfield wall was over 600 feet from home plate, a distance that was virtually impossible to reach on the fly. It was there that Willie Mays once made an amazing back-to-the-plate catch of a near 500+ foot fly ball that would have been an inside-the-park homerun, had he not caught up to it.

The left field foul pole was 270 feet away, a trivial distance that even an amateur like me could reach with a half decent swing. Ralph Branca, the ace of the Dodgers' staff, was pitching, and my Mother (by then an ardent Dodgers fan) and I were in our kitchen listening to the broadcast with the legendary Red Barber announcing for the Dodgers. Our vacuum tube radio was staring at us from a high shelf in the kitchen like the harbinger of doom it would soon turn out to be. The Dodgers were leading 4-2 with two outs in the bottom of the ninth. Giants runners were at first and second, and Branca was still pitching. Need I remind anyone of the outcome of that game. Bobby Thompson, a journeyman outfielder, hit a feeble pop fly to left field that barely cleared the fence just inside the foul pole only 260 feet from home plate. The Giants had won the game 5 to 4, and with it, the National League Pennant. Nothing could have been more devastating at the time. My Mom wept mostly in sympathy for me. Red Barber was not thrilled about this either, but Russ Hodges, the Giants' announcer, called it "the shot heard 'round the world." To this day, I wince whenever I hear an audio replay of that moment in 1951.

In 1955, the Dodgers finally beat the hated New York Yankees (who had beaten them every other time) in The World Series, and that afforded me a pleasant measure of retribution. A year later they departed Brooklyn for Los Angeles, and I progressively lost interest in the LA Dodgers and in baseball itself, as former Dodgers' players retired or were traded. Several years after moving back to SUNY Downstate in 1969 my interest in baseball was rekindled by the new baseball team in town, The New York 'Miracle' Mets. I had once again become a devoted, but better balanced, fan.

Brooklyn College and SUNY-Downstate Medical Center

At Brooklyn College I majored in Chemistry and minored in Biology and Physics. I was enthralled with Organic Chemistry, Biochemistry, and Biophysics. Had I not been admitted to Medical School I would have been just as happy to go to Graduate School to earn a PhD degree. Medical School, however, appealed to me more than graduate school because I wanted to gain the best possible perspectives on the pathophysiology of diseases. Nowadays with those goals, I would have opted for a combined MD/PhD program, but such programs were rare in those days. Most Physician-Scientists of my era had only an MD degree. The good ones had somehow 'bootlegged' their knowledge of basic or clinical science.

Throughout my time as a student I did not study for exams. I believed that examinations should test what I had learned, not what I could cram into my head immediately before an exam. That attitude notwithstanding, I achieved a 93+% overall score in the New York Regents Exams in High School (Erasmus Hall High School). At Brooklyn College, I had a 3.5+ GPA, and I graduated Magna Cum Laude from SUNY Downstate Medical School in 1959. Those grades, plus some other extra-curricular activities, landed me a much-coveted Internship at Boston City Hospital, II & IV Medical Services, Harvard Medical School Division. I was the first SUNY graduate to have been selected for Residency training on that service.

I had an intense interest in a Basic and/or Clinical Research career when I entered Medical School. To pursue those interests, I took several research electives during my third and fourth years. Professor *Victor Schenker*, a Biochemist in the Psychiatry Department, had been investigating a mood-altering substance that he had identified in saliva. He called it *Spitnik* (that name was coined in 1957 when the Russians had recently launched 'Sputnik'). I spent the better part of two years trying to develop a biological *assay* for identifying and measuring Spitnik's effects. Spitnik turned out to be a vasoactive amine compound, and although I had developed a workable assay using Rabbit Aortic Strips, the project was scrapped by the good Professor, who had found an easier way to measure Spitnik.

I also spent an elective Clerkship with *Dr. William Dock*, ('Doctor Dock' as we affectionately called him), a renowned self-styled cardiologist who had invented a device called the 'Ballisto-cardiogram,' capable of measuring normal and abnormal cardiac motion by accurately recording the directional forces imparted to a subject's body by the heart's contractions.

I especially valued the elective time I spent with *Clarence Dennis*, the Chairman of the Surgery Department, an excellent teacher, and meticulous and gifted surgeon. His surgical outcomes were outstanding with respect to his patients' rapid and relatively pain-free post-operative recoveries. Even more interesting for me was Dennis' research on The Bubble Oxygenator, a cardiac bypass device for carrying out open heart surgery while cardiac circulation had been bypassed and heart action arrested. Dennis was trying to extend the capacities of Johns Hopkins surgical greats Henry Blalock and Helen Taussig, who had developed surgical approaches for mitigating certain congenital heart disorders at a time when no cardiac bypass device existed. Such devices are now in routine use worldwide.

I told Professor Dennis that I was interested in becoming a surgeon and pursuing a research career that involved research projects like his on the bubble oxygenator. He was supportive and advised me on how to approach my goal: "Take residency training on a Medical service for two years, then come back to SUNY for a Surgical Residency under my direction." I immediately bought into that suggestion, a plan that led to me applying to the Boston City Hospital for a Medical Residency. I am certain that Drs. Dock and Dennis were players in pulling strings behind the scenes for me to obtain that premier Internship.

My Internship in Boston lasted for only one year and was followed by my move to NIH *(National Institutes of Health)* at The Division of Biologics Standards (DBS). I never returned for surgical training, although I maintained contact with Professor Dennis who was supportive of the new direction that I had taken.

Medical Residency at Boston City Hospital

When I started Residency training at Boston City, I did not have a working knowledge of patient care. I had not yet learned how to go about *working patients up*, as the saying went, writing orders, choosing diagnostic and therapeutic options, and so forth. Initially I received little guidance from my immediate supervisors, the Senior Residents, and sometimes felt I had been misled.

The second Resident I encountered in my second week, *Harry Jacob*, informed me that most patients admitted to our Medical Service were presumed to be malingerers. He encouraged me to *"try to sign them out"* AMA ('Against Medical Advice') regardless of their initial complaints or problems. His favorite ploy was to enter the hospital room with a Sigmoidoscope in his hand and suggest to the hapless and helpless patient that he was going to stick this instrument up someone's behind. Many patients did sign out rather than undergo what Harry was offering. Many patients must have been harmed by that behavior. I refused to consider such things, and we did argue about it. Fortunately for me, my time with Jacob lasted only a few days.

I next encountered *Thomas Merigan*, a self-aggrandizing second year Resident Physician who spent most of his time in the library reading when he should have been available to supervise and help us. He was always prepared with new *'to do lists,'* but was conspicuously absent when physical help was needed. On one notable occasion I was elbows deep trying to stabilize a sick patient who was vomiting blood. My working diagnosis was Alcoholism, bleeding Esophageal Varices, and Delirium Tremens (DTs). Merigan entered the room with a medical journal tucked under his arm. I looked at him pleadingly: "Do you have time to pull on the Sengstaken tube (*an inflatable nasogastric balloon catheter that is inserted into the stomach, inflated, and then pulled backwards in order to control bleeding at the esophageal-gastric junction*) while I start a blood transfusion?" He looked at me querulously: "You're doing really good guy. Keep it up! I'll be in the library if you need me. And don't forget to do a platelet count."

After about six weeks of experiences like those, I became disillusioned. While I was in that frame of mind, *Charles Davidson*, the Clinical Director of our service, invited me to his office for a meeting. Davidson was openly gay, as were many of the Staff on our Service. 'Charlie' had a distressingly loud laugh that usually emerged as: *"Ho! Ho! Ho!"* After we had exchanged a few pleasantries he asked me whether I would be interested in the second year of Residency at Boston City. I should have said YES immediately, of course. However, I had profited little from my first few weeks on the renowned Harvard service, which led to my reply, *"Dr. Davidson, I'll think about your offer and let you know in one week."*

As I found out later, he was hoping to replace one of the current First Year Residents with *Sandy Shapiro*, a former resident who had left BCH after one year's service to take a job at NIH in Bethesda, Maryland, and who now wished to return for a second Residency year.

One week later I informed Dr. Davidson that I had decided that I would like to stay on for a second year of residency, but he promptly replied that the position was no longer available to me. It had been offered to Sandy Shapiro. Our conversation ended with a hearty *"Ho! Ho! Ho!"* It would be an understatement to say that I was shocked and extremely dismayed.

A few days later, Professor *William B Castle*, The Chairman of our Medical Service, called me to his office. Castle had become famous for his discovery that the absence of *Gastric Intrinsic Factor* ('Castle's Factor'), led to a potentially fatal disease, *Pernicious Anemia*. He was a member of the prestigious 'National Academy of Sciences.' I had never spoken with him prior to that meeting but like most others, I held him in awe.

Castle was not at all imperious in his attitude as I had imagined he might be. He was polite and genuinely concerned with my predicament. He indicated that he could arrange for me to go to NIH to take Sandy Shapiro's position at The Division of Biologics Standards, a position that would require enlisting in the US Public Health Service to satisfy my military service requirement, in force at that time. He assured me that after I had completed my service at NIH, I would be welcomed back to Boston City to continue my residency training. That meeting had a magical elevating effect on my spirits, as I began to recognize a golden opportunity unfolding.

My First Real Romance

I shared a two-bedroom apartment in Beacon Hill, near Massachusetts General Hospital, with a former fellow summer camp co-counselor, tennis partner, and perpetual womanizing friend, *John Marshall (Jack) Frost*. Jack was in Boston studying Dentistry. Due to his gregariousness, I never felt like a stranger and acclimated easily to my new life in Boston. He introduced me to *Lorinda (Linda) Bleumer*, a charming, intelligent, caring, and quick-witted young lady. It was virtually 'love at first sight' for me, and we quickly became an item.

During that year Linda kept raising the subject of marriage. I was not at all averse to that idea. I brought her to Brooklyn to meet my parents. Linda did not make a hit with my parents entirely because she was not Jewish, and they let me know it. I was undaunted at first. A few weeks after our trip to Brooklyn my Mom sent my Father to Boston to dissuade me from considering marriage. He was an unwilling messenger and seemed uncomfortable representing something that he did not enthusiastically embrace. He and I sat together on a park bench in Boston Commons on a spring day while we went back and forth on the subject of marriage. I made it clear that coercion would not be effective and that I would make my own decisions. Nevertheless, their objections had raised doubts in my mind.

By the time I left Boston for NIH in July 1961 all I wanted was to simplify my life and postpone any decision concerning marriage. That did not sit well with Linda and our affair ended a few months after my arrival in Washington.[1] On the brighter side, the affair with Fibrinogen had now begun.

Michael Mosesson   May 24, 2015

---

[1] Linda has contacted me a few times during the past fifty years, by phone, once by Facebook, or by e-mail. These contacts were sometimes separated by twenty years or more. I was never offended or put off by her efforts because of the sincerity, warmth and charm she brought to each encounter. In fact, I looked forward to hearing from her and was flattered that she had not forgotten me.

CHAPTER II

FIBRINOGEN 101

THE PREPARATION OF HUMAN FIBRINOGEN FREE OF PLASMINOGEN

MICHAEL W. MOSESSON

*National Institutes of Health, Division of Biologics Standards,
Bethesda, Md. (U.S.A.)*

(Received July 4th, 1961)

SUMMARY

L-Lysine and ε-aminocaproic acid were shown to change the solubility characteristics of human fibrinogen and plasminogen in a manner that has been utilized to prepare fibrinogen free of this proenzyme.

When a solution of human fibrinogen in 0.3 M NaCl was diluted with lysine solution (pH 7.0) to a final concentration of 0.1 M lysine and precipitated at an ethanol concentration of 7%, fibrinogen containing less than one tenth of the original plasminogen was obtained in 95% yield. By repeating this procedure all detectable plasminogen may be removed. No loss of clottability or sensitivity to plasmin occurred, nor were there any detectable changes in the electrophoretic or sedimentation behavior of the fibrinogen.

INTRODUCTION

Fibrinogen and fibrin constitute the most sensitive substrates available for the assay of the plasma enzyme, plasmin. Most of the proteins which co-precipitate with fibrinogen during fractionation from plasma are relatively easy to remove by subsequent extraction or reprecipitation procedures. Plasminogen, the precursor of plasmin, has a great affinity for fibrinogen, as is evidenced by the great difficulty in removing completely all detectable amounts of the proenzyme. Even preparations of the highest purity[1] have appreciable amounts of plasminogen in the final product. This inability to separate plasminogen from fibrinogen has limited its usefulness as a substrate for plasmin in the presence of activators.

Some of the previous efforts at separation of these two proteins have been based upon the fact that plasminogen in the presence of fibrinogen is less soluble at low pH than is fibrinogen. Use has been made of this by KEKWICK *et al.*[2] in their ether fractionation method and by others[3] in applying the extraction procedure of LAKI[4] to achieve preparations which are relatively low in plasminogen. BLOMBÄCK AND BLOMBÄCK[1], on the other hand, employed glycine, which has a greater solubilizing effect on plasminogen than on fibrinogen to prepare fibrinogen low in proenzyme.

Abbreviations: ε-ACA, ε-aminocaproic acid; UK, urokinase; SK, streptokinase; HF, human fibrinogen.

The Division of Biologics Standards

In July 1960, I departed from Boston to fill Sandy (Sandor) Shapiro's vacated position at The Division of Biologics Standards (DBS) on the NIH campus. Sandy had effectively changed places with me by returning to Boston City Hospital to complete his medical residency. Although we did not meet each other until years later, I learned about him through John Finlayson and others, and I liked what I had heard. When we finally met several years later, he was at The Cardeza Foundation in Philadelphia and I had recently relocated to The Downstate Medical Center in Brooklyn, New York. Our friendship blossomed quickly and remained vibrant throughout our lives. Sandy, a brilliant violinist and superb scientist, was like a brother to me. Sadly, he left this world too soon (*see Photo*).

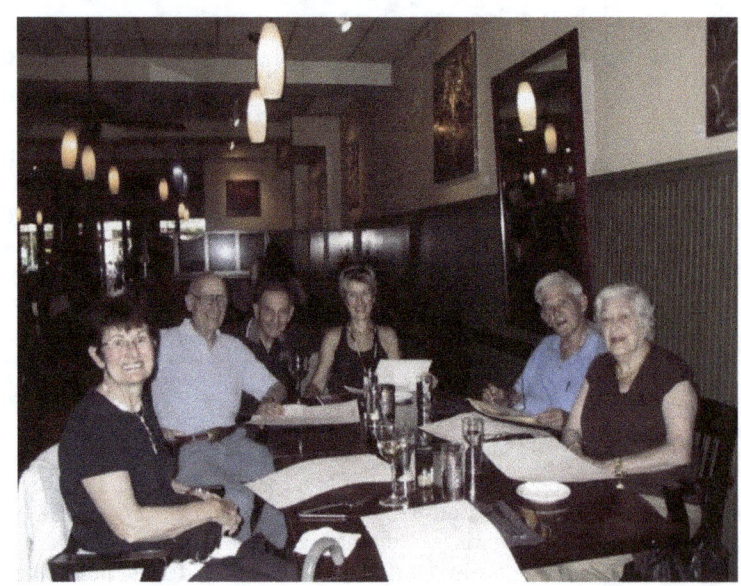

Photo (l-r): Shirley Mosesson, Sandy Shapiro, myself, Susan Rittenhouse Shapiro, David Aronson and his wife Doris Ménaché. A Memorial Day weekend 'DBS reunion' in 2007 in Burlington, VT, that took place a few weeks before Sandy's tragic 'sudden death' while bike riding.

The position at NIH served both as a primer for my research development that I call *'Fibrinogen 101'* and to also satisfy my military service requirement as a Senior Assistant Surgeon in the Public Health Service (PHS). My job titles at The Laboratory of Blood and Blood Products (LBBP) at DBS included *'Blood Bank Inspector.'* In that capacity I spent a lot of time traveling from one Blood Bank to another, tracking down and verifying the records of blood suppliers who had illegally updated time-expired blood units and then reissued them with new *'expiration dates'*, ostensibly to increase their profits. The results of such fraudulent activities were sometimes catastrophic for the recipients of outdated blood units and ranged from failure to raise the hemoglobin level, to severe kidney damage, or worse. But most of my time at DBS was spent in my LBBP laboratory or at the NIH library.

The important scientist/investigators at LBBP, from my perspective, were *David L. Aronson* (DL) and *John Finlayson*. Aronson was studying prothrombin and other vitamin K-dependent clotting factors, while Finlayson worked on immunoglobulins and plasma albumin. Most of the other staff dealt with blood product regulation or were designated blood bank inspectors. DL and I shared an office/laboratory and a makeshift desk. Our shared 'desk' consisted of a 2 by 3-foot pedestal across which a 2 by 6 foot 'tabletop' had been positioned, with DL on one side and me on the other *(see photo)*. Aronson kept virtually every document and most of his books on his desk, whereas I used my side of the tabletop for writing. That setup resembled an unbalanced seesaw. To compensate for the imbalance, I would slide the tabletop toward me, but David soon ran out of storage space. I then resorted to placing a water-filled four-liter bottle on my side to prevent the seesaw from tippling toward him. Eventually, DL agreed to move his 'filing cabinet' elsewhere.

DL was unkempt, seemed never to change shirts or wear clean pants. He had fathered four children with his wife Margie. At the time I arrived in Bethesda, their four children ranged in age from toddler to kindergarten age. I enjoyed playing with them and was a frequent visitor at their home. Margie had become an alcoholic, and their marriage fell apart. Eventually, DL changed his ways, most noticeably after he met *Doris Ménaché*, whom he married a few years after divorcing Margie. The *new* David Aronson dressed well, wore clean shirts and pants, a transformation that did not occur until after I had left at DBS.

DL earned his MD degree from Yale University and served a one-year internship at Mount Auburn Hospital in Boston. Shortly thereafter, he joined the Public Health Service as a commissioned Officer and wound up at DBS as a laboratory chief. Although he had a good understanding of the relevant regulatory problems facing DBS, he had developed few clinical skills, and removing stiches was not among them. I did not realize that until it was too late.

In 1962, while on a skiing trip in New Hampshire, I was struck in the mouth by a runaway ski and sustained a deep cut on my upper lip that required several stitches. A few days after returning from New Hampshire, I needed to have those stitches removed. DL volunteered and I accepted his offer. To my surprise he put on a pair of

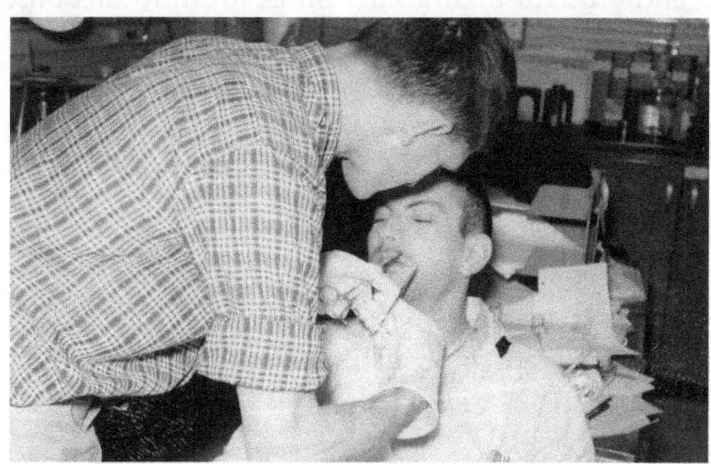

DL removing my stitches. Behind me is DL's side of our makeshift desk.

dishwashing gloves, picked up a forceps and scissors, and removed the stitches with only two painful miscues.

In contrast to Aronson, John Finlayson always dressed neatly, wore a clean lab coat, brought his lunch in the same brown bag every day, and was always well-organized. His office and laboratory were across the hall from mine. Despite their differences in style, they were intellectually well-matched and remained on good terms, at least as far as I could judge. I benefited from associating with them both, although I learned more about planning and executing experiments from John. When it came around to writing and organizing manuscripts, Finlayson's guidance and mastery of English grammar were invaluable. Over the years, I have continued to request that he read and critique many of my manuscripts, and he has never refused.

Finlayson had a keen sense of humor and was also a great storyteller. Still is! We spent hour after hour recounting and reworking stories about people we both knew, or people and situations from his days as a graduate student at The University of Wisconsin in Madison. To this day, I still retell some of his UW stories to anyone willing to listen.

This is one of my favorite Finlayson stories: I had been at DBS for about one year when an uncle of mine, Sidney Klausner, paid me a visit. I dutifully escorted him around the building, introducing him to my colleagues. Uncle Sid was not sophisticated as far as doctoral titles were concerned and so I tried to clarify each doctoral title. When it came time to introduce him to John, I said, *"Uncle Sid, this is Doctor John Finlayson, non-medical."* Finlayson cringed but did not reply. Some weeks later, John was escorting some of his own associates around the laboratory and brought them to my office for introductions. *"I would like to introduce you to Doctor Michael Mosesson, non-scientist!"* That was his belated but perfect response to my earlier introduction.

My First Publication, Plasminogen-Free Fibrinogen

The Division of Biologics Standards, which eventually became part of the Food and Drug Administration (FDA), was responsible for licensing and regulation of biologicals, including antisera and *'Fibrinolytic'* agents *(see John Finlayson's chapter)*. The first scientific problem assigned to me was to prepare purified plasma fibrinogen[1] that

---

[1]Glossary-

Fibrinogen- The blood protein that is the circulating precursor of fibrin clots that form in the circulation or at injury sites following conversion by thrombin.
Cohn methodology- EJ Cohn oversaw a research group during WWII which developed methods for 'fractionating' whole blood plasma into its major constituents
Precipitation- Causing an insoluble sediment to form in a solution.

was free of contaminating plasminogen. Having such material was deemed to be essential for solving a licensing issue at DBS, one concerned with measuring the composition and potency of fibrinolytic agents that were coming to market for treating intravascular thrombotic disorders, such as deep venous thrombosis (DVT) or Pulmonary Embolism (PE).

By 1961, there were several products being considered for licensure, each one intended as an injectable agent for producing an intravascular fibrinolytic state. This state could be achieved, 1) by infusion of the fibrinolytic enzyme plasmin, 2) by infusing a bacterial product called Streptokinase (SK) that converts inactive plasminogen to plasmin, or 3) by infusing some combination of these two agents. The problem was how to measure each component in the product itself to understand which one(s) were effective. The *'fibrinolytic'* potential of any agent was usually measured on a fibrin substrate that was invariably contaminated with plasminogen, the precursor of plasmin. In the presence of this contaminant, it was not possible to distinguish a plasminogen activator from the enzyme itself, plasmin.

SK itself is incapable of lysing fibrinogen, or fibrin, but when it combines with plasminogen (SK-plasminogen) the complex is then capable of converting plasminogen to plasmin. SK-containing products exhibit higher clot lysing *(fibrinolytic)* activity when measured on a fibrin substrate that contains plasminogen. The situation became more complicated when a product proposed for licensure contained both an activator and an enzyme, e.g., SK and plasmin. The solution to this problem was to prepare fibrinogen that was free of plasminogen, a feat that had not yet been accomplished.

During the first few months I learned how to separate plasma into its multiple constituent proteins, starting with reading published literature. These publications included the celebrated *'Cohn fractionation methodologies'* (1946-1951), John Ferry's fibrinogen/fibrin papers, John Edsel's and J. L. Oncley's books and articles dealing with biophysics and protein chemistry, Birger Blombäck's fibrinogen thesis (1956), and just about anything else I could find in the library about fibrinogen, plasminogen, or fibrinolysis. To further supplement my knowledge, I took evening courses at the US Department of Agriculture, including enzyme kinetics, protein chemistry, differential equations, and calculus.

Supernatant- The solution left behind after a precipitate is removed by centrifugation
Intravascular Fibrinolysis- Induction of a clot 'lytic' state within the vascular system
Streptokinase-a bacterial protein that activates fibrinolysis
FDA-The Food and Drug Administration
Trypsin-A pancreatic proteolytic enzyme that cleaves substrates like fibrin
Plasmin- A fibrinolytic blood enzyme produced from a precursor protein called plasminogen, by an activator like streptokinase.

Within a few weeks, I had devised a simple and effective procedure for preparing plasminogen-free fibrinogen, namely by precipitating plasminogen-contaminated fibrinogen in the presence of an amino acid, lysine, that competes with the lysine residues on fibrinogen that bind to plasminogen. The presence of lysine dissociates plasminogen from fibrinogen and permits fibrinogen to be precipitated with under standard conditions while leaving the plasminogen in solution. The title of the publication was: *'The Preparation of Human Fibrinogen Free of Plasminogen'* (1)(*see title page*). The product I had prepared provided a means for distinguishing unambiguously between activators and enzymes. I did not appreciate it at the time, but my research career had been launched based on that one discovery. I was invited to present my results on plasminogen-free fibrinogen at the 1962 annual meeting of the legendary Protein Foundation in Boston, and that same year I also presented my results in Mexico City, met Tony Fletcher, and after that eventful meeting, decided to move to St. Louis (*see 'My Search For The Structure of Fibrinogen'*).

Discoveries That Kept Me Busy

I soon came up with the idea that fibrinogen, once freed of contaminating plasminogen, could be used as an 'affinity reagent' to bind and remove plasminogen from plasma. Newly bound plasminogen could subsequently be separated from fibrinogen using my lysine dissociation procedure. The idea worked, but the amount of plasminogen that I recovered from plasma was exceedingly small, and I abandoned that approach. Only years later did I understand that failure to obtain larger amounts of plasma plasminogen using fibrinogen itself as an *affinity reagent* was because only *lys-plasminogen*, a minor component of the circulating plasminogen population, bound effectively to fibrinogen. *Glu-plasminogen*, the more abundant component, did not bind to fibrinogen. So much for that idea.

Since commercial preparations of *DEAE-cellulose* ion exchange resin were usually unsatisfactory, John Finlayson had synthesized his own resin. He guarded that DEAE (*diethylaminoethyl cellulose*) zealously, meticulously recovered every possible milligram of resin after using it for an experiment and regenerated its activity for future use.

In addition to applying *gradient elution ion exchange chromatography* for studying plasma albumin and immunoglobulins, John showed me how to use that technique for analyzing plasma fibrinogen. That collaborative work enabled us to distinguish two main chromatographic peaks containing what we termed 'Peak 1' and 'Peak 2' fibrinogen (2). We found similar chromatographic properties in several other species' fibrinogens (3). Further experiments led to stepwise elution methods for rapidly separating the fibrinogen peaks (4), and we identified other non-fibrinogen components in Peak 2 fibrinogen including factor XIII, and a plasmin inhibitory activity that I eventually identified as α2-antiplasmin (5). Later we would determine the unique fibrinogen γ chain amino acid sequences that accounted for the chromatographic properties of Peak 2 fibrinogen. That knowledge led me to the important discovery that Peak 2 fibrinogen was a potent thrombin inhibitor, an activity we termed *'Antithrombin I'*, and also that it bound and transported the Factor XIII in plasma *(see 'Antithrombin I')*.

Following our discovery of Peak 2 fibrinogen, John and I wondered what features might account for its behavior. The question we posed at the time was one we thought we could answer. Was it due to heterogeneity of the thrombin-cleavable 'fibrinopeptides'? Being located at NIH made it easy for us to get the help we needed, since we had only to walk across the campus to Harry Saroff's laboratory. Saroff, a well-known protein chemist, had the equipment and the know-how. He referred us to *Jules Gladner*, a member of his group who had worked on Bovine fibrinogen fibrinopeptides. Gladner was a Hobbit-like man (about 5' 2" and 110 pounds), whose bravado and boastfulness were inversely proportional to his diminutive size.

Gladner estimated that we would need 1 gram of peak 2 fibrinogen to properly analyze the fibrinopeptides, an unheard of quantity for us. We usually prepared milligram amounts, not grams. Nevertheless, John and I dutifully set about preparing that amount of fibrinogen. I fractionated fibrinogen from plasma day after day, and together we ran many DEAE chromatography columns to separate Peak 1 from Peak 2. After eight weeks we had prepared only 700 mg of peak 2 fibrinogen.

With that amount of fibrinogen in hand we sheepishly asked Gladner whether that amount of fibrinogen would suffice. "Don't worry," he said, "if it doesn't work on our first try, we can always collect the material from the chromatography paper and run the analysis again." We converted the entire 700 mg of Peak 2 to fibrin by adding thrombin, collected the fibrinopeptide-rich supernatant fraction, concentrated it, and placed the product in Gladner's hands. We did not learn until later that Gladner had turned our material over to *Robert Colman*, a post-doctoral Fellow, who I later came to know better in St. Louis at Barnes Hospital. I wish we had realized sooner that Colman had such limited laboratory 'bench' skills. Two weeks later Colman telephoned us: "I ran the material and the chromatogram did not come out. Do you have another gram of fibrinogen?" We pleaded, "Did you recover the peptide spots so we might run them again?" "Didn't Gladner tell you that you should have done that?" "No," he responded, "it was too much work and I threw the chromatogram paper away."

I had not seen John Finlayson, who ordinarily was even-tempered, become angry, but he did just that! He put down what he was doing, raced (he was a pretty good runner) across the NIH campus with me trailing behind, and entered Gladner's lab. At 5' 9" an enraged Finlayson towered over 5'2" Jules.

"You! You! You threw out the fibrinopeptides?" he gesticulated. "You didn't tell Colman to collect the material from that run?"

Gladner casually responded. "No, I forgot, and besides, I thought you guys could easily prepare more. After all, it's just fibrinogen."

I had to physically restrain Finlayson from annihilating Gladner on the spot. I am sure he would have extended that to dismembering Colman if I had not reminded him that murder could not resurrect our lost fibrinogen. We left in angry silence after considerable discussion and headed back to Building 29 (DBS). We did not attempt to repeat the monumental task that had consumed two full months of our time. As it turned out, Fibrinopeptide variants were not the answer to our problem, and we did not learn for several years that Peak 2 fibrinogen could be accounted for by a γ chain variant called γ' *(see 'Antithrombin I')*. That tale is told elsewhere.

In 1963, having completed 'Fibrinogen 101', I moved to St. Louis to complete my clinical training, and to work with *Sol Sherry*, the guru of fibrinolysis. I was not yet through with Colman, who happened to turn up there as one of Sol Sherry's Fellows. We had to share the laboratory's cold room space, and Colman soon proceeded to mess up several of my chromatography experiments as the designated *Klutz*. Somewhat later he was recruited to Philadelphia by Sol Sherry as a part of Sherry's move to become Chairman of the Department of Medicine at Temple University. Colman eventually became Director of *The Sol Sherry Thrombosis Center*, a position that Sol had first offered to me. Unfortunately, his offer came after I had become settled in my new position at SUNY and I felt obliged to refuse. C'est La Vie.

Michael Mosesson   May 8, 2015

References

1. Mosesson,M.W. 1962. The preparation of human fibrinogen free of plasminogen. *Biochim Biophys Acta* **57**:204-213.
2. Finlayson,J.S., and Mosesson,M.W. 1963. Heterogeneity of human fibrinogen. *Biochemistry* **2**:42-46.
3. Finlayson,J.S., and Mosesson,M.W. 1964. Chromatographic heterogeneity of animal fibrinogens. *Biochim Biophys Acta* **82**:415-417.
4. Mosesson,M.W., and Finlayson,J.S. 1963. Subfractions of human fibrinogen: preparation and analysis. *J Lab Clin Med* **62**:663-674.
5. Mosesson,M.W., and Finlayson,J.S. 1963. Biochemical and chromatographic studies of certain activities associated with human fibrinogen preparations. *J Clin Invest* **42**:747-755.

CHAPTER III

PILOT IN COMMAND, 1961-2013

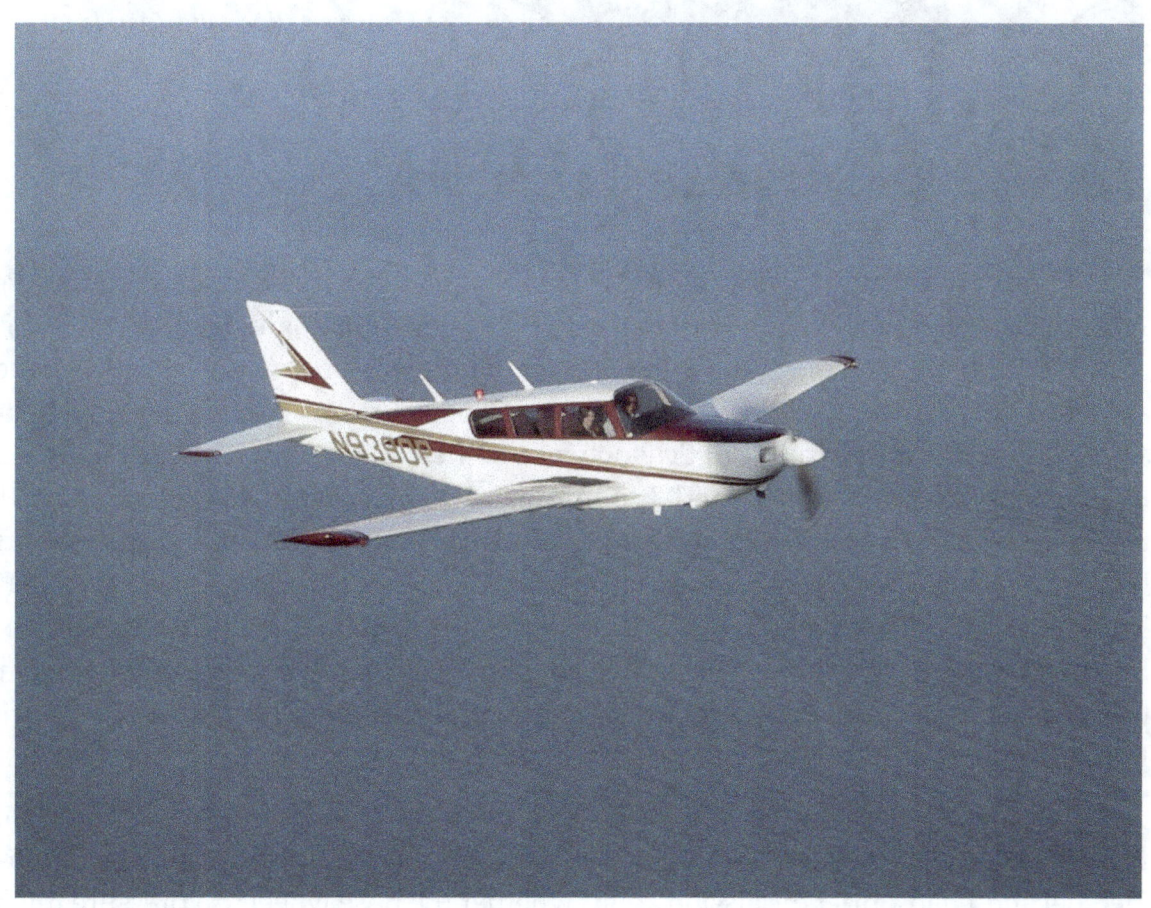

Piper Tripacer N8827C

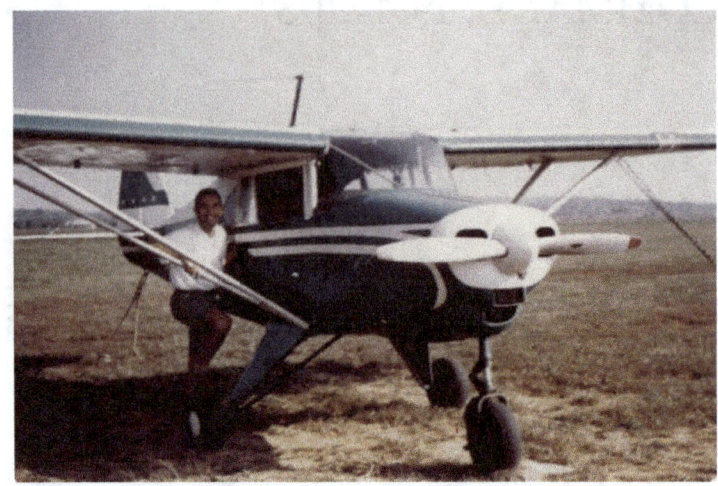

The author posing with his Piper Tripacer N8827C, Frederick Airport, Rockville, Maryland.

Both my piloting career and my career as a scientist lasted more than fifty years. A few weeks after I had begun working at The Division of Biologics Standards (DBS), one of my coworkers, *Bob Scheno*, dared me to take a flying lesson. I was up for the challenge and together we went to The Gaithersburg Airport for our first flying experience. I enjoyed that day immensely, but Scheno was terrified. He never went back for a second look or a lesson. On the other hand, I soon began taking flying lessons in a Cessna 150, a two-seater, and soloed after 20 hours of dual instruction. Shortly after that, I joined the Bethesda Flying Club and completed my pilot training in the club's green and white Piper *Tripacer* (N8827C) (see photo) at the Frederick Airport in Rockville, Maryland. My instructor was *Hershel Gibbs*, a decorated Korean War F-86 flying ace, whom I admired because he was so calm and unflappable, and an inspiring teacher. I passed my Private Pilot's license exam after having logged 74 total flying hours.

In March 1962, during a night training mission with Hershel and a new friend, Herb Rosenberger, we landed at the Harrisburg Airport in Pennsylvania. After landing, Hershel and I had a brief discussion about whether the nose wheel tire pressure might be low.

This was Rosenberger's first ride in a small airplane. He was seated behind us, listened to our conversation, and volunteered to inspect the nose wheel to see whether it needed air. Hershel and I both directed him to stay in the plane. Instead, he mindlessly unbuckled his seat belt, disembarked through the left rear door, ducked under the wing, and headed straight for the nose of the plane while the engine was idling and the prop turning.

We both shouted at him, but he was too focused on getting to the front wheel to pay attention to us. As soon as I recognized what he was intent on doing, I pulled the mixture control full back to starve the engine of fuel, but the shutdown process took more than five seconds to occur.

The engine did eventually quit, but not before Rosenberger had been struck by the rotating propeller blade. The upwardly rotating prop struck him first on the right wrist and the impact threw him backward, so that the following blade missed his head. We rushed to his aid immediately. I applied pressure to stop the profuse arterial bleeding from his arm while Hershel took off for the control-tower to notify the controller and summon help.

Hershel and I spent most of that night at the Harrisburg Hospital while Rosenberger was in surgery. After he was safely out of his surgery, we flew back just before dawn to Frederick Airport. Hershel piloted the plane because I was much too shaken to attempt that.

Rosenberger's wrist and hand had been permanently damaged, but he eventually recovered some wrist function. He sued me, Hershel Gibbs, and The Bethesda Flying Club for damages. A few months later, Gibbs and I flew back to Harrisburg to testify about the accident at the trial. Hershel and I roomed together the evening before the trial took place and we had a great time playing penny poker. Hershel was far better at flying than he was at poker, at least for pennies.

The trial proceedings took one full day and the judge awarded Rosenberger $15,000 for his injury, a relatively small amount even in those days, and a good deal less than the many thousands he had sued for. Fortunately, the amount awarded to him was within the limits of our insurance coverage. Altogether, it was an unnerving experience, but it did not diminish my enthusiasm for flying.

Billy Rosenblum

I met *Billy Rosenblum* at Blanche Barbaro's apartment on 16th Street in Washington, DC. Her apartment was near to Walter Reed Army Hospital. I met her by chance on a commercial flight from New York that was forced to make an emergency landing at the Baltimore Airport due to landing gear malfunction. As a result of that shared experience we became friends. She soon invited me to a bagels and lox brunch at her home. Besides befriending me, her primary motivation for the invitation was to find a husband for her daughter, preferably Jewish. I nicknamed her *The Balabuster*, (which is actually the Yiddish term for 'homemaker,' but to me, always seemed to be a useful term for a woman who seems to know about a lot of things, including a skill as 'matchmaker'). Billy Rosenblum had also been invited. I soon learned that he was a notorious womanizer, and he was charming and good-looking enough to be quite successful at that enterprise. Luckily for Blanche Barbaro, he never dated her daughter; nor, for that matter, did I.

Bill was enrolled in the Dental School at Howard University, nominally a school for African Americans. Bill was a committed racist who, for reasons that I could not explain, pursued his degree in dentistry at a school that he viewed as the 'enemy camp.' Perhaps it was the only school that had accepted him. He never changed his bigoted views, but we remained friends, nonetheless.

Shortly after obtaining my pilot's license, I took Bill for several rides in *Piper Tripacer N8827C*, including a memorable trip up the Atlantic coast to Teterboro Airport in New Jersey to visit our families in Brooklyn. Billy became enthused with flying, an enthusiasm that continued until the end of his life. After Washington, he and I went separate ways, myself to St. Louis, then to New York, and finally to Milwaukee. Billy moved from Washington to Los Angeles, intending to go into dual practice with his father. Unfortunately, his dad died of a stroke shortly after they had moved there, and Bill began a solo dental practice. He also pursued his chosen lifestyle as a womanizer and *bon vivant*. His flying achievements included an instrument rating and acrobatic flying skills. He was married twice. Neither arrangement worked out.

We maintained our friendship over the ensuing years, often renewing it when I visited California for one reason or another. Once he flew his Comanche N9390P to New York City to attend Matthew's Bar Mitzvah in Rockville Centre, New York, and he made several other trips in the Comanche to Wisconsin, where we would meet for a day or two at the Experimental Aircraft Association (EAA) fly-in in Oshkosh, Wisconsin. I had no expectation at that time that this airplane would one day become mine.

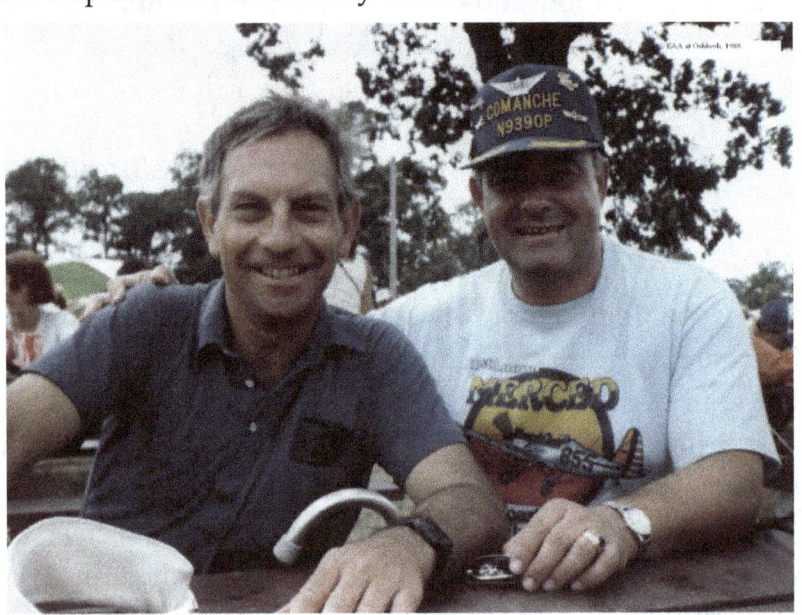

Billy and me at an EAA Fly-in at Oshkosh, Wisconsin.

While he was in dental school Bill dated a nurse named Joanna 'Jo' Reyes. She was raising two children through previous non-marital relationships, just his type of woman. Billy became infatuated with her and, insofar as he could do, professed his love.

During their torrid romantic affair, Jo abruptly departed on a trip to Italy accompanied by a former boyfriend. Under ordinary circumstances their affair would have ended in the same trivial way his other affairs had ended, except that Reyes made the mistake of getting killed in an automobile accident. Since Billy was usually the one to call things off, he had lost control of the situation and became despondent.

At the time of Reyes' death, I was at the Bethesda Naval Medical Hospital recovering from a pilonidal cystectomy. Billy visited me once and then phoned several times to discuss his suicidal intent, stating each time that he had no desire to go on living without Jo. He asked me whether Phenobarbital was an effective agent for suicide. I knew that it would be a bad choice for suicide, and I told him so, but I did not offer any alternatives. His threat gave me considerable concern, and so I called him from the hospital almost every day to speak with him.

One day, after an unanswered call, his cleaning lady discovered him in coma in his apartment and called the police. Unsurprisingly, he had not taken enough of the barbiturate to kill himself. Billy would try the same thing again thirty-four years later, again without success. After several days of sleeping it off in the hospital, he awoke, and by the time he was to be discharged, had become cheerful, and no doubt, happy to be alive. He never mentioned Jo Reyes to me again.

During his career as a pilot Billy owned a Waco, an acrobatic biplane, and the Piper Comanche (N9390P). He also had an expensive home in the Brentwood section of Hollywood, a Bughatti, two Porsches, and a garden complete with a lovely stream fed Koi pond. He had fathered at least one child and had one brief marriage in 1971, before his second marriage to Kim Rosenblum in 1995. Although they were married, Billy gave her no closet space in his bedroom. Instead, her clothes were housed in the 'guest room' which I usually occupied whenever I visited. I can only guess about their relationship, but based upon my later experiences, it was a tumultuous one.

Crossing America the First Time

On June 25, 1962, I departed The Frederick Airport in 8827C, and headed out for California to attend the wedding of a friend of mine in San Diego. I had logged a grand total of 110 hours flying, not very many considering the undertaking. My first stop was in Lancaster, PA, to pick up a new propeller for the plane, since the one that was installed on the plane was badly nicked and untrustworthy. After that I flew to the Hinsdale Airport near Chicago to pick up my friend *Newman Stevens* who would accompany me on this journey. I first met Steve in London during a third year Medical Clerkship at The

University College Hospital in London in 1957. He was the Registrar (Chief Resident) at the time. We developed a close and enduring friendship.

We departed for California the next morning at sunrise. Steve, who knew little about the vagaries of flying, had unwavering faith in my abilities. Most days we would leave before sunup to arrive at our day's destination before the afternoon thunderstorms had gotten started in earnest. Steve regularly fell asleep before the wheels had left the ground and did not awaken until I announced that we were arriving at a refueling stop, or at our destination for that day.

Using that type of self-preserving flight schedule, Steve and I made it safely as far as Winslow, Arizona without a significant weather problem. According to plan, we departed early the next morning from Winslow and climbed to 10,000 feet to be well above the terrain. This time the weather was not so perfect. A few minutes *en route* I spotted a huge bluish-black cloud directly in front of us. What was it doing there so early in the morning on an otherwise clear day?

There was high terrain on either side of that menacing cloud, and given the limitations of the *Tripacer*, I saw no way to go around, under, or over it. According to my thinking, it had no business being there that early in the day, and so I continued straight for it in disbelief for several more minutes.

Suddenly, there was a blinding cloud-to-ground lightning stroke a few hundred feet in front of me, issuing directly from the black mass ahead. The discharge was so bright that Steve awakened from his usual morning slumber. Having been raised as a proper Christian in India, Steve had never to my knowledge uttered a profanity. "My goodness!" was all that he could say. What I said was, "Oh Shit!" -- a more accurate reflection of his and my thinking.

We were over mountainous terrain in extremely dangerous weather for flying. I immediately executed a 180 degree turn and returned as fast as I possibly could to Winslow, where the weather had remained clear. A very sobering, nearly fatal, experience, to say the least.

After landing, Steve and I rented a car and spent the rest of the day visiting The Grand Canyon and its environs, as rain showers and thunderstorms broke out all around. The next day we had clear weather, and flew on to San Diego, California. With no further notable events, the beauty of the terrain beneath and before us, was just the experience that I had come for.

While we were in San Diego, we participated in the wedding ceremony of my friend from Washington, DC, Irving Herman. He had invited us to attend and participate, an invitation that had motivated me to make the trip in the first place. During Irving's

Jewish wedding ceremony, Steve and I each held one of the four corners of the *'Chuppah,'* the overhead canopy for a Jewish wedding. Such joy, and sweet memories!

A week or so later, Steve and I visited the 1962 World's Fair in Seattle, and after several days of enjoying that event, we headed back east. Several days later, I dropped Steve off at the Hinsdale Airport near Chicago and continued my journey home to Frederick. After two more hours flying, I landed for the day, refueled, and spent the night sleeping on a bench at the Findlay Airport in Ohio.

I awoke fatigued and hungry, and in no mental condition to fly that day. I dismissed those negative thoughts and started out for Frederick, MD, in anticipation of a triumphant reunion with my parents and Hershel Gibbs that evening, perhaps something like what Lindbergh may have experienced when he landed in France after crossing the Atlantic. My current flight was not nearly as ground-breaking as Charles Lindbergh's crossing of the Atlantic, but it was enough to satisfy me.

My decision to fly home that day was a bad one, an example of 'get-there-itis.' Knowing that my parents would be waiting for me at the Frederick Airport I just had to get there that day. What torment it must have been for them to have to wait expectantly as the sun was setting while I dithered over the Alleghenies.

After a mid-afternoon refueling stop near Pittsburgh, I continued east across the Alleghenies toward Frederick just before sunset. I first encountered scattered and broken clouds ahead of me with a few cumulus buildups in the distance. No worries, been there, done that. I climbed atop the broken cloud deck at about 7,000 feet. Very shortly, the clouds that billowed up in front of me made it quite clear there was some serious weather ahead. I climbed to 10,000 feet trying to stay on top, but the clouds ahead remained above me. I finally decided to turn back toward Pittsburgh.

Conditions were not any better toward the west than they had been toward the east. I continued heading west, away from the Alleghenies and my intended direction. The clouds continued to billow as rain showers broke out in every direction. Dusk and night flying were not my forte. In addition, I had a faulty radio transmitter that worked only some of the time. Ball-shrinking terror is closest to what I felt at that point. My response to the feeling of terror was to become more alert. Time seemed to slow down as I assessed the situation. I don't understand how this happens; however, this capacity has served me well throughout my life.

As I headed toward Pittsburgh over a solid cloud deck, I spied a small break in the clouds that was at most a few hundred yards in width. I chopped the power and dove for that opening like Jedi Luke in *StarWars*, using a steep descending bank to stay clear of clouds if possible. I had had no actual instrument flight experience at that time, and only minimal instrument training. Getting into clouds would have almost certainly produced a lethal *'graveyard spiral.'* I am now aware of that situation but was not so wise at that time.

At last, I broke out from beneath the cloud deck, and breathed an all too brief sigh of relief. My problems were not nearly over. There were medium to heavy showers in all directions, quite a bit of cloud-to-cloud lightning, and even cloud-to-ground lightning. Visibility was falling. I turned on the radio, which up to that point had been working off and on since we had left California. Thankfully, this time, it worked. I called the Pittsburgh area control frequency, revealed my desperate and deteriorating situation, and asked for help. They rapidly complied and directed me toward Pittsburgh's airport.

Just as the last rays of sunlight disappeared in the west, I located the Pittsburgh Airport, and a few minutes later, I landed safely. That had been a most terrifying flying experience. Once I had landed, I telephoned my parents and explained why I had been unable to make it to Frederick as planned. I nevertheless returned to Washington, DC that evening on a commercial flight and my parents met me at Washington National Airport. It was a pleasant reunion, but not nearly the triumphant one I had envisioned. I explained to them how challenging that last flying experience had been. My parents were overjoyed to see me still in one piece, and I was happy to be with them once again.

Flying in St. Louis

I completed my military service requirement as a PHS officer in 1963, and shortly afterward relocated to Barnes Hospital in St. Louis to continue Medical Residency training in Carl V. Moore's Department of Medicine. Sol Sherry was the Vice Chairman. While living in St. Louis, I did much flying, earned a Commercial Pilot's license, Multi-Engine rating, and most importantly, an Instrument Pilot rating, which I had coveted after my challenging experiences over the Rockies and the Alleghenies in 1962.

I completed that training with *John Williamson*, an accomplished pilot/instructor and, as I later discovered, a fearless one, as well. He was the exception to the rule that *'There are old pilots, and there are bold pilots, but no old, bold pilots.'* At least, it appeared that way to me. Simulated instrument training took place in Williamson's garage, which contained a *'Link Instrument Trainer.'* Most of those Link 'trainers,' even then, were out of commission, on their way to the Smithsonian Museum, or the refuse pile. To simulate thunderstorm turbulence, Williamson used to shake the tail of the Link trainer with me in the enclosed cockpit. When I had nearly completed the instrument training course, Jack announced that before he would endorse me for an FAA instrument flight check, I would have to experience flying in an actual thunderstorm situation with him along for the joyride.

When I first started flying in Washington, most of my instructors dismissed the dangers inherent to of flying near to, or into a thunderstorm, including Hershel Gibbs who had flown an F-86 fighter in Korea, where thunderstorms were the least of his concerns. As a result, I frequently took off in 8827C with thunderstorms breaking out all around me without worrying much about them. If I encountered a storm cell near me, I would simply turn away from it, fly around it, head for home, or land wherever possible, such as in a random farm field or another airport, to wait out the storm. But I had never flown into one of those dangerous cells.

Summertime thunderstorms in St. Louis were at least as frequent and severe as the ones I had experienced in Maryland. One particularly stormy afternoon, Williamson and I departed from Lambert Field in his Cessna 172. After flying a southbound course for several miles, we intentionally flew into a storm cell. After entry, I faced a virtual wall of water, electrical discharges all around, and severe turbulence. I could not control the plane's altitude, and it was a real struggle to fly straight and level.

Williamson calmly encouraged me to keep maintaining the attitude and a safe airspeed. It took about fifteen minutes to complete the passage through that storm cell, but it seemed like an eternity. When we emerged into smooth clear air, I was as shaken as Williamson had been calm. Shortly after that flight, he endorsed me for my FAA check ride, and I passed the flight exam with ease. Regardless, since then I have been terrified of thunderstorms, and have avoided them by as wide a margin as humanly possible. "Never again, I vowed to myself!" and I never have.

With my flying ratings now behind me, I had many more non-threatening flying experiences in St. Louis. After relocating to SUNY Downstate, I continued to fly actively for about a year from Teterboro Airport in New Jersey. Shirley and I had married, Matthew was born, and we eventually bought a house and two cars, a heavy new financial burden. Lacking funds to support my flying habit, I quit flying altogether in 1969, a pause that lasted twenty-seven years.

Piper N9390P

In November 1997, Billy Rosenblum telephoned me to announce that he had Cancer. A few weeks before then, he had noticed a swelling in his neck while he was shaving, went to see a physician who biopsied it, and informed him of the diagnosis. Bill was 59 years of age. Although his tumor was manageable and even potentially curable, he did not want to become a "cancer patient" under any circumstance, and instead, decided to end his life on his terms.

Billy explained that he had achieved all his life's goals and had no further ambitions. He would not consider disfiguring cancer surgery or radiation therapy. Then Bill abruptly changed the subject. "Would you like to have my Comanche?" I thought about his proposition for a moment before replying, "Yes Bill, but I haven't flown for more than 25 years; and besides, I would prefer that you receive treatment for your cancer, and that *you* keep flying that plane." He next said, "I've made up my mind and that's it! Do you want the plane or not?" He was adamant, leaving no room for a rejoinder. "Yes, I'd like to have it," I replied, "but I can't guarantee that I will ever go back to flying." My response was inconsequential. Bill had already made up his mind that I was to have his Comanche.

We had several more telephone conversations after that one, during which I pleaded with Bill to do something to treat his cancer. He refused to even consider it. I asked some of his other friends, like Roger Bick, an oncologist from California, to try to reason with him, but that led nowhere.

Late in March, Bill called to ask whether I would *help* him fly 9390P to Wisconsin. He was quite ill by then, and knew that he was ineligible to, if not incapable of, flying N9390P. He admitted that he had not piloted the Comanche, or any other of his airplanes, for at least two years, and that 9390P had not had its required annual inspection for even longer than two years. For my part, I had not piloted or flown in a small plane for years, and my knowledge of piloting and instrument navigation had slipped badly. I realized that I could be of no help to him as a co-pilot, or even as a passenger. Frankly speaking, I was fearful of the risks that I would be exposed to. I was hoping that my declination to accompany him might dissuade him from making the trip at all, or that perhaps we could hire a co-pilot to help him make that trip. Billy remained undaunted.

Upon departing LA on April 24, 1998 for Wisconsin in the Comanche, Billy reportedly flew through a significant amount of 'hard instrument' weather when departing Los Angeles until he broke out 'on top' and after that, was able to cross the Rockies uneventfully. It was a difficult task, considering that his instrument flying certification was long out of date, he was flying an airplane that was not airworthy, overdue for a major engine overhaul, and equipped with unreliable navigational equipment. En route, Bill made an intermediate stop in Durango, Colorado to refuel and telephone me with his ETA. He then flew non-stop to Timmerman field in Milwaukee. Quite an amazing feat for a dying man.

Later, Bill told me that he made the trip to Milwaukee to see me once more before he died. By that point in his life, Bill did not care much where or when he would die but cared more about how. A plane crash might even have been preferable for him. He lodged with us for three days, had difficulty keeping food or water down, and clearly had lost a significant amount of weight. We spoke endlessly with one another; I telephoned our mutual friend Roger Bick again, hoping that he could reason with him. But to no avail! The day before he returned to California by commercial air, Bill informed me of his intention to commit suicide as soon as he returned to Brentwood.

Before leaving Milwaukee, he signed ownership of 9390P over to me, and handed me $60,000 in cash in a brown paper bag. "You'll need this!" He was correct. N9390P was in poor condition with a long overdue Annual Inspection, a burnt-out engine, fading paint job, leaky cabin, outdated radios and navigation equipment, decaying upholstery, inoperative trim controls, defective fuel cells, and more.

Bill was quite right about how much it would take to fix 9390P. I spent much more than the $60,000 he had given me in making necessary repairs and upgrades, paying for an annual inspection, installing a quality rebuilt engine by 'Victor Aviation,' repainting, reupholstering, adding a one-piece windshield, replacing side windows, installing a Garmin 430 GPS and a reliable autopilot, and speed modifications, among several other items. By the time I was through I had spent more than $135,000. It took several months before I re-learned how to fly. My world had certainly changed.

Billy's Final Days

I flew to LA two days after Bill had left Milwaukee to be with him while he carried out his suicide plan. He again chose Phenobarbital as his 'drug of choice', mainly thru ignorance, just as he had done years before in Washington, DC following Jo Reyes' death. I pleaded with him to seek help, if not therapy or a hospice, or a more effective drug, but he was implacable in his resolve. "The last place I want to be when I die is in a hospital!" How disappointed he would be on that count. Phenobarbital was a poor choice for a suicidal agent since one had to ingest a large number of pills for it to be lethal, and he was having difficulty swallowing even water.

The night of his attempt at suicide, I lay in the bedroom next to his, but did not sleep for even a minute. The walls were thin, and every sound was audible. Just before he swallowed as many pills as he was able to swallow, I witnessed a violent argument between him and his then wife, Kim, concerning what he was about to undertake. It was as if I were not there, as far as their exchanges were concerned. I remember Bill shouting, "Listen to me! *Listen to ME!*" over and over with a mixture of abusive language thrown in. I was so mentally exhausted that I was unable to engage or disengage. I took a valium before I went to bed, and it had no effect.

After an hour or two, I lay awake listening to his stertorous breathing, hoping that he would die as he had wished. But, just as years before, it did not happen that night. He had not taken enough Phenobarbital. I was not sure where his wife Kim was, apparently somewhere in the house, but not with Bill. After two or three hours I left my room and went to the living room to sit and think. I investigated Bill's bedroom and saw him stretched out on the floor naked and comatose. Kim appeared and sat down beside me. "Would you please put a pillow over Bill's face so he can die?" she pleaded. "I can't do that", I responded. We ended up crying together for about twenty minutes. Shortly thereafter, I dressed and left the house. It was about 4:30 AM. Upon returning an hour or so later, Kim was gone, and Billy was still comatose. I had to leave. I packed my bag and left the house. Spent most of that day with *Sam Helgerson* at Baxter Healthcare in Duarte. I passed that visit off as a surprise consultation. I flew home the following day without knowing what had happened to Billy.

I found out some time later that Kim had returned home and called 911. Billy was taken by ambulance to a local hospital where he awakened from his stupor later that day. He was furious to still be alive and restrained in the place he least wanted to be. He signed himself out AMA and was taken home by Kim, who had hidden all the guns in the house.

When Bill could not find any of his guns, he became infuriated and went after Kim. She called 911 again for help and Bill was taken into custody stark naked in front of his house, barely coherent. He was then taken to a hospice under the care of a physician who mercifully administered an overdose of morphine. He died on May 10, 1998 and was cremated shortly thereafter.

A few days later I telephoned Kim. She explained certain things to me, and wrote a letter summarizing what Bill Rosenblum had meant to her:

"All things considered, if I were in his position, I could only hope to be one half as brave in facing death head-on…Your visits always meant the world to him and he cherished you as a friend and as a person… I'm lucky to have known him. He would often say to me, 'Well, Little One, how are we going to make today a fun day?' And you know what? He found some great answers."

I have not heard from Kim Rosenblum since then.

Shortly after I returned home from California, I composed a posthumous letter to Bill that I never sent.

'Dear Bill, ….I realize that we've reached the end of the trail with your illness…so now it's time say goodbye.'…..'Bringing 9390P to Milwaukee was courageous to the extreme, and I fully appreciate what you did for me and for you. You can be proud'….'I want to go beyond your gift of the Comanche to me, for which I will be ever grateful. Our relationship was extraordinary from the beginning. Although there were many differences between us, there were things we had in common. We were both focused in our interests, meticulous and hardworking, both of us loved flying, being with people we liked, and showing that we liked them.'

I learned to fly once again from basic ground school. I started flying a Cessna 172, until the Comanche had been rebuilt and was ready to fly again. It took many hours the second time, but I once again became a competent pilot. Eventually, I logged many more flying hours than I had logged before quitting flying 27 years earlier. Shirley and I made numerous trips around the USA and together we did an Australian 'Air Safari' in a Cessna 172 that lasted a month. The following year, *Mike Morris* and I visited many of the wine districts in southern Australia in a rented Piper Comanche. My longtime friend, *Bernie Sweet*, came along for the ride. I made some great friendships through flying, including one with *Mike Lynch* that was reinforced during a trip we flew together through the Rockies to San Diego in 2007.

In 2009, I sold 9390P to my friend *Jim Maroney*, a Delta Airlines pilot and acrobatic pilot in his famed *DeHaviland Super Chipmunk*. The Chipmunk had the same Lycoming engine as in the Comanche, and perhaps that was one reason he wanted to own 9390P. He also stated that he wanted the Comanche for his travels after he had retired from the airlines. I felt comforted knowing the Comanche was going to be with him, sort of 'keeping it in the family'. Tragically, Jim, the Pilot's Pilot, was killed in a crash of the Super Chipmunk in the 'The Great Smoky Mountains' of Tennessee on March 24, 2014 while en route to Florida to perform in an Air Show.

I used the proceeds from the sale of 9390P to partially fund the *Mosesson Library* at the BloodCenter of Wisconsin, to fund a collaborative research project with the BloodCenter Diagnostics Laboratory (See Chapter IX, 'The Fibrinolytic Potential of Blood'), and to purchase a partnership share in a Piper Lance (N7606C) owned by *Mike Elberson*. The Lance had a more comfortable seating arrangement as far as Shirley was concerned. Unlike the difficulties she had experienced in boarding 9390P, she had no problem boarding 7606P through its rear compartment door. We did indeed take a few trips in it. Not long ones, but enjoyable ones.

In a complicated series of administrative misadventures not worth detailing, my medical certification was challenged by the FAA, which maintained that I had coronary artery disease, as revealed by a CT scan that I had voluntarily disclosed during the course of a routine FAA flight physical for medical recertification. I was asymptomatic then and remain so even now. In any case, I fought for nearly a year to regain medical certification, finally achieved that goal, but in the end, decided it was not worth the effort any longer. I gave up flying on my own terms and withdrew from the partnership in N7606C.

In conclusion, I have had two flying careers admixed with a sparkling scientific career. Not nearly as exciting and compelling a story as Amelia Earhart's, but it is mine alone.

Michael Mosesson   *March 19, 2015*

CHAPTER IV

A POTPOURRI OF DISCOVERIES AND REMEMBRANCES

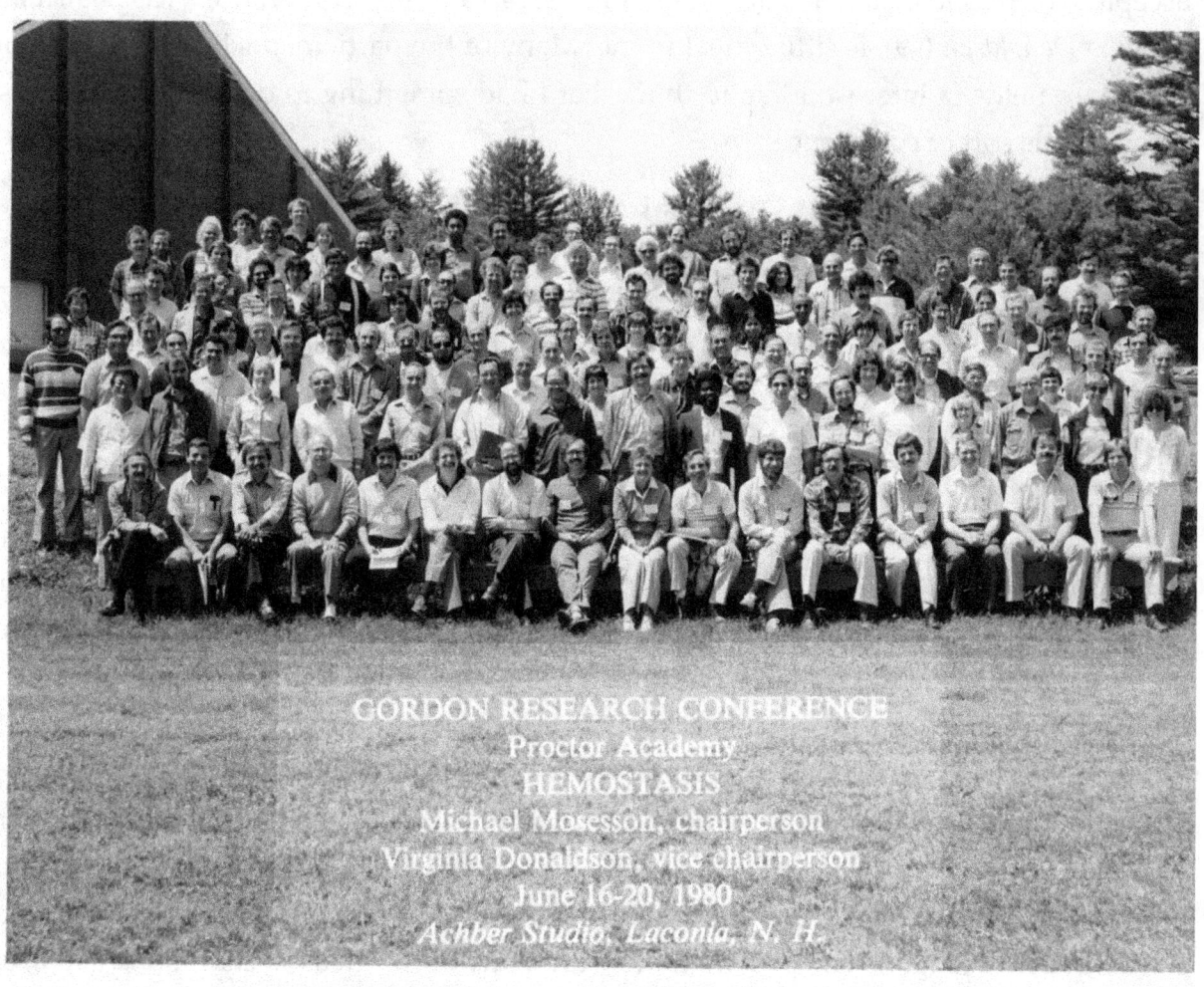

The photo on the face page of this chapter is from the Gordon Research Conference on Hemostasis in 1980, of which I was its Chairman. It was an honor and a pleasure to orchestrate the proceedings. Gordon Conferences were, and remain, great venues for introducing and exchanging new scientific ideas and concepts.

I knew most of the participants since as Conference Chairman I reviewed and accepted, or rejected, all applicants. I am number 10 and the Conference Vice Chairman, *Virginia Donaldson* (#9), is sitting next to me. Many of the participants became leaders in their own fields of interest. I like to think that I had something to do with their success through this sort of conference.

Notable participants were: *Gerd Greininger* (#1) and *John Shainoff* (#2), *Leon Hoyer* (#4), of factor VIII fame, *Ted Zimmerman* (#5) [factor VIII] who passed away prematurely from Ca Lung, my old friend *Fred Rickles* (#6) from U Conn and the CDC, *Gerry Fuller* (#7) who used to jog with me at his own peril at meetings of the American Heart association in Dallas, *Karen Kaplan* (#17) a developing clinical hematologist and investigator, *Alan Johnson* (#19) who was a charter member of *Ted Spaet's NY Clot Club*, *Uri Seligsohn* (#21), who became an important figure in Israeli Science, *John Hoak* (#27) who referred The Fish family ('*Fibrinogen Cedar Rapids*') to me for study and analysis, *Andrei Budzynski* (#27) who used to work in Victor Marder's laboratory, but eventually became a collaborator of mine who gave me the last of a rare enzyme, Hementin, use of which enabled me to prepare an undegraded form of Fibrinogen fragment E suitable for crystallization with thrombin by *Igor Pechik* and *Leonid Medved* [see #173 in *Annotated* Publications], *Eva Engvall* (#26) who invented ELISA, *Jacek Hawiger* (#30), *Susan Rittenhouse-Simmons* (#31), a renowned platelet metabolism investigator who eventually married my beloved friend, confidante and predecessor at DBS, *Sandy Shapiro* (#38), *Hymie Nossel* (#39), a prominent member of our *NY Clot Club* who died suddenly while jogging in 1983, *Elemer Mihalyi* (#45) a brilliant fibrinogen investigator who provided me with many of his ideas, *Victor Marder* (#55), an old adversary on the degradation products of fibrinogen issue-he turned out to be correct in that case, *Michael Bevilacqua* (#69) who was *Celso Bianco's* and my Graduate Student. Michael's dissertation was on "*Fibronectin Receptors on Mononuclear Phagocytes.*"

Other notable participants included *John Finlayson* (#119, who wrote a chapter for this present series and participated in many ways in improving my writing, as discussed elsewhere, *Dennis Galanakis* (#115), my first 'post doc' and a longtime friend, *David Amrani* (#72), who started out as my technologist, who I mentored for his PhD while we were are at SUNY, and who relocated to Milwaukee to became my associate in the Winter Laboratory at Sinai Samaritan Medical Center, *Larry Sherman* (#77), a longtime friend from St Louis whose seminal work on fibrinogen catabolism in rabbits is covered in this chapter, *Joel Bennett* (#123), a long time tennis playing buddy, *Gert Muller-Berghaus* (#91), who invited me to be on his 'Fachbeirat' [Research Advisory Committee] in Giessen and through whom I met *Eberhard Selmayr*, one of my heroes in the chapter on the *Fibrin Cross-linking Controversy*.

PHOTO IDENTIFICATION   HEMOSTASIS   PROCTOR ACADEMY   June 16-20 19

1 Gerd Grienger
2 John Shainoff
3
4 Leon Hoyer
5 Ted Zimmerman
6 Frederick Rickles
7 Gerald Fuller
8 Whyte Owen
9 Virginia Donaldson
10 Michael Mosesson
11 Johan Broekman
12 Marc Shuman
13 G. Vehar
14 G.M. Oosta
15 Michael Griffith
17 Karen Kaplan
18 Dominique Meyer
19 Alan Johnson
20 Margaret Rick
21 Uri Seligsohn
22 C. Marguerie
23
24 Fred Ofosu
25 G. Van Dieijen
26 Eva Engvall
27 John Hoak
28 Ken Mann
29 Andrei Budzynski
30 Jack Hawiger
31 S. Rittenhouse-Simmons
32 Robert Jesse
33 Soo Lee
34 Bob Rosenberg
35 Tom Edgington
36 James Maynard
37 Juan Chediak
38 Sandor Shapiro
39 H.L. Nossel
40
41 G.A. Jamieson
42 Mae Hultin
43 J.A. Donlon
44 T.J. Janus
45 E. Mihalyi
46 Howard Clark
47 John Kaplan
48 Alan Guarfoot
49 Euan Mac Intyre
50 John Bruno
51 Ed Nishizawa
52 Grace Boxer
53 Robert Wall
54 Jean Lue Wautier
55 Victor Marder
56 Charles Slattery
57 John Holt
58 Ingo Mahn
Thomas Duel

60 H. Hassouna
61
62 Sanford Shattil
63 A. Chadwick Cox
64 Annie Bezeaud
65 J.N. Shanberge
66 Hussain Saba
67 S.R. Saba
68 John Burch
69 Michael Bevilacqua
70 Randy Bell
71 Joseph Palascak
72 David Amrani
73 Judith Lahav
74 J. Niemetz
75 David Kosow
76 Thomas Detwiler
77 L. Sherman
78
79 Ira Sussman
80
81 Edward Kirby
82 M. Furlan
83 Tranqui
84 Amiram Eldor
85 Jim Halkett
86 Eduardo Lapetina
87 W. Holleman
88 Dennis Cunningham
89
90 Bruce Evatt
91 G. Muller-Berghaus
92 Barbara Alving
93 Jacob Rand
94 Andrewa Poggi
95 Lloyd Culp
96 David Crutchley
97 Babette Weksler
98 Ruth Ann Henriksin
99 Jan Sixma
100 Paula Tracy
101 Vincent Turitto
102 Fred Walker
103 Richard Clark
104 Rudy Haschameyer
105 Fred Grinnell
106 Zaverio Ruggeri
107 Lvigi DeMarco
108 Beatriz Dardik
109 Gary Levy
110 Andre Bagdasarian
111 Colvin Redman
112 Eric Jaffe
113 Dan Deykin
114 Robert Handin
115 D. Galanakis
116 Barry Coller
117

118 Andrew Schafer
119 John Finlayson
120 Harvey j Weiss
121 George Wilner
122 Roy Ittyerah
123 Joel Bennett
124
125 Stephanie Olexa
126 Claes Nilsson
127 Nils Bang
128 Walter Fowler
129 Christina Harbury
130 Stephen Prescott
131 Roy Hantgan
132 Klaus Lederer

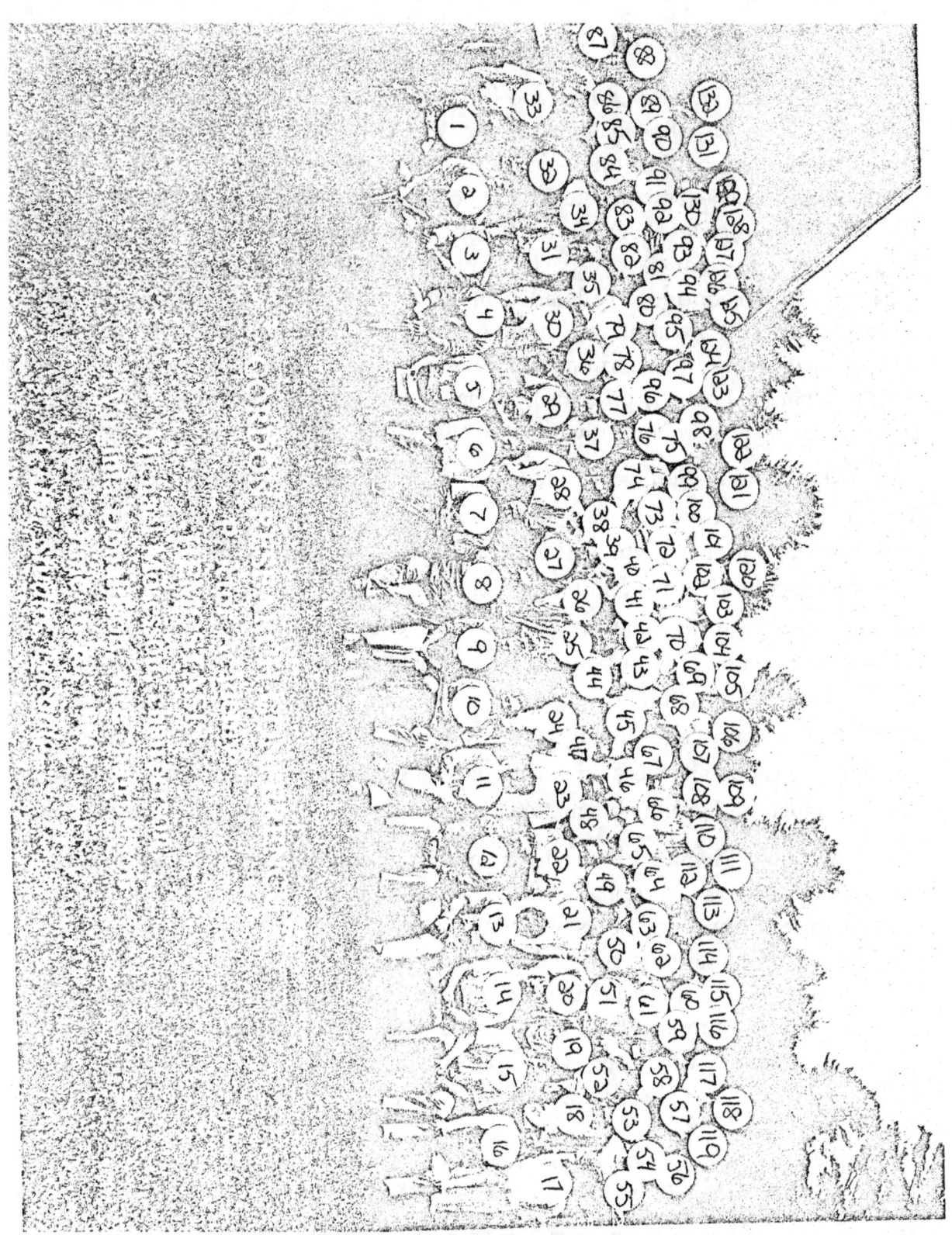

High Solubility Fibrinogens[3]

I moved to Bethesda, Maryland in 1960 to start service as a commissioned officer in The US Public Health Service at The Division of Biologics Standards (DBS) on the National Institutes of Health (NIH) campus. Like my predecessor, *Sandy Shapiro*, I was assigned to The Laboratory of Blood and Blood Products (LBBP) and officially became a 'Blood Bank Inspector' and 'Laboratory Investigator'. In that last capacity my first assignment was to prepare plasminogen-free fibrinogen [detailed in 'Fibrinogen 101']. At the time of my arrival I knew little about plasma fibrinogen, except that it circulated in blood and was the precursor of the fibrin clot. I approached this situation by first learning how to separate the many proteins in plasma by a general process called 'Plasma Fractionation,' most importantly the one called 'Cohn Ethanol Fractionation.'

That investigation was launched at the beginning of World War II at The Protein Foundation in Boston under the direction of Edwin J. Cohn, a Boston Aristocrat and Scientist, who earlier in his career had studied the conditions for protein solubility. The most important objective of this 'Top Secret' project was to prepare stable, purified plasma proteins that could be used under battlefield situations. Several of the products that emerged from the plasma fractionation project, such as fibrin film and plasma albumin, came into field use during WW II (also see the fibrin cross-linking chapter). Because it was highly classified, the methodological details were published only after the war had ended. Several of these products and production methods are still in use.

In Cohn 'Method VI' the least soluble plasma protein, fibrinogen, was precipitated first as 'Fraction I.' I made the surprising discovery that about 30 percent of the fibrinogen in plasma had remained soluble following precipitation of *'Fraction I.'* The fibrinogen remaining in the supernatant plasma solution was recovered in the next precipitating precipitated fraction called 'Fraction II + III.' I did not begin to understand why some of the fibrinogen in plasma was present in 'II+III', and since I was fully occupied with other projects, I deferred further

---

[3] Terminology:
Catabolites-These are intermediate *breakdown* products, in the case of fibrinogen, they are produced by a process involving cleavage of peptide bonds and release of cleaved peptide material from the parent protein.
Coagulate (adj, coagulable)-v. To form an insoluble fibrin clot after thrombin cleavage of fibrinogen to form fibrin.
Dysfibrinogenemia- a congenital abnormality of fibrinogen structure causing *dys*function.
Fractionate-v., to separate into constituent parts or subfractions
Precipitate-v., to render insoluble

inquiries on that subject until after I had moved to St. Louis to complete my residency training (1963-65). My investigations of 'Higher Solubility Fibrinogens' began during my stay in St. Louis and continued for years afterward at SUNY, as detailed in another section.

The Barnes Hospital Ward Medical Service

On July 1, 1963 I began year two of Medical Residency on the 'Ward Medical Service' at Barnes Hospital. In those days 'The Ward Service' contained and admitted all indigent and virtually all African-American, patients, whereas Caucasians and wealthier folks wound up on the so-called 'Private Service' in a more luxurious and racially selective part of the hospital called *Queeny Tower*, named after the former Chairman of Monsanto Chemicals.

The House Staff were divided up as well. Practice-oriented Residents were assigned to the Private Service, whereas the 'Academically-oriented' Residents, like me, were selected for the 'Ward Service.' Private Service patients were supervised by their own admitting physicians who were aided by the Resident Staff. In contrast, Ward Service residents were officially supervised by the 'full-time' faculty member who had been assigned to that team, and they usually were given considerable independence in managing their assigned patients. On one very special occasion, The Chief of Medicine, Professor *Carl V. Moore*, asked me to consult on a Ward Service patient with a very low platelet count, a consultation that launched a new subject of inquiry for me.

Discovering 'The Cold-Insoluble Globulin of Plasma'

Moore was a highly regarded clinician, hematologist, teacher, and renowned clinical investigator. He knew a great deal about blood platelet disorders, some of it from a first-hand experience that had nearly cost him his life. His experience had to do with a serious clinical disorder now known as 'Auto-Immune Thrombocytopenia' (AIT)[4], Hearing that story had become a right-of-passage for new Residents.

Several years before my arrival, Moore and his colleague, *William Harrington*, had been baffled by a patient with a low blood platelet count (*thrombocytopenia*). Moore suspected that the thrombocytopenia was due to a factor in the blood, possibly an antibody, that caused depletion of circulating platelets.

---

[4] *Auto-Immune Thrombocytopenia* (AIT) is a disorder characterized by a low platelet count (*thrombocytopenia*) due to circulating antibodies directed against platelets, causing the platelets to be removed from the circulation. Thrombocytopenia is often associated with punctate hemorrhagic lesions (*petechiae*) on the skin and in other organs including the brain.

To test their hypothesis, he and Harrington decided to have blood serum obtained from the affected patient injected into their veins to monitor its effects on their blood platelet levels. Given what was known about AIT, their plan was innovative and resourceful, but also highly risky.

According to plan, they were admitted to The Ward Medical Service, and came under the care of the house staff. Soon after patient serum had been administered, both Moore's and Harrington's platelet counts dropped precipitously. The Resident physician assigned to Moore's case came to his bedside to examine him for the possible effects of thrombocytopenia. He requested that he lie flat. Moore, whose head had been resting in an elevated position on several pillows, consented to the examination but refused to lie flat. Ever the teacher, Moore said, "If I'm going to develop *petechiae* because of a low platelet count, I'd prefer that they occur in my skin and not in my brain." He was, of course, referring to increases in intracranial pressure that occur when lying in a recumbent position. The resident understood immediately and dutifully conducted his examination with Moore's head well above chest level.

Harrington's clinical status deteriorated to the extent that, reportedly, he was given the last rights of the Church. Nevertheless, they each recovered fully from their dangerous experiment. Whatever the risk may have been, they had discovered a plausible mechanism for immune-mediated thrombocytopenia (AIT).

With that inspiring story as background, I was pleased and surprised that none other than Carl Moore had asked me to consult on Mrs. *Alma Beene*, the patient with severe thrombocytopenia who had also experienced several episodes of transient cerebral ischemia (*'mini-strokes'* or *TIAs*). Initially, the thrombocytopenia was believed to be due to AIT but, paradoxically, it had not responded to an often-effective treatment, steroids. I went immediately to visit Mrs. Beene, and after reviewing her record and examining her, I began by studying her plasma in my laboratory.

In addition to a low platelet count, I found a reduced plasma fibrinogen level (*'hypofibrinogenemia'*). When I placed her plasma in a refrigerator (2-4° C), a precipitate formed that resembled a fibrin clot. Unlike a fibrin clot, the precipitate promptly dissolved when re-warmed at 37° C. This fibrinogen-rich precipitate was called *Cryofibrinogenemia*. Based upon these initial observations, I suggested to Professor Moore that Mrs. Beene was suffering from a chronic form of a syndrome known as Disseminated Intravascular Coagulation (DIC) or *Chronic Consumption Coagulopathy*.[5]

Chronic Consumption Coagulopathy was known to be associated with an underlying malignancy, but our main problem was to find a way to manage her thrombocytopenia, hypofibrinogenemia, and ischemic attacks, if not also to find the underlying basis for her illness. I suggested a trial of intravenous heparin, a potent anti-coagulant, a therapeutic avenue that had not previously been considered. Once we began a heparin infusion, Mrs. Beene's platelet count and fibrinogen level rose within hours, a response that confirmed the presence of *Chronic Consumption Coagulopathy*.

It took several more weeks to establish an appropriate type and dose of anti-coagulation, but once we had achieved that we sent Mrs. Beene home to the care of her family. Later tests revealed a disseminated Ovarian Carcinoma, a malignancy that accounted for the Coagulopathy. Although her platelet counts remained in the normal range, and TIAs were no longer an issue, she succumbed to the underlying cancer within a few months.

I continued to investigate Mrs. Beene's cold insoluble precipitate. The components included, as expected, fibrinogen and fibrin, but in addition, there was another major component that amounted to ~50% of the total protein. By electrophoretic analysis, this component migrated more rapidly than fibrinogen, and fit an earlier description by Morrison et al. [1] of a protein found in the least soluble fibrinogen fraction. They named it *'Cold-Insoluble Globulin'* and suggested that it was an altered form of fibrinogen[6]. Even though that terminology was vague, I retained that designation and soon showed that Cold-Insoluble Globulin ('CIg') was a unique and previously uncharacterized component of normal plasma, now known as *Plasma Fibronectin*.

I wrote a detailed 'Case Report' about Mrs. Beene, including my characterization of *CIg* as a constituent of normal plasma as well as a component of her *cryofibrinogen* precipitates. That now famous report entitled *'Chronic*

---

[5] <u>Consumption Coagulopathy</u> or <u>Disseminated Intravascular Coagulation</u> (DIC) is caused by increased activation of blood coagulation that results in consumption of plasma fibrinogen and platelets.

[6] *<u>Cold-Insoluble Globulin</u>* (CIg) was first identified in studies of human plasma fractionation that at the Protein Foundation in Boston under EJ Cohn during World War II. This component of a cold insoluble fibrinogen-rich fraction (termed 'Fraction I-1') was believed to be a modified form of fibrinogen, perhaps even a dimer that had somehow been rendered insusceptible to the action of thrombin [2]. That belief was dispelled by my studies on Mrs. Alma Beene's Cryofibrinogen precipitate.

Intravascular Coagulation Syndrome' was published in The New England Journal of Medicine [3] (Addendum 1).

What had started out in St. Louis as a laboratory curiosity relating to the composition of a cold-insoluble fibrinogen-rich precipitate, had evolved into a burgeoning investigative field covering many subjects including cellular adhesion, morphology and spreading, cell matrix formation and function, cytoskeletal organization, phagocytosis, embryogenesis and embryonic differentiation, wound healing, and malignant transformation. *Richard Hynes* (MIT) wrote an excellent account of the history and expansion of the fibronectin field that is well worth reading [4].

Shortly after I arrived at SUNY, I developed a simple and reliable method for purifying Plasma CIg and then investigated the physical, biochemical, and immunological properties of the purified material. Those results turned into a landmark paper [5] that left little doubt that CIg was a unique plasma protein. Its relationship to a cellular and cell matrix protein termed *Fibroblast Surface Protein* was soon clarified.

During that same period there were numerous groups that were investigating a *fibroblast surface protein* that was also a component of the intercellular matrix. Among its names were: LETS (large, external, transformation sensitive), SFA (surface fibroblast antigen), FSP (fibroblast surface protein), CSF (cell spreading factor). These cell surface/intercellular matrix proteins were all immunologically and structurally related to plasma CIg, and the situation was clarified at a Cold Spring Harbor Symposium in 1973. Over the next several years collaborations that had originated at that conference led to many new studies that were elegantly summarized at a New York Academy of Sciences Symposium organized by *Anti Vaheri, Erkki Ruoslahti*, and *Deane Mosher* entitled: *'Fibroblast Surface Protein'* [6]. I contributed a chapter on Plasma CIg [7].

Tony Chen joined my group as a Post-Doctoral Fellow in 1974, and we soon improved the purification procedure for CIg [8]. We also drew attention to its ubiquitous nature by identifying it in amniotic fluid [9], in synovial fluid [10], and, with *Marge Zucker*, even in platelet α-granules where it was stored with its erstwhile companion Fibrinogen [11].

A few years later, *Gene Homandberg* and I prepared functionally intact monomers of CIg [12], and in collaboration with my friend *Rolf Huseby*, a biophysicist, we investigated its conformation using circular dichroic spectroscopy [8]. Sometime later *Michael Benecky* joined my group, and after several false starts we clarified the roles of the heparin binding sites on Fibronectin on its heparin interactions [13]. Benecky and I also published our results on steady state fluorescence analyses of CIg [14], and ionic-strength- and pH-dependent conformational states of human plasma fibronectin [15].

I sometimes collaborated with outside groups in studying the tissue forms of fibronectin [16;17], and in identifying a receptor for Fibronectin on Fibroblasts [18]. *Bob Colvin* and I had previously collaborated in studying Afibrinogenemic subjects, investigations that had clarified the role of fibrin deposition in causing induration in the *'delayed hypersensitivity skin reaction'* [19]. I followed that with a study on Fibronectin deposition in normal subjects and in an Afibrinogenemic subject in delayed-type hypersensitivity. That project was carried out with the help of *Richard Clark* (#103, Cover Picture) who headed The Dermatology Department at SUNY Stony Brook campus on Long Island [20].

My interest in Fibronectin began to wane even as outside interests were burgeoning. These groups were moving in the direction of neoplasia and cell proliferation, subjects that were important but tangential to my expanding interest in Intravascular Thrombosis. It also did not help when I hired three marginally competent people: *Nancy Tooney, Gene Homandberg*, and *Michael Benecky*, to work on this subject. Tooney had very few useful ideas and did not communicate well. After spending two unproductive years in Milwaukee Nancy Tooney returned to her tenured position at Pace College in New York. Homandberg was undisciplined, moody, often paranoid. Simply stated he did not 'work and play well with others. After three years of antagonizing just about everyone on my staff, he departed without fanfare or farewell. Benecky was impressed with himself as a cutting-edge physical chemist, but his technical and intellectual skills did not match his own self-assessment. Small wonder that these experiences led me to return to my first love, Fibrinogen.

My Associates at SUNY

Dennis Galanakis, MD, was my first 'Post-Doctoral' student at SUNY. He was living in New York City and sought me out at *The Federated Society* meetings in Atlantic City knowing that I was about to move to SUNY. He wanted to learn how to do research in the Coagulation Field and although he had no laboratory or research skills whatsoever, I took him on. Those were stressful times, especially for Dennis, but his intense desire to succeed led him to success. I taught him research skills from the ground up, assigned him library research projects and then quizzed him, required him to write draft manuscripts and worked with him on every word and sentence. He was a slow learner but an indefatigable worker. We failed on some research projects and succeeded on others, but eventually we completed two projects concerned with the High Solubility Fibrinogens. By then I referred to them as *'Fibrinogen Catabolites'* [21;22].

Because of that research training, Dennis found a job in the Pathology Department at SUNY and eventually accepted a more permanent position in The Pathology Department on the SUNY campus at Stony Brook on Long Island. His writing skills improved to the extent that he could fashion his own manuscripts from start to finish, which he eventually did. He perfected his laboratory skills, especially as they concerned plasma protein fractionation. Using those skills, he completed and reported, many credible research reports on Dysfibrinogenemias, including the effects of Albumin on fibrin structure. He's also turned the 'tables' on me in that I had of late requested him to send me some of his Fibrinogen subfractions that I had shown him how to prepare.

Celso Bianco was in The Pathology Department at SUNY and the Director of the Blood Bank. He became my closest scientific colleague and a very close friend. We joined forces, Celso the Cell Biologist, and me, the Protein Chemist, to mentor a MD/PhD candidate, *Michael Bevilacqua* (#69, cover picture), whose thesis research involved identification of a *'Fibronectin Receptor on Human Monocytes'* [23]. We were successful in that endeavor. Michael's accomplishments at SUNY launched a meteoric career as a medical scientist, inventor, and business executive. Michael and I and Celso remain in touch.

Ruth Umfleet had worked for me for a few months while I was in St. Louis and at my invitation, relocated with me to SUNY as my Senior Research Technologist. She was instrumental in helping me complete the research for our 1970 CIg paper, so much so that I made her a co-author [5]. After five years in New York, Ruth married her longtime boyfriend and moved to Texas. *David Amrani* (#72, cover picture) filled the vacancy she had left. After several years working as a Laboratory Technologist, he indicated his desire to obtain a PhD degree with me as his mentor. I liked that idea, and together we decided that his Thesis research project would be about Fibronectin and he would carry out the project in my laboratory. He was accepted into the Graduate program at St. John's University and was assigned by his thesis advisor to my care according to plan.

During the next three years David proved capable of designing, conducting, and interpreting his experiments. He characterized the components that co-precipitated with Fibronectin in forming the so-called cold-precipitable *"Heparin Precipitable Fraction of Plasma"* (HPF), most notably Factor VIII and von Willebrand factor [24]. His studies significantly bolstered *Nick Stathakis's* work that defined the interactions among the major components of HPF, Fibrinogen, CIg, and Heparin [25]. He also studied the heterogeneous forms of Plasma Fibronectin found in the circulation [26] and, in cooperation with *Tony Chen*, a Post-Doctoral Fellow, determined the covalent structure of fibronectin dimers and the basis for its heterogeneity in plasma [27]. As an exercise in developing his writing skills we wrote a comprehensive review article on fibronectin structure and its biological activities [28]. Collectively, that body of work earned him the PhD degree. When I decided to relocate to Milwaukee at Sinai Samaritan Medical Center in 1981, I invited him to move with me as an 'Associate Scientist' on my team, and he accepted that challenge. He stayed at SSMC for several more years and eventually moved on to extend his career at Baxter Healthcare.

During that same period, I took on a new post-doctoral fellow from Athens, Greece, *Nick Stathakis*, to whom I had been introduced by Dennis Galanakis, his 'compatriot' of Greek origin. Since Nick's intended stay in the USA was short, he drove himself night and day to complete his projects. He developed hyperthyroidism, including a moderate opthalmopathy. That hypermetabolic state seemed to provide him with additional energy. He refused remedial treatment and continued working at a frenetic pace. Once his projects had been completed, he returned to Greece and his symptomatology abated. I verified that he was euthyroid on a subsequent trip to Athens to visit him and his family.

Nick successfully addressed all the experimental challenges in less than a year. He developed a method for separating fibrinogen gamma (γ) chains from the gamma-prime (γ') chains in plasma [29]. He delineated the role of Plasma Fibronectin in forming the Heparin Precipitable Fraction of Plasma (HPF) [25], and he demonstrated the central role of Plasma Fibronectin in causing precipitation of Fibrin-Fibrinogen complexes [30]. This last project provided a plausible explanation for the *Cryofibrinogen* precipitates we had observed in Mrs. Beene's plasma, the St. Louis 'Chronic Intravascular Coagulopathy' patient, study of which resulted in the discovery of Plasma Fibronectin (CIg)[3].

Although Nick completed these projects in less than one year, writing the manuscripts and publication took place over a considerably longer period, long after he had returned to Athens. We had many written exchanges. He would describe his results in a meticulously hand-written 'manuscript.' I would then examine his ideas and eventually would return a heavily edited script, much in the style I had so often experienced with John Finlayson's analyses of my own manuscripts. (*Sample documents are on file in the Mosesson Library*).

Sol Sherry, The Crown Prince of Fibrinolysis

Plasminogen becomes activated to plasmin by exogenous agents, including a bacterial agent called Streptokinase (SK), or an endogenously produced agent like tissue plasminogen activator (tPA). By the time I arrived in St. Louis, physiological and clinical aspects concerning the Fibrinolytic System (Figure 1) had been comprehensibly reviewed by Sherry in a *Physiological Reviews* article [31]. That article was required reading for everyone in this field, certainly for me, and it helped propel Sherry to national prominence.

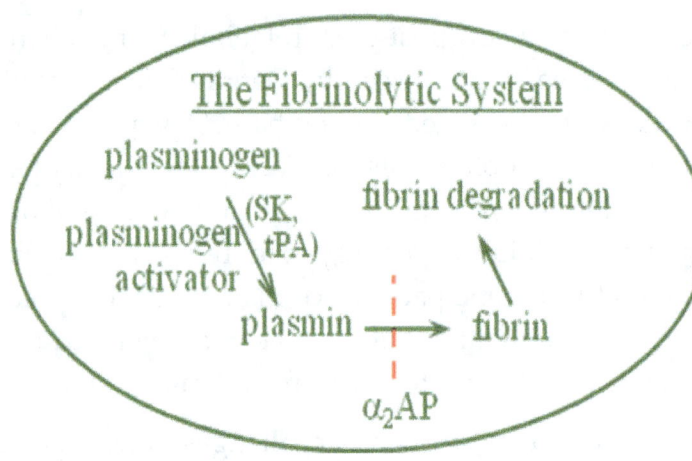

Figure 1. *The Fibrinolytic System-Plasminogen is converted to the enzyme plasmin by activators such as streptokinase (SK) or tissue plasminogen activator (tPA). Plasmin then degrades fibrin or fibrinogen and can be inhibited by α2-antiplasmin (α2AP).*

In the 1940's, while he was at NYU, the birthplace of *Fibrinolytic* therapy, Sherry became involved in clinical studies of fibrinolytic activators like streptokinase (SK) for managing *Empyema*, an infectious process forming in the pleural space (i.e., the space between the lungs and the chest wall). In that pre-antibiotic era, Empyema was managed by inserting tubes into the chest to facilitate drainage of the bacterial exudates. That procedure was often ineffective because infectious exudates became loculated (walled-off) in pockets created from fibrin clots, and healing was greatly delayed. By instilling a fibrinolytic activator, SK, directly into the chest cavity, dissolution of loculated fibrin pockets was accelerated, and drainage became more effective. Sol was at the center of these investigations and was working with some of the early leaders in the field, *William S. Tillett* and *Alan Johnson* (#19, cover picture). I like to think of him in those times as the nascent 'Prince of Fibrinolysis'.

From his position at NYU, Sol moved to The University of Cincinnati (1951) as head of the May Institute for Medical Research and extended his activities toward developing synthetic substrates for measuring the activity of plasmin and other proteolytic enzymes. In 1954, he moved to Washington University to become Chief of the Medical Service at The Jewish Hospital of St. Louis. In 1958, he moved 'across the street' to become Co-Chairman of Carl Moore's Department of Medicine where, with *Tony Fletcher* and *Norma Alkjaersig*, he further expanded his clinical research to fibrinolytic activators, SK or UK, as potential agents for dissolving intravascular thrombi such as those occurring in deep venous thrombosis (DVT), pulmonary embolism (PE), or even myocardial infarction (MIs) and stroke.

Sherry was also an excellent clinician, a clear and analytical thinker. He orchestrated many of the weekly 'Grand Rounds' Clinical Pathology Conferences (CPC's) that almost everyone attended. In staging these Clinical Case Presentations, the Moderator would call upon faculty and residents to dissect and analyze specific aspects of the patient's condition or the disease process. Under his able baton, Sol would eventually pull together all the necessary threads and orchestrate them into a coherent diagnosis and solution. CPC proceedings were transcribed and published in the prestigious 'American Journal of Medicine ('*The Green Journal*'), the official Journal of the 'Association of American Physicians' (AAP).

Fletcher and Alkjaersig

Shortly before my arrival in St. Louis to begin my Residency Tony Fletcher, a straightlaced Brit, married his long-time co-worker, Norma Alkjaersig, PhD, a straightlaced Danish lady. Norma supervised all laboratory operations in Sherry's group, whereas Tony spent his time leading clinical trials of fibrinolytic therapy. They were a formidable team. I officially joined the group as an '*Enzymology Fellow*' after my second year of Residency although I had been carrying out laboratory experiments on my own well before that (Figure 2).

Although I would have preferred it to be otherwise, Tony came to regard me as a rival, rather than a colleague. I soon learned that Fletcher and Sherry had a very toxic relationship. Since I had come on as Sherry's Fellow and shared my ideas and progress with him, I became 'untouchable,' effectively excluded from details concerning any of Tony's and Norma's experimental protocols or results. He never disclosed anything concerning the product of fibrinolysis he called 'First Derivative,' but it was clear that we were working on the same subject.

My laboratory was located just down the hall from Tony's and Norma's. My laboratory space contained a weird and bulky contraption called a 'Robot Chemist.' This semi-automated machinery had been acquired by Tony Fletcher without any clear plan for its deployment. Its' 'tracks' took up most of the laboratory space like an oversized Lionel train setup. It had not been fully assembled and tested, and I wasn't inclined to do that. After a short time, I discretely disassembled the apparatus, piled it neatly in a corner of the lab, and placed my own equipment in its place. Because of our toxic relationship, Tony never set foot in my laboratory, and probably never knew what I had done. The contraption remained undisturbed in the same corner during my entire stay at Barnes Hospital, and for all I know it remains there still.

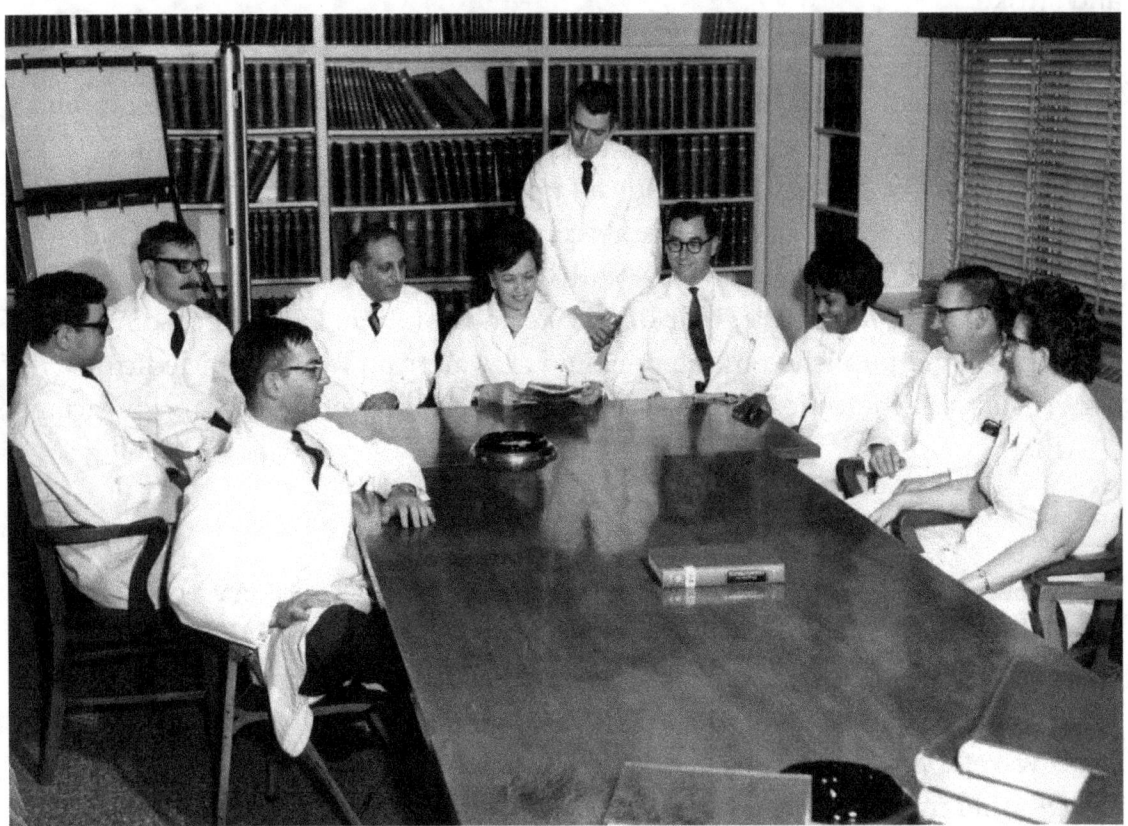

Figure 2. *The Enzymology Group (1965). Clockwise from the left: MWM, Bernie Sweet, Chester Kucinski, Sol Sherry, Norma Alkjaersig, Ed Genton (standing), Tony Fletcher, Odessa (Norma's assistant), Larry Matler (Tony's lab assistant), the laboratory diener. Missing: Jack Hirsch and Larry Sherman (#77, cover picture)*

Back to The High Solubility Fibrinogens

To recover a high proportion of plasma fibrinogen in a single precipitation step, I used glycine-saturated solutions as described by *Louis Kazal* who was from the University of Pennsylvania [32]. More than ninety percent of the plasma fibrinogen precipitated in that step, and by repeating the same procedure I obtained fibrinogen that was more than 95% coagulable. I then worked out procedures for subfractionating the fibrinogens according to their solubility using

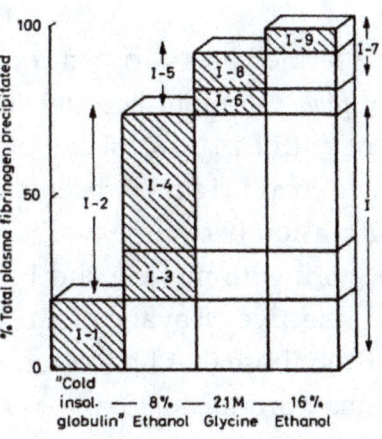

Figure 3. *A diagram showing fibrinogen subfractions numbered according to increasing solubility (Fractions I-1-to Fraction I-9). The vertical axis indicates the proportion of each subfraction in plasma [35].*

terminology that had been introduced by *Birger Blombäck* in 1956 for lower solubility subfractions ('I-1' to 'I-4') [33]. Accordingly, I assigned higher numbers ('I-5' to 'I-9') for the more soluble fractions (Figure 3). As a testimonial to the adversarial relationship between Fletcher and Sherry, Sol and I were the only authors of that investigation of high solubility fibrinogens [34]. Our findings raised new and important questions about how such fibrinogens had arisen.

The changes in structure accounting for increasing solubility turned out to be an inverse function of the Aα chain sizes. The higher the solubility of any given subfraction, the smaller its Aα chains [21;22;36]. Aα chain shortening came about through proteolytic cleavage and release of peptides from the C-terminal region, the so-called αc domain (Figure 4), an event, I reasoned, that must have occurred in the circulation. Based upon that surmise, I coined the term *Fibrinogen Catabolites* to suggest that degraded fibrinogens were *in vivo* derived metabolic intermediates.

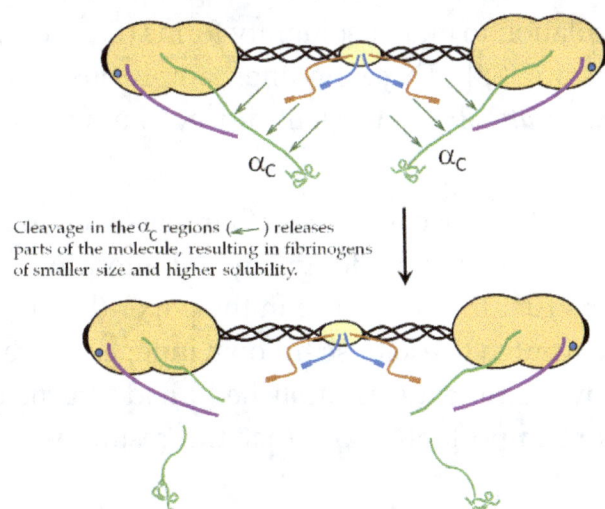

Figure 4. *The upper drawing represents an intact fibrinogen molecule containing intact terminal portions of its Aα chains, termed 'αc' (green). The green arrows indicate sites at which cleavage results in derivatives lacking portions of its αc regions (lower drawing).*

My initial thinking was that catabolic intermediates arose through the Fibrinolytic System, namely that proteolysis by *plasmin* might account for such derivatives (see Figure 1). I pursued that concept with *Larry Sherman* (#77, cover picture), a newly arrived post-doctoral fellow who had originally been slated to work with Tony Fletcher. Because of mounting tension between Sol Sherry and Tony Fletcher, Larry was re-assigned by Sol to work with me. He and I showed that early phases of plasmin digestion involved selective cleavage of Aα chains, but the plasmic cleavages differed significantly from those that I had found in the plasma products [37], making it unlikely that *Catabolic Intermediates* in the circulation had arisen through the Fibrinolytic System.

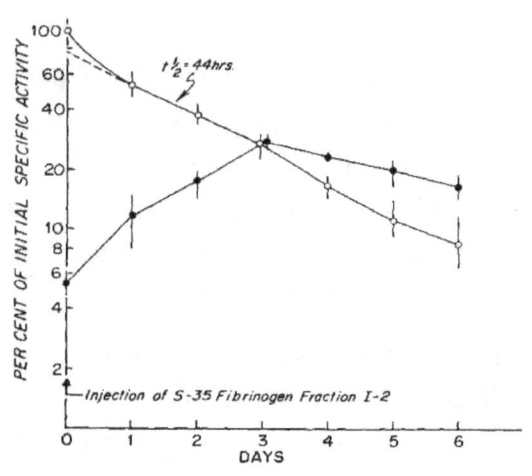

Figure 5. *These results showed that high solubility fibrinogen (open circles) were transformed from lower to higher solubility forms (solid circles) [38].*

To further pursue these findings, *Larry Sherman* and I designed a fibrinogen *'turnover'* experiment in rabbits. Their fibrinogen is similar in most respects to that of humans, including the existence of high solubility intermediates. Our experiment examined whether fibrinogen intermediates arose *in vivo*. Using radioactively-labeled low solubility rabbit fibrinogen, Larry could show that precursor high solubility fibrinogen was transformed in the circulation to higher solubility forms (Figure 5), a so-called *precursor-product* relationship [38]. These findings amply justified terming human fibrinogen derivatives 'Catabolites.' We still did not know how these intermediates had arisen.

It surprised me that I was not included as a co-author of Sherman's seminal 1972 paper. As his supervisor I had been involved in designing and interpreting the experiments, and I helped him construct the key figure in the paper (below). Perhaps, as a newcomer to this field he wanted to establish his own independence. Whatever the basis for that decision, by the time it was published I had returned to New York. In the end, it was more important to me that the results were published in a reputable Journal.

During these St. Louis days Fletcher remained uncommunicative and inscrutable, even though I had always shared my findings on high solubility plasma fibrinogens with him, particularly those showing that they were catabolic intermediates. I understood using molecular sieving chromatography he had identified the lower molecular weight fibrinogens that he termed 'first derivative.' They were the same as *Fibrinogen Catabolites.*

Shortly after my return to SUNY, I met *Peter Harpel* from Cornell Medical School in Manhattan, and we soon were friends and collaborators. Peter was very bright and a seemingly self-effacing person who frequently asserted to me with bravado, *"Imagine me, a Jewish boy from Bangor, Maine, getting this far."* At that time, he was studying a proteolytic enzyme inhibitor in plasma called alpha 2-macroglobulin ($\alpha 2M$) in concert with his faithful laboratory sidekick, 'Mr. Chang.'

The mechanism by which $\alpha 2M$ functions as an enzyme inhibitor is that it encloses plasmin-like enzymes within its cage-like structure without impairing the enzyme's catalytic site. 'Entrapment' does not interfere with the enzyme's capacity to cleave small substrates, but it reduces the enzyme's ability to cleave larger structures like proteins. Peter and I wondered whether entrapment in $\alpha 2M$'s 'cage' might still allow plasmin to cleave fibrinogen Aα chains. In our experiments, we prepared $\alpha 2M$-entrapped plasmin, and then examined the degradative cleavage profile on fibrinogen. The fibrinogen products forming in the presence of plasmin-$\alpha 2M$ complexes were similar to plasmin-cleaved fibrinogen products, but qualitatively different from the catabolic fibrinogen products we had previously identified. We concluded that circulating fibrinogen catabolites had formed through a proteolytic mechanism that was not related to plasmin cleavage [39]. Peter and I holed up together for three days and two nights in a Dallas hotel during an American Heart Association meeting to write the report. In the end, we were successful, although we had to resist would-be hookers and intrusive cleaning maids.

My interest in identifying the culprit enzyme continued, a search that lasted several more decades. During that period, I conducted many experiments designed to reveal an enzyme or a cell-mediated enzymic process that could account for 'Fibrinogen Catabolites.' None was forthcoming unfortunately. I collaborated with many investigators, including *Alvin Schmaier* (University of Michigan), and even with a former adversary, *Patrick McKee* (University of Oklahoma). Identification of the specific process by which Fibrinogen Catabolites form remains a mystery that nowadays seems to be of little interest to others in this field. Hopefully that indifference will change.

Marriage

I met *Shirley Ann McDowell*, a staff nurse on the Barnes Surgical Service, while I was doing a clinical rotation as 'Consult' to her service. Ours was not at first a comfortable situation. Shirley seemed interested in me as a fill-in for her recent and hopefully future boyfriend, John Hatly, which was okay with me in the beginning. Sometimes she met with Hatly clandestinely in the hope that their relationship would improve. It never did. Our relationship blossomed and I was happily left with 'My Shirley.' Our developing relationship coincided with my decision to return to New York at SUNY-Downstate Medical Center. That decision was strongly influenced by my father's recent colon resection for carcinoma. I wanted to move closer to home to deal with any contingencies that might arise.

We decided to get married while we were attending *Marilynn Anderson's* wedding in Effingham, Illinois in April 1966. Marilynn was Shirley's closest friend and remained so until she died in 2003. Shirley and I were married on July 23, 1967 in a Reform Jewish Ceremony on Long Island. Our son, Matthew, was born on January 1, 1968. During his ritual circumcision (*'The Bris'*) one week later, my mother, Esther, was asked (in Yiddish) by the Rabbi, what was Shirley's Hebrew name. She had none, of course. Always fast on her feet, my Mom created the name "Sarah Hannah" and that name stuck. My Mother eventually accepted Shirley despite the fact she was not Jewish. Eventually I moved her from Brooklyn, which had been home for her entire life, to the Chai Point Senior Residence in Milwaukee. Her initial rejection of Shirley as a 'daughter' evolved to an enduring love, and eventually to total dependence. My father died from a myocardial infarction (MI) in 1974. That event further intensified my interest in intravascular thrombosis, a focus that has lasted throughout my career.

A Sabbatical Year in Paris At Hôpital Beaujon

After spending a few years assembling a reliable and productive research team at SUNY, I decided to spend a leave-of-absence in Paris with *Doris Ménaché*, an old friend, who at that time was the director of clinical laboratory services at Hôpital Beaujon in Clichy, a suburb of Paris. I first met Doris at The Federated Society meetings in Atlantic City while I was at NIH and heard her present a case of *Congenital Dysfibrinogenemia*[1], an abnormality that came to be known as *Fibrinogen Paris I*. By the time I had moved to St. Louis, we had begun a collaboration.

Over a period of several years we had not gotten much closer to a solution. It seemed to me that spending a year in her laboratory focusing on that problem would materially advance our collaboration. Thus, 'Fibrinogen Paris I' became my official reason for requesting a leave. There were, of course, other reasons for wanting to do this, including my desire to master the French language, to live like a Frenchman in Europe while experiencing French culture, and lastly but not least, to learn Electron Microscopy.

Once I had made my decision, preparation for the Sabbatical was easy. I enrolled at Alliance Française to learn French, formally requested a leave-of-absence from SUNY, applied for and was awarded a Josiah Macy Faculty Scholar award that materially helped to defray my reduced income while I was away from New York. In July 1977 after one and a half years of studying at Alliance Française, Shirley and I plus our three children (Matthew, 10, Marni, 8, and Aimee, 3 years of age) embarked on The Queen Elizabeth II, bound for Le Havre.

Upon our arrival, we took possession of a Peugeot 504 that I had previously purchased in Rockville Centre, and then drove directly to our rented apartment in Paris at Rue de L'Abbé Groult in the 15th Arrondissement (District). I also bought a second car, a Peugeot 305 that was on its last legs, from *Edwin Franklin*, (a renowned immunologist from NYU), who had just completed his own Sabbatical leave in Paris. He had occupied that same apartment the previous year and recommended it to me.

We enrolled Matt and Marni in a bilingual School called École Bilingue, and Aimee went to a French-only Nursery School. The French language soon became a necessity for her as a means for self-defense, and she answered the call. Reportedly, the first French word she uttered at her school was 'Arrête' (literal meaning "Don't come any closer mister!") directed at a pesky little boy who had been bothering her in some way. After the school day, at home, she would repeat that word over and over, making sure it was pronounced correctly. A few years later when she was in High School in Shorewood, she spent several weeks in Paris with our friends *Marie-Helêne* and *Patrick Denninger* to improve her French and experience the French lifestyle.

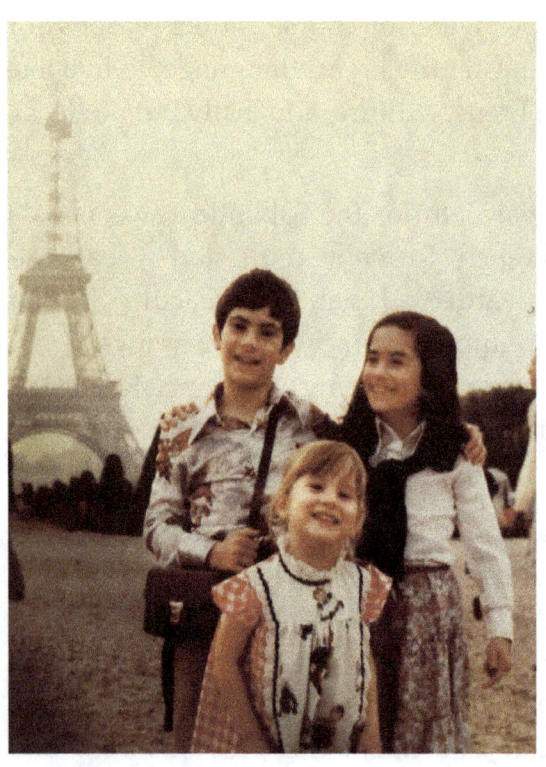

(L to R) Matt, Aimee, and Marni in front of the Eiffel Tower

I have kept in touch with Marie-Helêne over these many years and so has Aimee. During a memory-lane trip to Paris in 2011, Shirley and I visited the Denningers and were treated to a delightful round of golf at their country club, Les Chênes. I played with Marie-Helêne, while Shirley and Patrick followed along in a golf cart.

I began to learn about electron microscopy from *Gerard Feldmann* and subsequently *Jacques Escaig* [40;41]. The knowledge I gained enabled me to devise ways of using microscopy to develop evidence bearing on the γ chain cross-linking controversy (see *Chapter VI*). I also studied an unrelated disease syndrome known as *Familial Mediterranean Fever* (FMF), an inflammatory disease of unknown origin. Many of the subjects we studied lived in France, but most of them had roots in North Africa and The Middle East. In collaboration with *Jan Luc Wautier* (#54, cover picture), who obtained the samples for our study, we showed that FMF plasma from FMF subjects almost always contained significant amounts of *soluble fibrin* manifesting as *cryofibrinogen* precipitates [42]. I knew of no other disease in which such abundant amounts of circulating fibrin occurred in almost all subjects.

Fibrinogen Paris I

Platelet fibrinogen is situated in its α-granules, but how it got there was a mystery at the time. Was fibrinogen synthesized in the platelet progenitor cell, the megakaryocyte, and then passed on to budding platelets in their own α-granules? I was not alone in believing that the source of the fibrinogen in platelets was plasma fibrinogen. The question was how to prove or disprove that conjecture. Studying Paris I fibrinogen gave us some answers.

Paris I fibrinogen supported platelet aggregation poorly and I began to suspect that fibrinogen recognition at the platelet surface was a requirement for its ingestion into platelets. With *Martine Jandrot*, then a student in Doris Ménaché's group, we isolated the fibrinogen from Paris I platelet α granules and found only normal fibrinogen molecules. There was no evidence that any mutant Paris I fibrinogen molecules were present [43]. In earlier studies, we had found that Paris I γ chains were unable to cross-link with one another to form γ dimers, nor could they incorporate amine donors such as *dansyl cadaverine* [44;45]. On the basis of these observations we suggested, correctly as it turned out, that the structural defect in Fibrinogen Paris I molecules had impaired their binding and uptake by platelets, a surmise that was amply confirmed by *Elizabeth Cramer*, who showed that the Fibrinogen in platelets came from circulating fibrinogen that was identified for eventual ingestion into platelet α granules by binding to the platelet fibrinogen receptor ($\alpha_2\beta_3$).

A few years later we showed that the Paris I abnormality was due to an amino acid insertion upstream from the otherwise normal C-terminal platelet-binding and cross-linking site [46]. Why the normal platelet recognition sequence was not recognized by the platelet fibrinogen receptor, has still not been settled. *Igor Pechik* (University of Maryland) attempted to model the Paris I sequence in the context of known crystal structures, but unfortunately his project got sidetracked by mundane things such as putting bread on the table.

Looking Back

A few years passed (1985) before *Professor Jacques Caen*, a benefactor and enabler throughout all my visits to France, (and an indefatigable tennis and ping pong player), invited me to be a Visiting Professor of the Collège de Paris VII, and charged me with delivering four lectures during a one month stay. I chose to deliver all of my lectures in French. I believe that I was the first American at Paris VII to have delivered my lectures in French and, as well, to have responded to all questions and comments in French. To prepare myself for this task, I spent nearly the entire month holed up in my hotel room, preparing my presentations with a Scientific French dictionary always at my side.

In retrospect, my many visits to Paris were enormously successful and gratifying. They were also great for my family, then, and even now. During these visits I advanced my investigative skills, skills that enabled me to make valuable contributions and pursue new avenues of inquiry. The effects of the knowledge and expertise I gained pervade several chapters of this book. The friendships I made were among the most genuine and enduring of my life.

Michael Mosesson April 14, 2015

CHRONIC INTRAVASCULAR COAGULATION SYNDROME*

Report of a Case with Special Studies of an Associated Plasma Cryoprecipitate ("Cryofibrinogen")

Michael W. Mosesson, M.D., Robert W. Colman, M.D., and Sol Sherry, M.D.

Abstract In a patient with a chronic intravascular coagulation syndrome characterized by depletion of fibrinogen and platelets, participation of other clotting factors or secondary fibrinolysis were not demonstrable. Heparin was effective in controlling the syndrome, which was evident 10 months before discovery of a primary ovarian carcinoma. Warfarin did not prevent thrombotic complications.

A plasma cryoprecipitate ("cryofibrinogen") was constantly present. Physicochemical studies demonstrated, in addition to fibrinogen, a β_1 globulin amounting to approximately 50 per cent of the total protein. The β_1 globulin, presumably an "incomplete cryoglobulin," formed a reversible, cold-precipitable complex with the fibrinogen and was immunochemically related to a normal serum protein. The reason for the association of the cryoprecipitate with the intravascular coagulation process was not determined, but its presence helped to establish the diagnosis and reflected the intensity of intravascular coagulation during heparin and other therapy.

CONSUMPTION coagulopathy is an example of excessive intravascular coagulation characterized by marked reduction in some or all coagulation factors ordinarily consumed during clotting of blood in vitro.[1] This report describes a chronic case of this syndrome in which the manifestations preceded the appearance of an ovarian carcinoma by many months. Several interesting and important aspects are emphasized: heparin is the therapy of choice, both acutely and in long-term management; "secondary" fibrinolytic phenomena are not necessarily present; and a cryoprecipitate ("cryofibrinogen"), present in plasma but not in serum, served as an aid in diagnosis and in following the course of the illness. Detailed studies of the composition and nature of the cryoprecipitate suggested that in this case the cryoprecipitate represents a reversible, cold-insoluble complex between fibrinogen and a β_1 globulin. The β_1 globulin has the characteristics of an "incomplete cryoglobulin."[2]

Case Report

A.B., a 55-year-old Negro houseworker, was admitted to Barnes Hospital on December 10, 1965, for evaluation of previously undescribed heart murmurs and subungual splinter hemorrhages. She had been in good health until several weeks previously, when she experienced increasing lassitude. Three weeks before admission she noticed subungual hemorrhagic spots. In addition, she described 3 episodes of throbbing pain in the left shoulder, subscapular area and upper arm and an episode characterized by transient disorientation, confusion and dysphasia.

On admission the vital signs were normal. Several subungual splinter hemorrhages were observed in both fingers and toes, as well as 3 small ecchymotic lesions on the right heel. The heart was not enlarged; a Grade 2 to 3 of 6 systolic murmur was audible along the left sternal border, and a Grade 2 of 6 diastolic murmur along the left sternal border and at the aortic area. An electrocardiogram showed the pattern of diaphragmatic lateral ischemia. Subsequently, only nonspecific abnormalities of the T waves were seen. Five blood cultures taken between the 1st and 3d days in the hospital were sterile. The initial platelet count on the 3d hospital day was 36,000. Sternal bone-marrow aspiration and biopsy were both within normal limits. The megakaryocytes were slightly increased in number. Platelet agglutinins, measured against patient and normal platelets, were not detectable.

Prednisone (60 mg per day) was initiated on December 17. Because of a lack of platelet response, the dose was raised to 100 mg per day on December 28. Throughout this period the daily platelet count ranged between 8000 and 30,000. The heart murmurs persisted. On January 1 and 2, 1966, the patient had a transient episode of disorientation and slurring of speech. Diminished stereognosis and mild weakness of the right hand were noted on the 2d occasion. The diagnosis of a consumption coagulopathy syndrome was considered; the fibrinogen level,[3] determined on 3 successive days was 46, 62 and 45 mg per 100 ml (normal, 200 to 400 mg). A cryoprecipitate was observed when plasma was cooled to 2 to 4°C. No serum cryoprecipitate was present. Additional coagulation assays had the following results: 1-stage prothrombin time, 16.6 seconds (50 per cent of normal); silicone clotting time, 70 minutes (normal, 60 to 90 minutes); glass clotting time, 8.5 minutes (normal, 5 to 15 minutes); and partial thromboplastin time[4] 43 seconds (control, 45 seconds). The euglobulin lysis time was 105 minutes (normal, more than 240 minutes). An unheated fibrin plate test showed no lysis at 18 hours. The plasminogen level was 3.1 casein units per milliliter (normal 2 to 4 units); immunoelectrophoresis of the patient's serum against rabbit antihuman fibrinogen serum on this and several subsequent occasions gave no evidence of fibrinogen or fibrin breakdown products.

Subsequent Course, Including Studies of Heparin and Related Therapy

Steroid administration was discontinued, and a trial of intravenous heparin (75 mg every 6 hours) was initiated on January 8, 1966. Blood was oozing from all venipuncture sites although no other evidence of bleeding was apparent. The response to heparin administration was prompt and dramatic (Fig. 1). During the 3d week heart murmurs were no longer audible.

On January 31 heparin was discontinued, and this was

---

*From the Department of Medicine, Washington University School of Medicine, St. Louis, Mo. (address reprint requests to Dr. Mosesson at Downstate Medical Center, Department of Medicine, Brooklyn, New York 11203).

Supported by grants (H-3745, TI AM 5312, K3-HE-32,569, and HE-11409) from the National Institutes of Health, Bethesda, Maryland, and by a United States Public Health Service research grant (FS-36) from the General Clinical Research Centers Branch, Division of Research Facilities and Resources.

References

[1] Morrison PR, Edsall JT, Miller SG. Preparation and properties of serum and plasma proteins. XVIII. The separation of purified fibrinogen from fraction I of plasma. J Am Chem Soc 1948;70:3103-9.

[2] Edsall JT, Gilbert GA, Scheraga HA. Non-clotting component of human plasma fraction I-1 ("cold insoluble globulin"). J Am Chem Soc 1955;77:157-61.

[3] Mosesson MW, Colman RW, Sherry S. Chronic intravascular coagulation syndrome 1. N Engl J Med 1968;278:815-21.

[4] Hynes RO. Fibronectins. New York: Springer-Verlag; 1990.

[5] Mosesson MW, Umfleet RA. The cold-insoluble globulin of human plasma. I. Purification, primary characterization, and relationship to fibrinogen and other cold-insoluble fraction components
1. J Biol Chem 1970;245:5728-36.

[6] Fibroblast surface protein. 312 ed. NY: Ann NY Acad Sci; 1978.

[7] Mosesson MW. Structure of human plasma cold-insoluble globulin and the mechanism of its precipitation in the cold with heparin or fibrin-fibrinogen complexes. Ann NY Acad Sci 1978;312:11-30.

[8] Mosesson MW, Chen A, Huseby RM. The cold-insoluble globulin of human plasma: Studies of its essential structural features. Biochim Biophys Acta 1975;386:509-24.

[9] Chen AB, Mosesson MW, Solish GI. Identification of the cold-insoluble globulin of plasma in amniotic fluid
1. Am J Obstet Gynecol 1976;125:958-61.

[10] Carsons S, Mosesson MW, Diamond HS. Detection and quantitation of fibronectin in synovial fluid from patients with rheumatic disease. Arthritis Rheum 1981;24:1261-7.

[11] Zucker MB, Mosesson MW, Broekman MJ, Kaplan KL. Release of platelet fibronectin (cold-insoluble globulin) from alpha granules induced by thrombin or collagen; lack of requirement for plasma fibronectin in ADP-induced platelet aggregation
1. Blood 1979;54:8-12.

[12] Homandberg GA, Amrani DL, Evans DB, Kane CM, Ankel E, Mosesson MW. Preparation of functionally intact monomers by limited disulfide reduction of human plasma fibronectin dimers. Arch Biochem Biophys 1985;238:652-63.

[13] Benecky MJ, Kolvenbach CG, Amrani DL, Mosesson MW. Evidence that binding to the carboxyl-terminal heparin-binding domain (Hep II) dominates the interaction between plasma fibronectin and heparin
3. Biochemistry 1988;27:7565-71.

[14] Benecky MJ, Kolvenbach CG, Wine RW, DiOrio JP, Mosesson MW. Human plasma fibronectin structure probed by steady-state fluorescence polarization: evidence for a rigid oblate structure
2. Biochemistry 1990;29:3082-91.

[15] Benecky MJ, Wine RW, Kolvenbach CG, Mosesson MW. Ionic-strength- and pH-dependent conformational states of human plasma fibronectin
1. Biochemistry 1991;30:4298-306.

[16] Chen LB, Moser FG, Chen AB, Mosesson MW. Distribution of cell surface LETS protein in co-cultures of normal and transformed cells
4. Exp Cell Res 1977;108:375-83.

[17] Chen LB, Gudor RC, Sun TT, Chen AB, Mosesson MW. Control of a cell surface major glycoprotein by epidermal growth factor
6. Science 1977;197:776-8.

[18] Colvin RB, Gardner PI, Roblin RO, Verderber EL, Lanigan JM, Mosesson MW. Cell surface fibrinogen-fibrin receptors on cultured human fibroblasts. Association with fibronectin (cold insoluble globulin, LETS protein) and loss in SV40 transformed cells. Lab Invest 1979;41:464-73.

[19] Colvin RB, Mosesson MW, Dvorak HF. Delayed-type hypersensitivity skin reactions in congenital afibrinogenemia lack fibrin deposition and induration. J Clin Invest 1979;63:1302-6.

[20] Clark RA, Horsburgh CR, Hoffman AA, Dvorak HF, Mosesson MW, Colvin RB. Fibronectin deposition in delayed-type hypersensitivity. Reactions of normals and a patient with afibrinogenemia. J Clin Invest 1984;74:1011-6.

[21] Mosesson MW, Finlayson JS, Umfleet RA, Galanakis DK. Human fibrinogen heterogeneities. I. Structural and related studies of plasma fibrinogens which are high solubility catabolic intermediates. J Biol Chem 1972;247:5210-9.

[22] Mosesson MW, Galanakis DK, Finlayson JS. Comparison of human plasma fibrinogen subfractions and early plasmic fibrinogen derivatives. J Biol Chem 1974;249:4656-64.

[23] Bevilacqua MP, Amrani D, Mosesson MW, Bianco C. Receptors for cold-insoluble globulin (plasma fibronectin) on human monocytes
1. J Exp Med 1981;153:42-60.

[24] Amrani DL, Mosesson MW, Hoyer LW. Distribution of plasma fibronectin (cold-insoluble globulin) and components of the factor VIII complex after heparin-induced precipitation of plasma. Blood 1982;59:657-63.

[25] Stathakis NE, Mosesson MW. Interactions among heparin, cold-insoluble globulin, and fibrinogen in formation of the heparin precipitable fraction of plasma. J Clin Invest 1977;60:855-65.

[26] Amrani DL, Homandberg GA, Tooney NM, Wolfenstein-Todel C, Mosesson MW. Separation and analysis of the major forms of plasma fibronectin. Biochim Biophys Acta 1983;748:308-20.

[27] Chen AB, Amrani DL, Mosesson MW. Heterogeneity of the cold-insoluble globulin of human plasma (CIg), a circulating cell surface protein
5. Biochim Biophys Acta 1977;493:310-22.

[28] Mosesson MW, Amrani DL. The structure and biologic activities of plasma fibronectin. Blood 1980;56:145-58.

[29] Stathakis NE, Mosesson MW, Galanakis DK, Menache D. Human fibrinogen heterogeneities. Preparation and characterization of γ and γ' chains. Thromb Res 1978;13:467-75.

[30] Stathakis NE, Mosesson MW, Chen AB, Galanakis DK. Cryoprecipitation of fibrin-fibrinogen complexes induced by the cold-insoluble globulin of plasma
3. Blood 1978;51:1211-22.

[31] Sherry S, Fletcher AP, Alkjaersig N. Fibrinolysis and fibrinolytic activity in man
6. Physiol Rev 1959;39:343-82.

[32] Kazal LA, Amsel S, Miller OP, Tocantins LM. The preparation and some properties of fibrinogen precipitated from human plasma by glycine. Proceedings of the Society for Experimental Biology and Medicine 113, 989-994. 1963.
Ref Type: Generic

[33] Blombäck B, Blombäck M. Purification of human and bovine fibrinogen. Arkiv Kemi 1956;10:415.

[34] Mosesson MW, Sherry S. The preparation and properties of human fibrinogen of relatively high solubility. Biochemistry 1966;5:2829-35.

[35] Mosesson MW. Fibrinogen Heterogeneity. Ann NY Acad Sci 1983;408:97-113.

[36] Mosesson MW, Alkjaersig N, Sweet B, Sherry S. Human fibrinogen of relatively high solubility. Comparative biophysical, biochemical and biological studies with fibrinogen of lower solubility. Biochemistry 1967;6:3279-87.

[37] Sherman LA, Mosesson MW, Sherry S. Isolation and characterization of the clottable low molecular weight fibrinogen derived by limited plasmin hydrolysis of human fraction I-4. Biochemistry 1969;8:1515-23.

[38] Sherman LA. Fibrinogen turnover: demonstration of multiple pathways of catabolism
J Lab Clin Med 1972;79:710-23.

[39] Harpel PC, Mosesson MW. Degradation of human fibrinogen by plasms alpha2-macroglobulin-enzyme complexes
1. J Clin Invest 1973;52:2175-84.

[40] Mosesson MW, Feldmann G, Menache D. Electron microscopy of fibrin Paris I. Blood 1980;56:80-3.

[41] Mosesson MW, Escaig J, Feldmann G. Electron microscopy of metal-shadowed fibrinogen molecules deposited at different concentrations
1. Br J Haematol 1979;43:469-77.

[42] Mosesson MW, Wautier JL, Amrani DL, Dervichian M, Cattan D. Evidence for circulating fibrin in familial Mediterranean fever. J Lab Clin Med 1982;99:559-67.

[43] Jandrot-Perrus M, Mosesson MW, Denninger M-H, Ménaché D. Studies of platelet fibrinogen from a subject with a congenital plasma fibrinogen abnormality (fibrinogen Paris I). Blood 1979;54:1109.

[44] Mosesson MW, Amrani DL, Ménaché D. Studies on the structural abnormality of fibrinogen Paris I. J Clin Invest 1976;57:782-90.

[45] Denninger MH, Jandrot-Perrus M, Elion J, Bertrand O, Homandberg GA, Mosesson MW, et al. ADP-induced platelet aggregation depends on the conformation or availability of the terminal gamma chain sequence of fibrinogen. Study of the reactivity of fibrinogen Paris 1. Blood 1987;70:558-63.

[46] Rosenberg JB, Newman PJ, Mosesson MW, Guillin M, Amrani D. Paris I Dysfibrinogenemia: A Point Mutation in Intron 8 Results in Insertion of a 15 Amino Acid Sequence in the Fibrinogen γ-chain. Thromb Haemost 1993;69:217-20.

CHAPTER V

MY SEARCH FOR THE STRUCTURE OF FIBRINOGEN

The cartoon above was drawn by Russ Doolittle at the time of an intense debate concerned with fibrinogen structure. He caricatured each of the 'players' (see Figure 5 for details).

Round Two at SUNY Downstate

Although pleased with my prospects in St. Louis, I nevertheless decided to return to New York in 1967. My father had recently undergone surgery for colon cancer and I knew I would be valuable to him in New York. Sol Sherry provided glowing recommendations on my behalf to *Ludwig Eichna*, a former colleague of his at NYU Medical School, and currently Chairman of The Department of Medicine at SUNY. Eichna offered me a faculty appointment as Assistant Professor, and without hesitation I accepted it.

The scene at SUNY had changed from my days as an undergraduate. Eichna was an old-school cardiologist/clinician/teacher/academician. Being in his department was an outstanding experience to sample his clinical acumen, leadership, and dedication to purpose. When he retired as Chairman of the Department eight years after my arrival, instead of simply ending his medical career he reapplied to SUNY-Downstate for entry into the Medical School, and he was accepted. The reason for recycling his medical education was to experience first-hand the medical educational environment in the 1970's from start to finish, compare this experience with his previous medical education in the 1930's, report his findings, and make recommendations for modifying medical education in the 1980's and beyond. He did that in great style [1].

Ike, as he was affectionately called by fellow classmates, asked no favors or special treatment, took and passed (some barely) all the courses, exams, and clinical clerkships, and was awarded a second medical degree in 1979. He was thereafter referred to as Ludwig Eichna, **MD**^{2}. During his 'Sophomore' year, I gingerly approached him in one of the lecture halls to request that he sponsor me for membership in The Association of American Physicians, a prestigious medical honor society, of which he was a past President (1971). He graciously agreed to do this after first reprimanding me for interrupting his attention to the lecture. I was elected to membership the same year Ike earned his second MD degree.

The Conundrum About Fibrinogen's Shape

Between the 1940s and 1970s, hydrodynamic measurements, such as flow birefringence, sedimentation velocity, viscosity, diffusion, and light scattering, were used to determine the shape of plasma fibrinogen. Some reports suggested a rod-shaped molecule with an axial ratio ranging from 5:1 to 18:1, while others proposed shapes that were ellipsoidal or even globular.

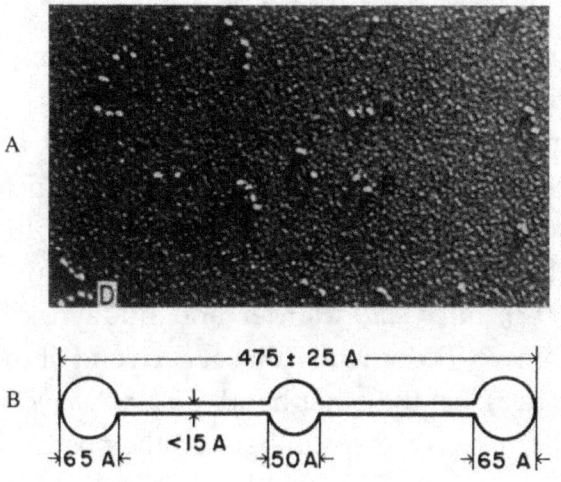

Figure 1. *Hall and Slayter's 1959 'shadow cast' images of bovine fibrinogen that they interpreted as indicating an elongated multi-nodular structure [7]. Shadow Casting is explained below in the section on 'STEM at The Brookhaven National Laboratory.'*

Electron microscopy (EM) entered the structural picture at about the same time. EM reports, like hydrodynamic ones, supported just about any shape or length, ranging from globular to elongated to ellipsoidal to needle-like [2-6]. Hall and Slayter's EM images, published in 1959, suggested that it was an elongated multi-nodular molecule [7] (Figure 1). Köppel [8] painted a different picture. His model was globular in shape (Figure 2). For me at least, existing EM studies could not resolve the confusion that hydrodynamic measurements had introduced.

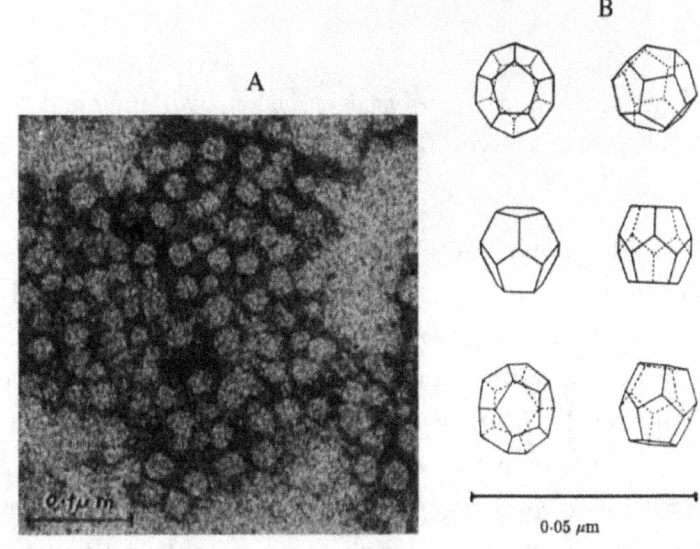

Figure 2. *Köppel's specimens had been 'negatively stained' (an imaging technique described in the section on 'STEM at the BNL'). His interpretation of fibrinogen's shape is on the right [8].*

When I first became involved in this issue around 1972, I knew little about electron microscopy, and determining molecular structure from hydrodynamic measurements was even more esoteric. Despite that setting of ignorance I nevertheless decided to join the controversy. Biochemical approaches for determining the structure of the fibrinogen molecule had included immunological identification of the degradation products of fibrinogen by Nussenzweig [9;10], electrophoretic, biophysical, and biochemical delineation of the pattern of fibrinogen degradation by plasmin [11;12], *inter alia*, Marder and Budzynski's model as well as Pizzo's was comprised of two 'D domains,' one at each end of the molecule, plus a central 'E domain' (Figure 3). On the other hand, *Birger Blombäck*, a highly regarded investigator, mistakenly reversed the number and the positions of these core domains (i.e., two outer E domains and a middle D domain [14].) There were other variations of that theme. Confusion reigned.

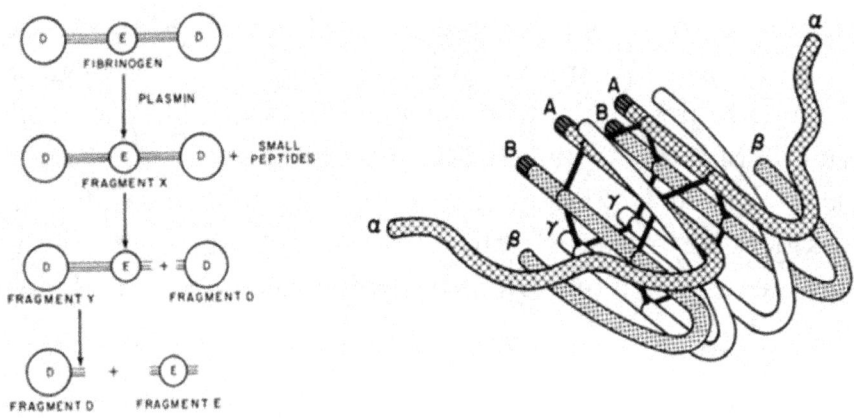

Figure 3. *The elongated model proposed by Marder and Budzynski (left) [11] and the more globular shape (right) that we proposed [13].*

To resolve some of the confusion, in a collaboration with John Finlayson, we conducted fibrinogen degradation experiments, the results of which led us to propose a more globular shape for fibrinogen, a dimeric structure containing a single E domain and two D domains. The D domains in our model, unlike the one proposed by Marder and Budzinski were bound together by disulfide bonds [13]. We opted for a more globular shape since our data suggested that there were disulfide bonds that bridged between the D domains causing the molecule to assume a more globular shape, resembling the structure that had been proposed by Köppel [8] *(compare Figures 2 and 3)*. Our proposal engendered considerable backlash, to say the least, and eventually led me to conduct additional investigations.

I first presented our results at a Gordon Research Conference in 1973 without having recruited many (if any) converts to my view (Figure 4). Doubt crept into my mind because there were so many people holding a view opposite to my own. I felt increasingly isolated but heartened by the aphorism: *'Consensus does not constitute proof'*, and I bravely soldiered on.

The following year *Russ Doolittle* organized a symposium on 'Fibrinogen Structure' that took place at an American Heart Association meeting in Dallas, TX in 1974. Speakers included Doolittle, *Victor Marder*, *Andrei Budzynski* and *Pat McKee*, as well as John and me. He and I took everyone on that afternoon with considerable trepidation for my part and alacrity for John's.

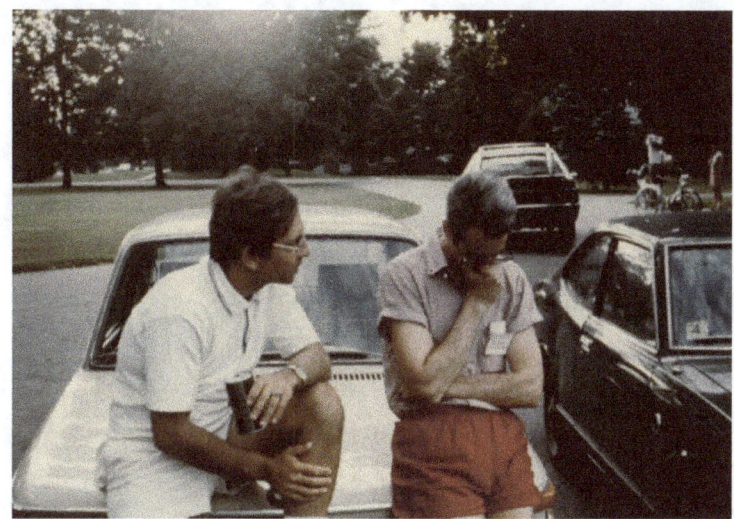

Figure 4. *John Finlayson and me discussing fibrinogen at a 1973 Gordon Research Conference. By 1976 we had published a comprehensive review detailing the issues up to and beyond the conference in Dallas [15]*

Doolittle opened the symposium by flashing his now fabled *'Blind Man and the Elephant'* drawing that detailed each of the personalities he had caricatured (Figure 5). He depicted my relationship with Finlayson as "*Mosesson sitting on the shoulders of a real biochemist*" and that might not have been far from the truth. His diagram also captured the roles played by Marder, Budzynski, Blombäck, Takagi, Mihalyi, and McKee. In particular, he lambasted Lazlo Lorand (LL), his favorite culprit, who had had little to do with the fibrinogen structure controversy, as a buffoon sorting through dung at the elephant's hind end.

Doolittle's animosity toward Lorand reflected earlier fiery encounters between the two involving accusations of plagiarism and poor science. For anyone interested, Doolittle was always more than pleased to provide mimeographed documentation detailing Lazlo Lorand's transgressions. In Doolittle's account, Lorand had served as a peer reviewer of one of his manuscripts. Lazlo must have liked what he had read, and he transplanted Doolittle's observations to a footnote in one of his own forthcoming publications, and then claimed them as his own original observations. Lorand denied that accusation of course, but at least once he self-convicted himself by pilfering incorrect conclusions.

Doolittle's feathers remained eternally ruffled though. In my opinion, Russ should have been pleased to share the onus of his own error. Their fight did not end there. They continued to rehash those episodes and argue about them for the next thirty or so years. Hence the 'unidentified' character 'LL' on Doolittle's diagram.

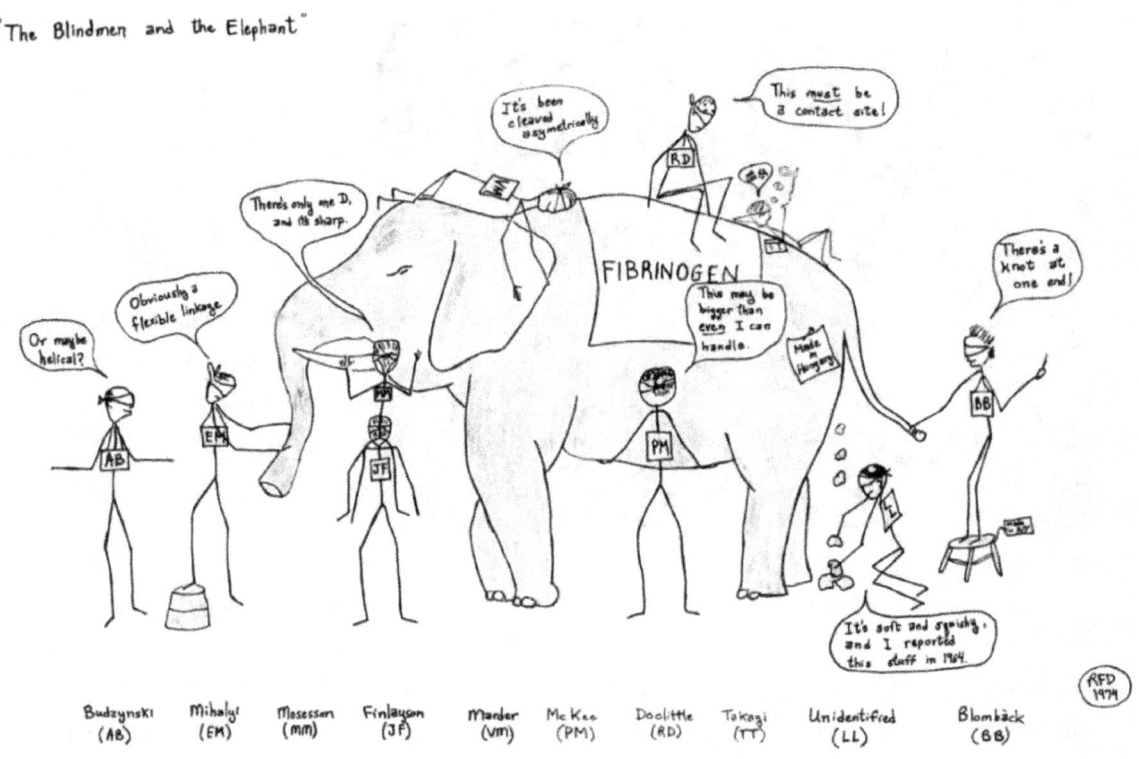

Figure 5. *'The Blind Man and the Fibrinogen Elephant', drawn by Russ Doolittle. 'BB' is Birger Blombäck, 'LL' Laszlo Lorand', 'MM' and JF' (myself and John), 'PM', Pat McKee, etc.*

Presentations that day were lively, animated, and mostly one-sided. John Finlayson, with his usual aplomb, mocked all of us with his French bakery depiction of fibrinogen models (Figure 6). Although I represented my position well, at the end of the symposium few participants were in my corner. The best I could say was that I was at no risk of being accused of plagiarism! I also showed a humorous slide or two (Figure 7).

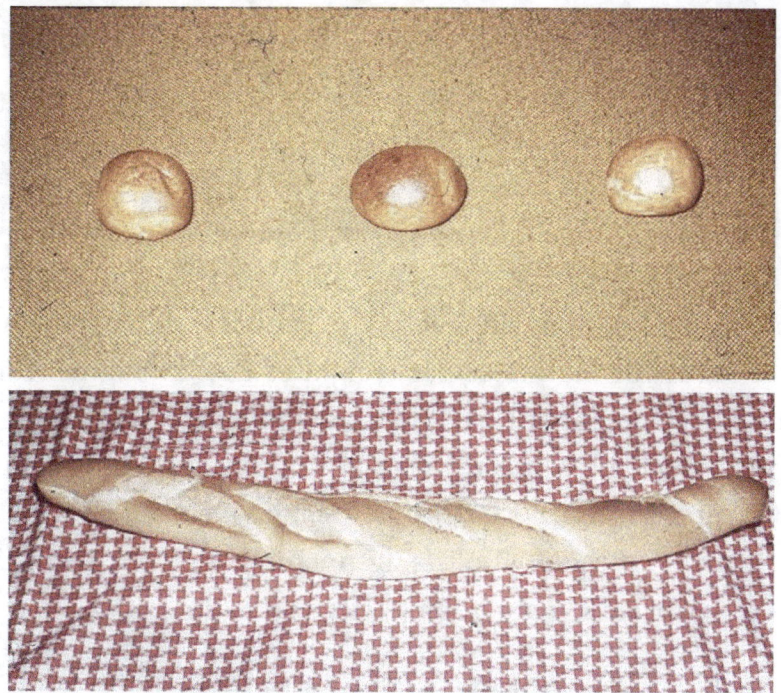

Figure 6. *John Finlayson's French bakery slide.*

Doolittle capped the symposium by remanding "Anyone who agrees with Mosesson, please exit to the left; those who do not agree, exit to the right." I, of course went 'left' and I believe that John Finlayson did so too, more out of loyalty than conviction. In fact, having listened to all the presenters and the raucous discussion that day, doubt was now lodged firmly in my mind. I finally began to realize that I had been incorrect about the existence of disulfide-linked 'D Domains' that had led to suggesting a globular shaped molecule.

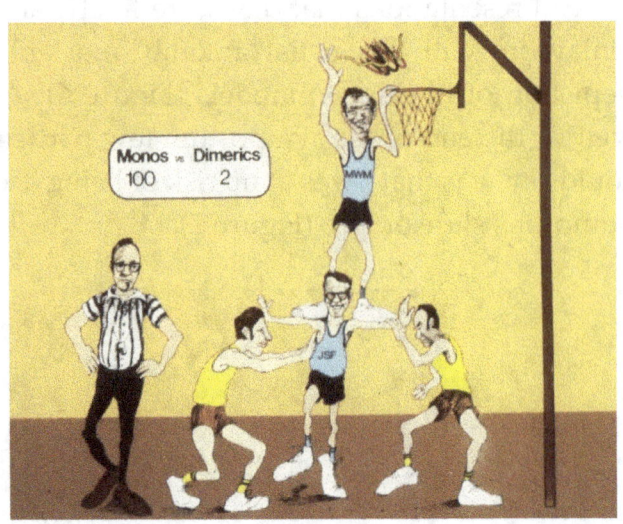

Figure 7. *The author standing on John Finlayson's 'broad' shoulders in a basketball game and scoring with his model of fibrinogen. Victor Marder (on the right) and Andrei Budzynski (on the left) were defending against Finlayson. Russ Doolittle, the referee, was paying little attention to goings on.*

Following the Dallas meeting it seemed possible to me that an accurate and unambiguous value for the molecular weight of the 'D fragment' isolated from early plasmic digests might settle the fundamental issue of whether fibrinogen D domains were covalently linked. Mainly I used sedimentation equilibrium analyses in the analytical ultracentrifuge. Despite a sustained and robust effort, the results fell short of the goal of being unambiguous, as detailed in a review article [15]. I then turned my attention to electron microscopy.

A Sabbatical Leave in France

During the months that followed the Dallas meeting, I arranged a leave-of-absence, meaning a sabbatical year in France on sabbatical. The ostensible reason for requesting that leave was to investigate the first described congenital *Dysfibrinogenemia*, 'Fibrinogen Paris I,' an inherited dysfunctional fibrinogen. The designation 'Paris I' had been assigned by the convention of naming congenital abnormalities after the city in which it had been discovered.

Doris Ménaché, the 'Chef de Services Laboratoires' at Hôpital Beaujon in Clichy had reported that abnormality in 1963. She had made limited progress in characterizing the abnormality and even less in locating the region in the molecule that accounted for its anomalous behavior. Doris agreed to sponsor my visit to Paris and to support my application for a *'Faculty Scholar Award'* from the Josiah Macy Foundation, an award that helped supplement the salary I had relinquished at SUNY-Downstate. My leave began in the spring of 1977 and lasted until the end of summer the following year.

I had in mind other reasons for wanting to spend that year in France. Foremost among them was a desire to learn French and experience French culture, education, and living, and provide those same opportunities to Shirley and our three children (then 9, 7, and 3 years of age). Naturally, as stipulated in my *'Faculty Scholar Award'* application I intended to help elucidate the structural defect in 'Fibrinogen Paris I' and study its effects on Paris I fibrin structure and function. Finally, I wanted to become a competent Electron Microscopist, as detailed a bit further on.

Imaging by Negative Staining or Metal Shadowing

'Negative staining' is a contrasting technique that involves depositing protein specimens on a grid surface, then embedding them with an electron dense solution (typically Uranyl Sulfate), removing excess solution from the grid by 'wicking' with filter paper and lastly, freeze-drying the grid under high vacuum. The electron dense solution deposits around and within the proteins on the grid, and the 'stained' objects are subsequently imaged in a transmission electron microscope (TEM). Numerous pitfalls and artifacts are encountered with this technique, and there always remains the uncertainty as to whether any given object represents one, or more than one, molecule.

Gerard Feldmann from the Liver Disease Section at Hôpital Beaujon in the Paris suburb of Clichy taught me how to operate his TEM and how to process proteins by *'negative staining'* for imaging. Because he was most adept at imaging sectioned specimens, he could not help much in showing me how to distinguish 'staining' artifacts from real proteins. Without such guidance I floundered at first. After several weeks without making progress, Gerard sent me across town to learn *'shadow casting'* with Jacques Escaig, an engineer who at the time we met was working on an improved version of the high vacuum apparatus that we would use for shadow casting.

The most significant problem Jacques and I encountered with this technique was the large variety of shapes we encountered as a function of the protein concentration at which fibrinogen had been deposited (Figure 8). Figuring out which object(s) represented fibrinogen molecules seemed to be a guessing game, and as it turned out, I was a poor guesser. More than once during our almost daily sessions at the microscope, Jacques pointed out multi-nodular shapes that corresponded to what Hall and Slayter had described (Figure 8, yellow ovals).

I resisted those ideas since I was still hoping to find globular shaped fibrinogen molecules. When Jacques and I had completed the study, I wrote in our report that the globular shapes that were common only in highly diluted specimens (green circles) were likely to represent fibrinogen molecules [16]. That turned out to be incorrect.

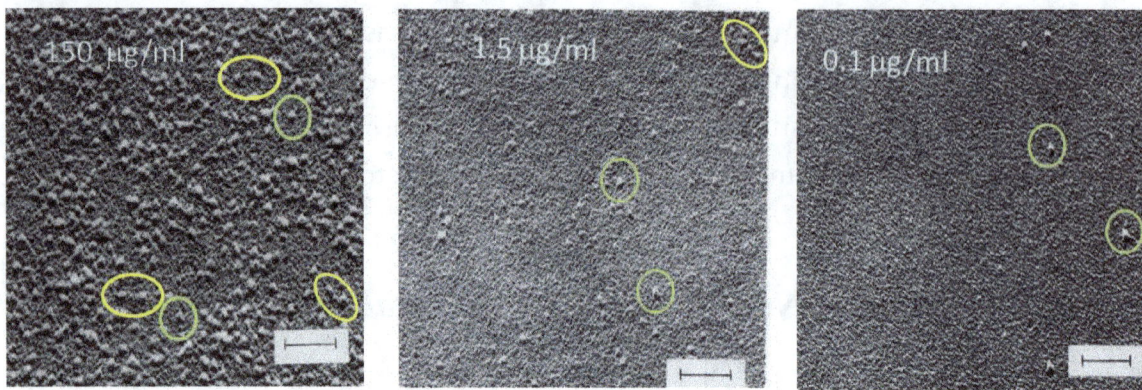

Figure 8. *Data from our 'shadowing casting' EM study of varying the concentration of fibrinogen on the appearance of objects. Adapted from [16]. The concentration at which fibrinogen was applied to the grid is indicated in each panel. Elongated multi-nodular structures that corresponded to a fibrinogen molecule in length are shown within the yellow ovals. Globular objects (green circles) were observed at all concentrations but were most common at the higher dilutions.*

Scanning Transmission Electron Microscopy (STEM) At Brookhaven National Laboratory

A few months after returning from my Paris sabbatical I presented a seminar to the Biochemistry Department faculty at SUNY. I first summarized arguments for and against elongated or globular shapes and then showed my EM studies from Paris. I concluded that my results were consistent with a globular shaped molecule, but they were by no means conclusive. More needed to be done and I would be the first to say so.

At the end of the seminar *Eliot Shaw*, a friend and colleague, approached me. Shaw was an accomplished scientist who was widely acclaimed for his discovery of a new class of synthetic enzyme inhibitors called chloromethylketones. [He would soon leave SUNY for an executive position at Ciba-Geigy Pharmaceutical in Switzerland.] He urged me to contact *Joseph S. Wall* in the Biology Department at The Brookhaven National Laboratory (BNL) on Eastern Long Island, about a 60-mile drive from SUNY. He explained that Wall had recently moved to the BNL and was developing a new kind of analytical microscope called STEM that might be helpful in addressing the fibrinogen shape issue. Although I did not fully comprehend the impact of what he was telling me,

I was wise enough to take his advice, but not before I had carried out new studies at SUNY on platinum shadowed fibrinogen specimens.

These images showed to my satisfaction that at high dilution (for example, the right panel in Figure 8) fibrinogen molecules were so sparse that few, if any, of them were likely to have been imaged. Instead, the objects that I had previously believed to represent fibrinogen molecules were 'artifacts' attributable to microparticulate contaminants ('dust') in *Jacques Escaig's* vacuum apparatus. And to my chagrin multi-nodular shapes showed up again in the more concentrated specimens. Where to go from here?

Joseph Wall and 'Scanning Transmission Electron Microscopy'

Joseph S. Wall obtained his PhD with Albert V. Crewe, a physicist at the University of Chicago who was instrumental in developing *Scanning Transmission Electron Microscopy* (STEM). Following Wall's doctoral stint with Crewe, he moved to the Biology Department at Brookhaven National Laboratory (BNL), (part of the 'US Department of Defense'), where he set about designing and building his own version of STEM. Joe's version was to be dedicated to biological problems. By the time I showed up, his microscope had been built and was operational. Wall was looking for biological problems to address and my problem fit that bill perfectly.

On my first visit Joe explained STEM to me. In turn, I exposed him to the existing issues concerning fibrinogen structure. Over the ensuing weeks I learned much more about STEM and how powerful that technique would be for addressing my issues. Over the next few months, we carried out a series of closely coordinated biochemical and STEM analyses that culminated in a landmark publication [17].

The Power of STEM

STEM has several methodological advantages over TEM. The STEM electron beam is of lower intensity than that employed for TEM imaging, and results in minimal radiation damage to the proteins being imaged. Images are generated by collecting and processing the electrons scattered by carbon-rich protein molecules, eliminating the need for contrasting techniques like 'shadow casting' or 'negative staining' to produce visible images. The images are of higher resolution than can be obtained with TEM. More importantly, the number of electrons scattered by any object is directly proportional to the object's mass. By using internal mass calibration standards (e.g., Tobacco Mosaic virus particles) an absolute value for any object's mass can be obtained, a value that can easily be compared with a protein's known molecular weight to ascertain unambiguously whether the computed mass corresponds to one, or more than one, protein molecule.

The first images of fibrinogen that we obtained at BNL made it clear that my former idea that fibrinogen molecules had globular shapes due to internal disulfide bridging was simply not correct. Fibrinogen molecules were predominantly elongated, multi-nodular structures as had first been suggested by Hall and Slayter some twenty years earlier (Figure 9). In retrospect, the multi-nodular elongated objects that Jacques Escaig had pointed out to me now appeared to be the same ones we were imaging by STEM. There also were more compact shapes, some of them globular in shape (green circles). STEM mass measurements confirmed that they also were single molecules of fibrinogen.

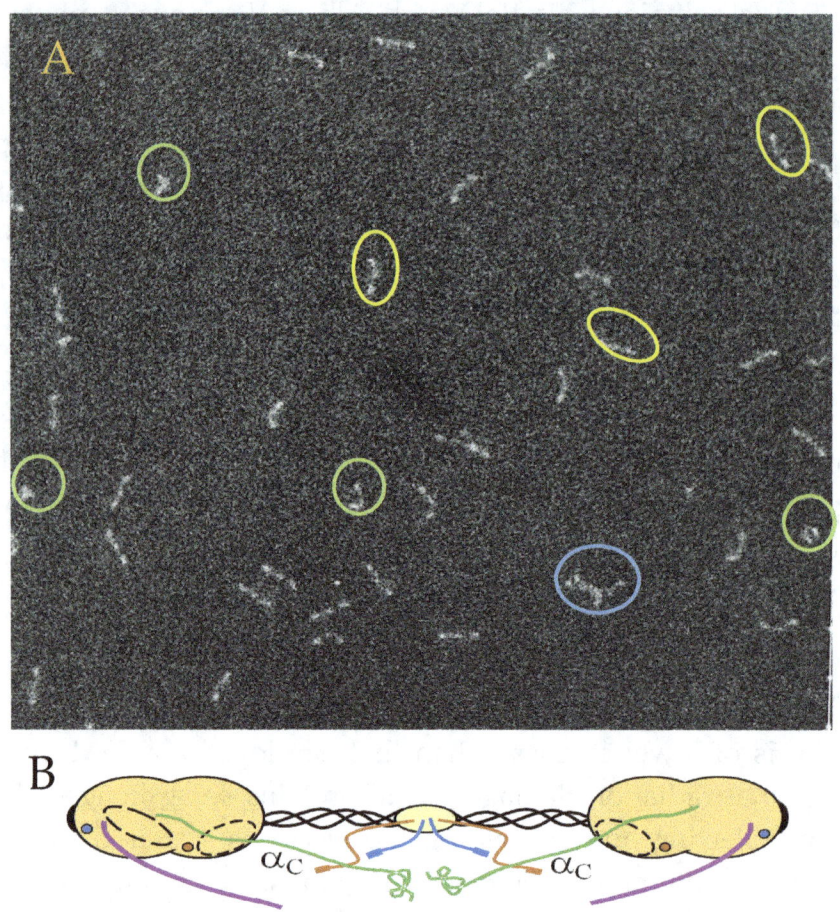

Figure 9. *STEM image of a field containing fibrinogen molecules [panel A]. The mass of each object in the field was determined and its value compared with the known mass of a single fibrinogen molecule (340 kiloDaltons). Panel B is an illustration of a single fibrinogen molecule such as those imaged by STEM image. In most cases the mass value obtained corresponded to that of a single fibrinogen molecule. In one case, the mass value was twice that of one fibrinogen molecule*

(blue circle) and therefore consisted of two fibrinogen molecules. Elongated 'tridomainal' (trinodular) structures predominated, as exemplified by the objects circled in yellow and illustrated in panel B. Some fibrinogen molecules were 'folded' into more compact, sometimes 'globular' shapes (green circles).

To expand these findings, we treated fibrinogen with *glutaraldehyde* prior to specimen preparation for imaging. Glutaraldehyde is a divalent reagent that 'fixates' (i.e., introduces intramolecular covalent cross-links between structures that are contiguous (e.g., an adjacent central and outer domain), thereby 'fixating' what might otherwise be a transient undetected configuration. Following the glutaraldehyde treatment, partially and fully folded shapes were more common, illustrating the flexibility of native fibrinogen molecules.

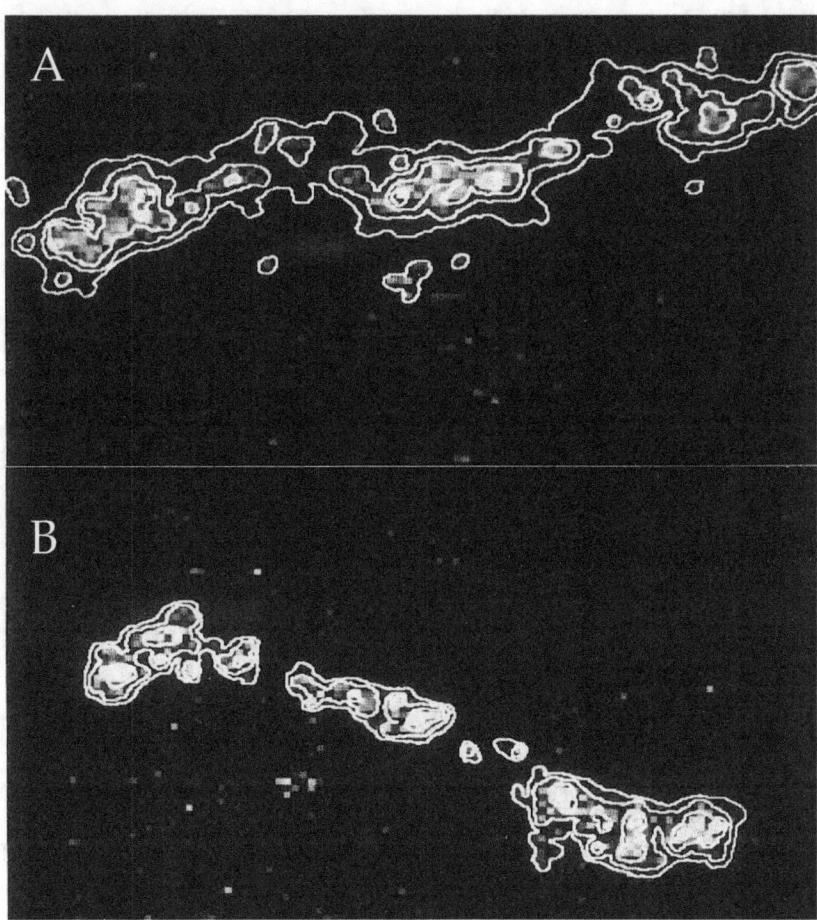

Figure 10. *Density contour maps of single fibrinogen molecules based on pixel intensities (i.e., mass distribution). The map in 'A' was from an intact fibrinogen molecule (mass, 340 kDa) whereas 'B' was from a molecule that lacked its 'αC' domains (mass, 290 kDa). After comparing the distribution of mass in these molecules it was clear that αC domains were disposed along the axis of an intact molecule and extended to its central domain, as illustrated in fibrinogen diagram in Figure 9. This figure was adapted from [17].*

In addition to definitively settling the existing controversy regarding fibrinogen's shape, our study provided the highest resolution images of fibrinogen that had yet been obtained. They revealed new aspects of fibrinogen substructure and allowed us to integrate microscopic detail with biochemical data. For example, we mapped individual molecules in a topographical density format that allowed us to locate the mass attributable to the 'αC' domain which was disposed along the long axis of fibrinogen and extending as far as the central domain (Figure 10). The αC domain was not 'flailing about' randomly in space as Doolittle's earlier conjecture had suggested [18]. Our findings were later substantiated by Veklich et al. [19] using TEM imaging of platinum shadowed specimens.

Our STEM studies were eventually published in the Journal of Molecular Biology [17] and included a formal retraction of my former assertions relating to a covalently linked closed or globular structure for fibrinogen. My search had finally ended.

Michael Mosesson   May 30, 2015

References

[1] Eichna LW. Medical-school education, 1975-1979: a student's perspective 6. N Engl J Med 1980;303:727-34.

[2] MITCHELL RF. The examination of some plasma proteins by electron microscopy
1. Biochim Biophys Acta 1952;9:430-42.

[3] Krakow W, Endres GF, Siegel BM, Scheraga HA. An electron microscopic investigation of the polymerization of bovine fibrin monomer. J Mol Biol 1972;71:95-103.

[4] Gorman RR, Stoner GE, Catlin A. The adsorption of fibrinogen. An electron microscope study
10. J Phys Chem 1971;75:2103-7.

[5] Pouit L, Marcille G, Suscillon M, Hollard D. [Electron microscopy study on the various stages of fibrin formation]
2. Thromb Diath Haemorrh 1972;27:559-72.

[6] Blakey PR, Groom MJ, Turner RL. The conformation of fibrinogen and fibrin: an electron microscopy study.
1. Br J Haematol 1977;35:437-40.

[7] Hall CE, Slayter HS. The fibrinogen molecule: its size, shape, and mode of polymerization
9. J Biophys Biochem Cytol 1959;5:11-6.

[8] Koppel G. Electron microscopic investigation of the shape of fibrinogen nodules: a model for certain proteins
1. Nature 1966;212:1608-9.

[9] NUSSENZWEIG V, SELIGMANN M, PELMONT J, GRABAR P. [The products of degradation of human fibrinogen by plasmin. I. Separation and physicochemical properties. 2. Ann Inst Pasteur (Paris) 1961;100:377-89.

[10] NUSSENZWEIG V, SELIGMANN M, GRABAR P. [The degradation products of human fibrinogen by plasmin. II. Immunological study: existence of native anti-fibrinogen antibodies possessing different specificities]
1. Ann Inst Pasteur (Paris) 1961;100:490-508.

[11] Marder VJ, Budzynski AZ. The structure of the fibrinogen degradation products
89. Prog Hemost Thromb 1974;2:141-74.

[12] Pizzo SV, Schwartz ML, Hill RL, McKee PA. The effect of plasmin on the subunit structure of human fibrin
67. J Biol Chem 1973;248:4574-83.

[13] Mosesson MW, Finlayson JS, Galanakis DK. The essential covalent structure of human fibrinogen evinced by analysis of derivatives formed during plasmic hydrolysis. J Biol Chem 1973;248:7913-29.

[14] Blombäck B. The N-terminal disulphide knot of human fibrinogen
1. Br J Haematol 1969;17:145-57.

[15] Mosesson MW, Finlayson JS. The search for the structure of fibrinogen. In: Spaet TH, editor. Progress in Hemostasis and Thrombosis. Vol 3. Orlando: Grune and Stratton; 1976. p. 61-107.

[16] Mosesson MW, Escaig J, Feldmann G. Electron microscopy of metal-shadowed fibrinogen molecules deposited at different concentrations.
1. Br J Haematol 1979;43:469-77.

[17] Mosesson MW, Hainfeld JF, Haschemeyer RH, Wall JS. Identification and mass analysis of human fibrinogen molecules and their domains by scanning transmission electron microscopy. J Mol Biol 1981;153:695-718.

[18] Doolittle RF. Structural aspects of the fibrinogen to fibrin conversion. Adv Protein Chem 1973;27:1-109.

[19] Veklich YI, Gorkun OV, Medved LV, Niewenhuizen W, Weisel JW. Carboxyl-terminal portions of the α chains of fibrinogen and fibrin. J Biol Chem 1993;268:13577-85.

CHAPTER VI

FIBRIN, THE PERFECT BIOELASTOMER

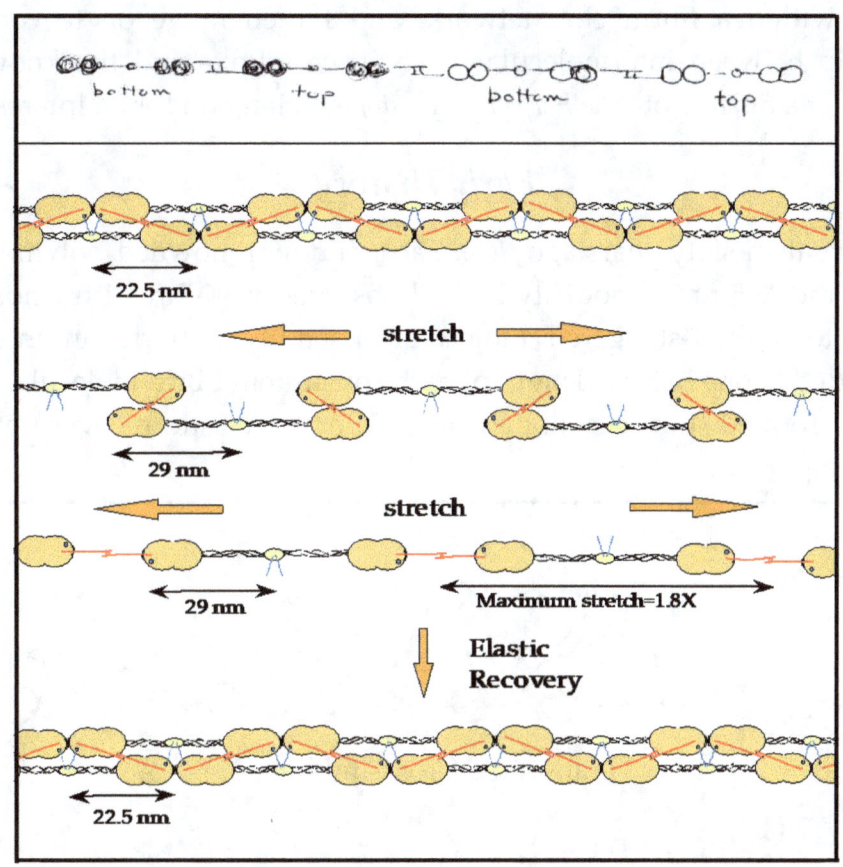

The above diagram ('Figure 8; reproduced here) illustrates the structural basis for this chapter's title, 'Fibrin, The Perfect Bioelastomer'. The drawings show the effects of stretching an assembled fibrin polymer to its limit and the result of releasing the imposed stress on its final form. In the article that follows I support the title's assertion by reviewing the history, the controversies, the experimental evidence, and the personal interactions that preceded and eventually resulted in my explanation for the nearly perfect elasticity of an assembled fibrin polymer. The pencil diagram (top) is from John Ferry's letter to me by which he drew what he believed to be the explanation for the elastic properties of fibrin.

"What gets us into trouble is not what we don't know. It's what we know for sure that just ain't so." ~~Mark Twain

In the first part of this monograph I examine the basis for the controversy that developed in the 1980's and 1990's over the orientation of 'cross-linked fibrin γ chains' within a fibrin clot network, and I then move on to consider the relationship between intermolecular γ chain crosslinks and the known elastic properties of a fibrin clot, *The Perfect Bioelastomer*. Hang on for an interesting tale.

Early History

More than sixty years ago, *John Ferry*, a now renowned polymer chemist, attributed the 22.5 nm periodicity he had observed in X-Ray diffraction patterns of fibrin, to a -half-staggered molecular assembly pattern, an interval that corresponded to one half the length of each constituent fibrin molecule, 45 nm [1]. Once fully formed, fibrin exhibited nearly perfect elastic recovery after being stretched (Figure 1).

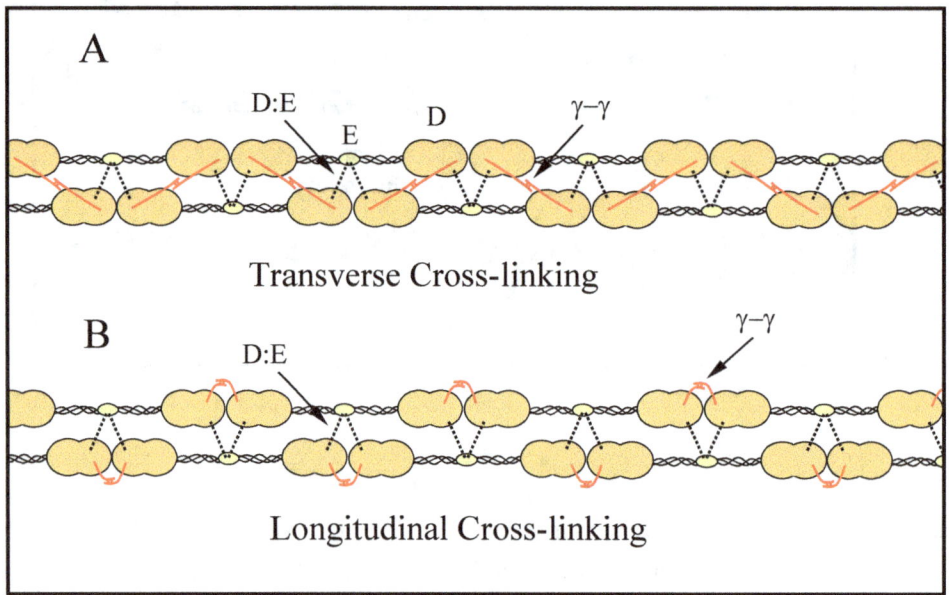

Figure 1. *Transverse vs. Longitudinal Cross-linked Fibrils-* The diagram depicts half-staggered overlapping assembly of fibrin molecules [⬭-⬭] that results in formation of fibrin fibrils. There are two possible locations for the covalent bonds [⊥] that link adjacent molecules through their γ chains: In 'A', they are situated **'transversely'** between fibril strands; in 'B', they are situated **'longitudinally'** along each fibril strand.

Ferry's contributions to this saga began in the 1940's in Boston at 'The Protein Foundation,' a topic that is also covered in Chapter IV. Research at the Protein Foundation was focused on separation, purification, and characterization of the proteins in human blood. That body of work included development of stable blood products for use in battlefield conditions. The studies were conducted in a 'top secret' setting, and findings were not published until after the end of World War II. One of Ferry's contributions was 'Fibrin Film' (Figure 2).

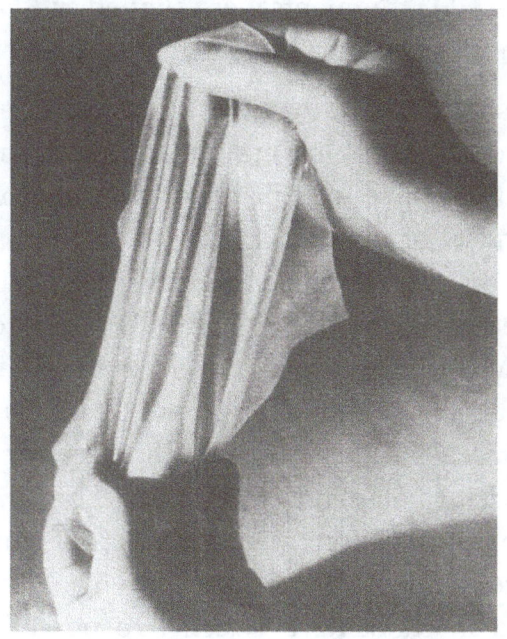

Figure 2. *The fibrin film shown was used during World War II under battlefield conditions to seal bleeding or gaping wounds, until injured soldiers could be transported to a field hospital for further management. Since then many new 'fibrin sealant' products have been developed, and many are currently in clinical use. (Photograph reproduced from John Ferry's Keynote Address in 1982 at the New York Academy of Sciences meeting on 'The Molecular Biology of Fibrinogen' [2]).*

Cross-Linked Fibrils

Fibrin clots are deposited at wound or injury sites after having been converted from fibrinogen to fibrin by the enzyme *thrombin*. The resulting fibers are comprised of double--stranded fibrils, as illustrated in Figure 1. Each fibrin 'unit' is comprised of two D domains (orange) connected through 'coiled coil' sections to a central E domain (yellow), ⬭−⬭. Double-stranded fibrils form through 'end-to-middle' 'D:E' associations between fibrin units (dotted lines, ….,). A separate enzymatic process mediated by factor XIII, results in the formation of covalent 'cross-link' bonds between γ chain pairs (γ-γ, ⌐).

Origins of the Cross-Linking Controversy

Until the mid-eighties, there was no credible evidence for either possible cross-linking arrangement, although early on (1973) in his comprehensive review on the fibrinogen to fibrin conversion [3], *Russ Doolittle* depicted the cross-linking portions of γ chains as protruding from the ends of D domains, and interacting with a neighboring γ chain in a *'longitudinal'* alignment, a reasonable speculation at the time. Perhaps Doolittle had opted for that alignment because it was consistent with his earlier finding that cross-linked γ chain pairs themselves were in an anti-parallel orientation [4], although there was no basis for linking his finding to the orientation of γ chain pairs in a fibrin clot.

That was how matters stood until 1981 when Walter Fowler [5] published electron micrographs of D-dimers that had been purified from proteolytic digests of cross-linked fibrinogen. The covalently linked D fragments were aligned *end-to-end* in a so-called 'D-D long' alignment, as illustrated (⊂⊃⊂⊃).

Fowler inferred from this that the structures he had observed were an accurate representation of the intermolecular cross-linking arrangement in assembled fibrin fibrils. He did not reckon with the effects of fibril assembly (or the lack thereof) on positioning of these bonds. For my part, I still had no reason to question that conclusion, and I remained disinterested until shortly after I had relocated from SUNY to Sinai Samaritan Medical Center (SSMC) in Milwaukee to become Co-Chairman of the Department of Medicine and Director of the Research Program (1981). During that period, I had accepted an invitation from *Gert Müller-Berghaus* (University of Giessen, West Germany) to join his Scientific Advisory Committee (*'Fachbeirat'*). During my third visit to Giesen in 1984, I met *Eberhard Selmayr*, who was completing his 'research' rotation in fulfillment of the requirements for earning a Veterinary Doctor's degree. Selmayr's chosen subject introduced me to the ambiguities involved in choosing between two possible cross-linking arrangements. His work eventually kindled an intense and long-lasting interest on my part.

Selmayr had designed a most clever experiment to unambiguously evaluate the different outcomes of *'longitudinal'* (*'DD-long'*) versus *'transverse'* cross-linking, as depicted in his diagram (Figure 3) [6]. He first immobilized fibrin or fibrinogen on Sepharose beads, and then he mixed these beads with fibrinogen, and added factor XIII to produce cross-linking. Following that, he measured the extent to which the fibrinogen had become cross-linked to fibrin- or fibrinogen-bound beads. He presumed, quite correctly, that the D domains of fibrinogen would form 'D:E' contacts with bead-bound fibrin E domains and that would promote *transverse* γ chain cross-linking (as illustrated on the left side of Figure 3). In the case of bead-bound fibrinogen (not shown in the diagram), fibrinogen D domains would form only *DD-long* contacts with bead-bound fibrinogen, and therefore γ chain cross-linking would be measurably less.

The results were clear and unambiguous, at least as far as I was concerned. Many more cross-links formed between fibrinogen and fibrin than between fibrinogen and 'control' fibrinogen-beads. Selmayr concluded, based upon these observations, that the γ chain cross-linking arrangement must be transverse. These conclusions were at odds with Fowler's proposed 'D-D long' arrangement and they were also at odds with Doolittle's earlier conjecture.

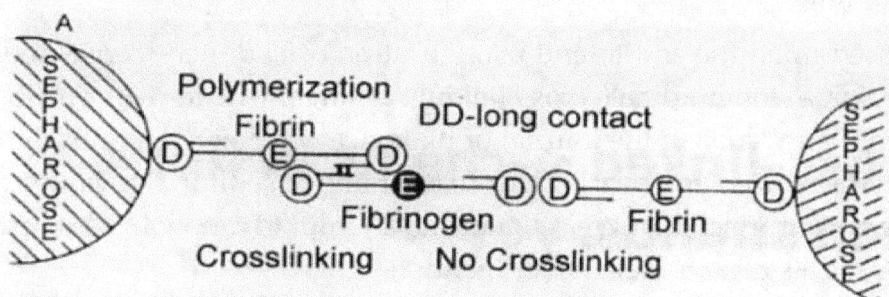

Figure 3. *Selmayr's Diagram [6].*

That year, I returned home from Giessen naïvely believing that once Selmayr's report was published it would not take long for other investigators, including Doolittle, to revise their views of the γ chain cross-linking arrangement. Three years later, Selmayr published another set of results on the ultrastructure of urea-dissociated cross-linked fibrin clots [7]. His observations and interpretation supported earlier conclusions on a 'transverse' cross-linking arrangement[7]. I tried several times to contact Selmayr to urge him to continue his studies, but he had disappeared into his veterinary practice. He had effectively left the issue in my care.

One year after Selmayr's final report, *Kevin Siebenlist* and I reported our own investigation on time-dependent fibrin γ chain cross-linking [8]. We demonstrated that higher ordered forms of cross-linked γ chains (e.g., trimers, tetramers, etc.) were produced during prolonged incubation periods with factor XIII. These findings supported but did not offer rigorous proof for a 'transverse' arrangement.

Some New Players

Four years later, in a publication that was aimed at challenging Selmayr's conclusions, John Weisel fired the first salvo in the evolving controversy when he reported his observations on the ultra-structure of digestion products from a proteolytic digest of cross-linked fibrin [9]. After the digestion phase of their study had been completed, they added a solvent, acetic acid, that caused non-covalently linked digest fragments (including the E- and cross-linked D fragments) to disassociate. They then imaged the products by transmission electron microscopy (TEM). Under those conditions they found that cross-linked D dimers were end-

---

[7] Several years after Selmayr's report had been published, John Ferry told me that he had refereed that manuscript and, despite some reservations, he had recommended its publication.

to-end linked doublets (⚬⚬) similar to the shapes that Fowler had previously observed with D dimers derived from digestion of cross-linked fibrinogen [5].

Based upon the end-to-end configuration of D dimers Weisel took this as evidence for a 'longitudinal' cross-linking arrangement in a fibrin fibril. They published their results in the Journal of Biological Chemistry, a publishing venue that I had disavowed years earlier due to their uneven editorial review style. I was therefore not surprised that Weisel made no attempt to rationalize his results with Selmayr's, as his reports were never mentioned.

Weisel had little insight into the design flaws built into his experiments. Like Doolittle and Fowler before him, he never considered the role that the non-covalent D:E interactions in fibrin networks played in orienting γ chains for cross-linked. It was evident to me that their experimental approach could not distinguish 'longitudinal' from 'transverse' positioning. At that point, I decided to re-enter the argument.

In our first reported experiment, Kevin Siebenlist and I produced cross-linked D:fibrin:D complexes by cross-linking fibrin molecules ●–•–● to isolated fibrinogen D domains ● under two sets of solvent conditions: 1) those conducive to fibrin assembly, or 2) the dissociative conditions previously used by Weisel [10]. We isolated the complexes and then examined them by Scanning Transmission Electron Microscopy (STEM), including mass analysis of every discrete object [11]. [For more detail on STEM and STEM mass analysis see: *'My Search for the Structure of Fibrinogen'*.]

Under solvent conditions conducive to fibrin D:E interactions, the cross-linked D-fibrin-D complexes were folded like this: ●●●, a configuration demonstrating that cross-linked γ chains were positioned 'transversely.' Under dissociative solvent conditions like those used by Weisel, the D-fibrin-D complexes had unfolded and looked like this: ●●–•–●● That was a clear demonstration of the role that non-covalent D:E interactions play in promoting transverse positioning. I was not nearly finished.

Cross-Linked Fibrinogen Fibrils

Several years before the cross-linking controversy had begun, John Shainoff reported that factor XIII could mediate *fibrinogen* cross-linking [12]. With his report as a stimulus, we tried to produce and evaluate the structure of factor XIII cross-linked fibrinogen fibrils at the Brookhaven STEM facility [13]. We combined our

STEM images and mass analyses with detailed biochemical analyses and standard TEM imaging of assembled fibrinogen polymers.

It is important to re-emphasize that the 'D:E' interactions that are critical for fibrin assembly are not available in fibrinogen molecules because E domains are unaltered and therefore unreactive. Despite the absence of D:E interactions, double-stranded fibrils formed in the Factor XIII-fibrinogen mixtures (Figure 4). They had assembled in a half-staggered molecular arrangement that was the same as those found in assembled fibrin fibrils: . *What did that mean?*

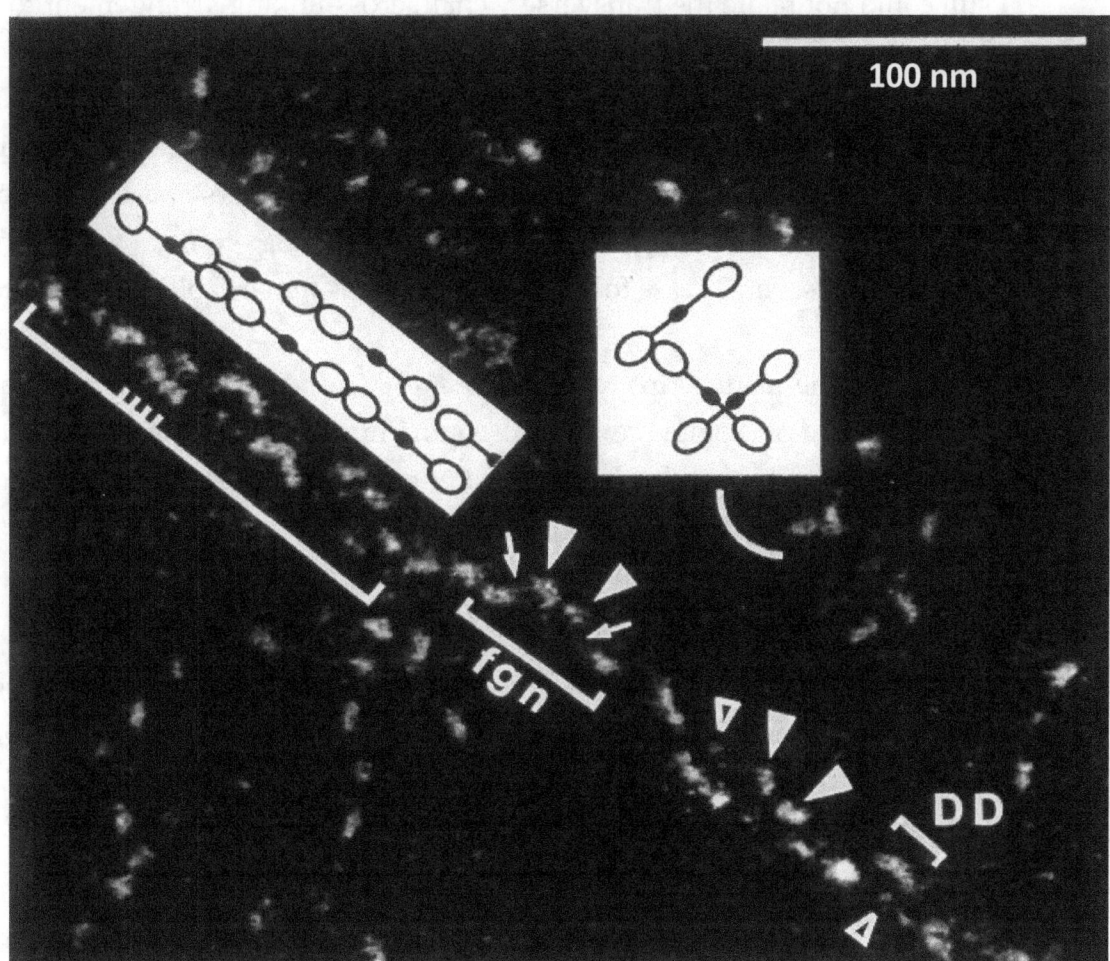

Figure 4. *STEM image of fibrinogen that had been incubated with FXIIIa to produce cross-linked molecules. A double-stranded fibrinogen fibril lies in a diagonal position, a diagram illustrates the molecular arrangements. The arrows point to strands ('filaments') representing cross-linked γ chains that extend between fibril strands. The white bar (top right) represents 100 nm. Reproduced from Ref. [13].*

It took me weeks of patiently examining and re-examining the images before I figured out what was going on. What a striking revelation it was. Image resolution was so good that we often identified filaments extending between the D domains of fibril strands. They represented the intermolecular portions of cross-linked γ chains. Over time, cross-linked fibrils coalesced to form ribbon-like fibers having the same periodicity found in the fibrils. When I finally arrived at a rational interpretation of these results, I was exuberant! We had discovered a persuasive, meticulously documented result unequivocally supporting transverse cross-linking! At least, in my mind.

I still could not relate the transverse γ chain cross-linking arrangement to a property or function of fibrin. John Ferry provided the connection shortly after I had sent him drafts of our manuscript on cross-linked fibrinogen fibrils (1994). He explained in his letter [Addendum 1] that years earlier he had studied the elastic properties of stretched cross-linked fibrin or fibrinogen polymers and found that they were nearly *perfectly elastic* [14]. He linked those findings to our own recent observations. It took several years for me to integrate his remarkable insights into my own thinking.

I submitted the manuscript to *The Journal of Molecular Biology*, and it was quickly rejected based on a single reviewer's comment: "*The specific details….fail to make a conclusive molecular correlation, and must be considered at best as supportive of one model….Lack of a firm conclusion on a molecular level…severely limits its interest to the readership.*" It was a non-sequitor, as far as I was concerned. Undaunted, I resubmitted the very same manuscript to *The Journal of Structural Biology*.

One of two peer reviews was positive and constructive. The second amounted to a soliloquy that ignored the power of our arguments based on STEM.[8] The last sentence was slavish, "*I still believe the previous evidence for the*

---

[8] The full commentary: "*This paper presents electron microscopic evidence and arguments that γ chain cross-links produced by factor XIII are transverse rather than longitudinal. There has been some controversy over these two possibilities for the last decade, with the most direct evidence seeming to favor the longitudinal bond arrangement. After reading the Introduction, I approached the present paper with two questions. First, would it provide compelling evidence that the cross-links are transverse, and a convincing explanation of previous data indicating a longitudinal crosslink? My conclusion is that the paper fails completely on both counts. Second, I asked whether the new data and arguments here, although perhaps not compelling, are sufficiently interesting to merit publication, with the goal of fanning the flames of a controversy most of us thought to be dying or dead. I regret to say that in spite of the obviously extensive effort and the high quality of the micrographs, I cannot generate the necessary enthusiasm to recommend publication. I still believe the previous evidence for the longitudinal crosslink is completely convincing, and publication of a report*

longitudinal crosslink is completely convincing, and publication of a report claiming otherwise, especially one based on electron microscopic images that are too complicated for most people to interpret on their own, will needlessly confuse a well-established scientific conclusion." The JSB editor, Robert Glaeser, appreciated the nonsensical quality of that review and he accepted the manuscript for publication, but only after I had replied to all comments. Rightly or wrongly, I assumed that Russ Doolittle (or his alter ego) had written those comments.

A Visit to San Diego

Doolittle was a member of the Chemistry Department at UCSD in San Diego. He was a respected authority in those days, plus he had become a member of The National Academy of Sciences, most likely based on contributions he made before the cross-linking issue became so controversial.

Doolittle and I had had other collegial interactions. We had organized a New York Academy of Sciences (NYAS) conference entitled the 'Molecular Biology of Fibrinogen' (1983), and then compiled the proceedings for publication in the NYAS volume [16]. The book was reverently referred to as 'The Fibrinogen Bible.'

I was still not fully aware of Doolittle's intransigence on the cross-linking issue; I invited myself out to his laboratory for a two day visit early in 1995. I wanted to share my latest findings and get some feedback from him.

Doolittle's interests were wide ranging and included studies comparing the structure of human fibrinogen with that from a primitive fish, the Lamprey Eel [15]. His interest evolved into what turned out to be an aborted collaboration.[9] My visit had been puzzling. Previously we had had an open and cordial relationship. Instead, Russ now was barely interested in data I showed him, did not engage in discussion, productive or otherwise, and handed me off for most of the visit to a pleasant but deferential Post-Doc named *Ed Shipwash*. In an annoying offhand

---

claiming otherwise, especially one based on electron microscopic images that are too complicated for most people to interpret on their own, will needlessly confuse a well-established scientific conclusion."

[9] In the 1990's Russ suggested that we compare the structures of fibrin prepared from Human and Lamprey Eel (a primitive jawless fish) plasma. I enthusiastically accepted that offer, and shortly after receiving Lamprey plasma and thrombin from him I prepared and analyzed the fibrinogens and fibrins by TEM and STEM. The images were superb! There were notable similarities and some differences between them. Several times I offered to draft a manuscript, but Russ declined for reasons that were never made clear. I decided not to publish those findings and have instead placed a summary of this work in the Mosesson Library.

way, Doolittle informed me before my departure that he had succeeded in crystallizing the fibrin D fragment, but he did not share any results or insights.

The following year he published an article on the structure of crystallized monomeric D fragments and the cross-linked D-dimers that he termed 'double-D' [17]. The two D domains were in contact with one another, ⬬⬬ , an arrangement that could easily have been anticipated from numerous prior investigations including ours (see [13]) The γ chain segments that bridged between the D domains were not visualized, but it was easy to infer that they were situated between two D domains. He extrapolated these observations to conclude that this positioning was the same as that in an assembled fibrin fibril. He summarily dismissed all prior reports on this subject from Selmayr to Mosesson with this statement: "...*the crystal structure now demonstrates that γ chains are connected end to end*" [17].

I was incensed by that self-serving rhetoric and wrote a 'Letter-To-The-Editor' of Nature to point out flaws in his reasoning [Addendum 2]. Both reviewers of that submission were evidently convinced that Doolittle's conclusions were true beyond doubt, and that contrary opinions challenging that dogma were not worth considering. Doolittle's response to that submission echoed those of the reviewers, and my submission was rejected.

I was so frustrated by that decision, I emailed Russ directly, saying "...One thing I will admit about you is that you are a clever and persuasive writer. However, the existing experimental facts in this matter will not go away simply because you decided to dismiss them all in favor of X-ray crystal data, or because you have invoked a one word rebuttal, namely 'distance/' "

The following day he replied angrily, "*Let me start by saying that I found your comments to be tasteless and insulting. If you were nearby, you'd be risking a punch in the snoot.*" Given his rather scrawny physique I had little fear that he might ever land such a blow with authority (Figure 5).

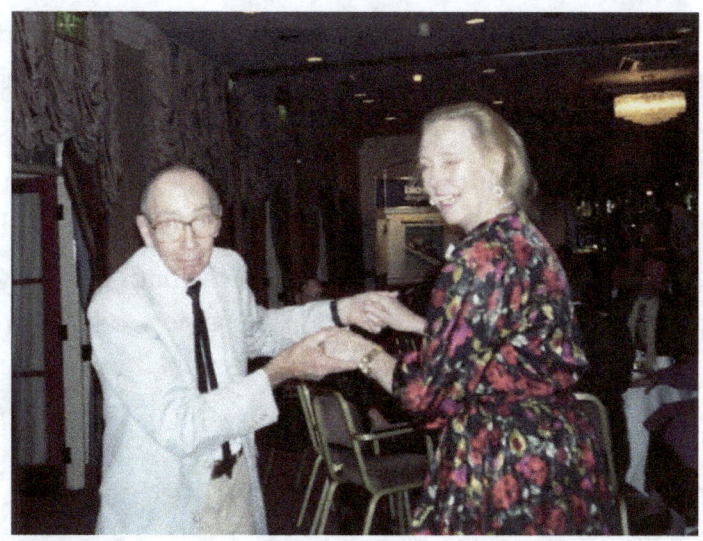

Figure 5. *Doolittle did not tolerate well opinions that were different from his own. Here he is 'dancing' with his nemesis, Agnes Henschel, at the 13th meeting of The International Fibrinogen Research Society in Cheshire, UK, 1994. He mischaracterized her as 'A German Panzer Division' because she had accurately determined the amino acid sequence of fibrinogen before he had, and because she had pointed out the errors in his own sequencing work [Addendum 3].*

New Evidence, Same Tired Rebuttal

Kevin Siebenlist and I designed an experiment that exploited the difference in size between fibrinogen γA and γ′ chains. When fibrin/fibrinogen mixtures containing these chains undergo intermolecular cross-linking in the presence of factor XIII, they form three types of γ dimers, γA-γA, γA–γ′, or γ′-γ′ that are distinguishable by differences in their electrophoretic migration rates. The quantitative distribution of the different γ dimers in these experiments hinged upon whether the chains had been positioned 'longitudinally' or 'transversely' prior to cross-linking, permitting us to distinguish between the two arrangements. Our results showed that cross-linking had taken place between 'transversely' positioned γ chains [18]. Despite their authenticity, and despite the fact that our experiments did not utilize electron microscopy, Doolittle indiscriminately lumped them as "opposing electron microscopic observations" and then summarily dismissed all of them [19].

While we were working on that experiment, *Yuri Veklich* from Weisel's group reported results from having assembled fibrinogen molecules on a fibrin fragment E template before cross-linking the mixture with Factor XIII. After cross-linking had taken place, they processed the digest with their usual solvent, acetic acid, and then imaged the products [20]. Under such dissociative conditions they found only single-stranded fibrinogen fibrils that were aligned end-to-end. Once again, they concluded incorrectly that such a finding constituted evidence for longitudinal cross-linking. Once again, we set to work to refute their conclusions.

We used an experimental format similar to theirs, except we did not dissociate the cross-linked products with acetic acid before imaging them [21]. It was no surprise to us that we found numerous transversely cross-linked double-stranded fibrils, just as we had several years before in our fibrinogen cross-linking experiments [13]. These new results were conclusive since they pointed unequivocally to a *transverse cross-linking* arrangement. But that seemed to make no difference.

Unfolding The γ-Module

Doolittle's canonical interpretation of the D-D crystal structures left no room for any cross-linking arrangement other than a 'longitudinal'. He bolstered his conjecture by arguing that the folded chains in the γ module of the D Domain could not extend far enough for cross-linking to occur in a transverse arrangement, his so-called 'Distance Argument.' Although we had no rejoinder at the time, it was clear that γ chains must somehow become unfolded for bridging transversely between fibril strands to occur.

There was no evidence at that time for such unfolding, and we once again turned to the BNL STEM to provide that evidence. To locate the tails of the γ chains by STEM we tagged those chains with an electron dense gold cluster (O) [22]. It worked! Most of the gold-tagged ends of γ chains were found near the middle of the molecule. They could not have been located that far away from the D Domain without significant unfolding of the γ modules. Hard evidence for reversible unfolding of the D Domain γ module would become available about a year later (Figure 6).

Leonid Medved's group identified a hairpin-like structure in the γ-module (called a 'β-strand insert') that could be reversibly 'pulled out' without disrupting the overall structure of the γ-module [24]. This led to their hypothesis that unfolding of the β-strand insert would accommodate the distance required for transverse cross-linking. Subsequent experiments [23] showed unfolding of the γ-module exposed previously cryptic sites that resided in that region. Doolittle's 'distance' argument was in tatters, or so I believed, but he continued to disseminate his dogma.

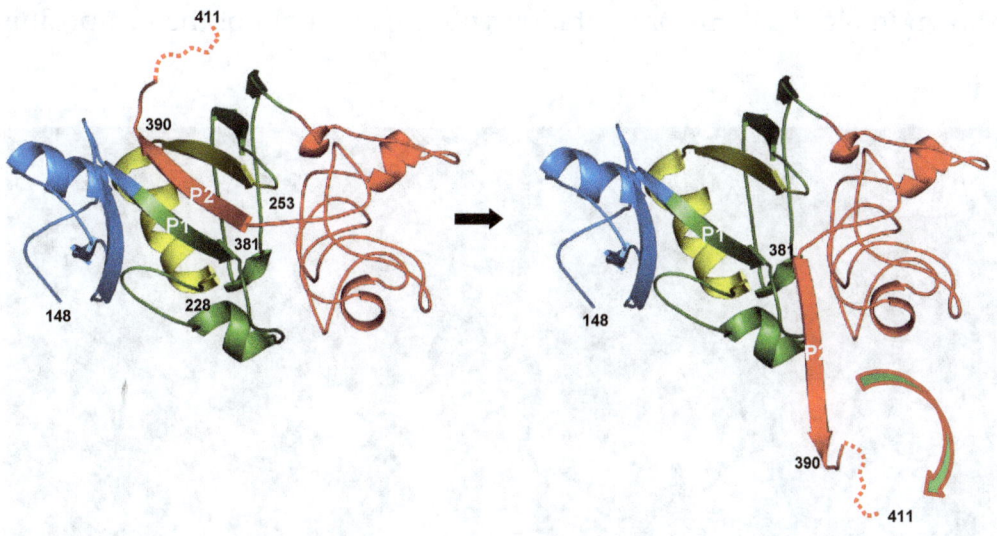

Figure 6. *The 'pull out' hypothesis explains 'transverse' cross-linking. A folded γ module is at the left. It contains a β-strand insert ('p2', in red) lying next to an anti-parallel β-sheet ('p1', in green). P2 can be 'pulled out' (right, curved arrow), extending the terminal γ chain region that contains the cross-linking site. Adapted from [23].*

John Ferry to the Rescue

Shortly after relocating to Wisconsin from SUNY in 1981, I met *John Ferry*, shortly before he had retired as Chairman of the Department of Chemistry at the University of Wisconsin in Madison (1982). Until his death in 2002, he remained actively engaged in dialogue with colleagues, he continued to mentor notable Post-Docs like *Michael Müller*, and collaborated on fibronectin and fibrin projects with *Marsha Bale* and *Deane Mosher*.

John Schrag, his longstanding associate in the Chemistry Department, told me that when Ferry was close to his death, he managed to send his regrets to *John Weisel*, who had recently sent him a manuscript for review, stipulating that he would not have time to respond. That tale exemplified the intense intellectual engagement that characterized John Ferry's life and entire career.

Shortly after meeting this great scientist in 1981, I invited him to be the Keynote speaker at the forthcoming New York Academy of Sciences Fibrinogen Symposium in [16]. Ferry accepted the invitation and he did not disappoint—he presented an authoritative, comprehensive, and well-balanced review of the fibrinogen to fibrin conversion dating from 1942 [2], including a picture of a fibrin film shown in Figure 1. His presentation was the highlight of the symposium for me.

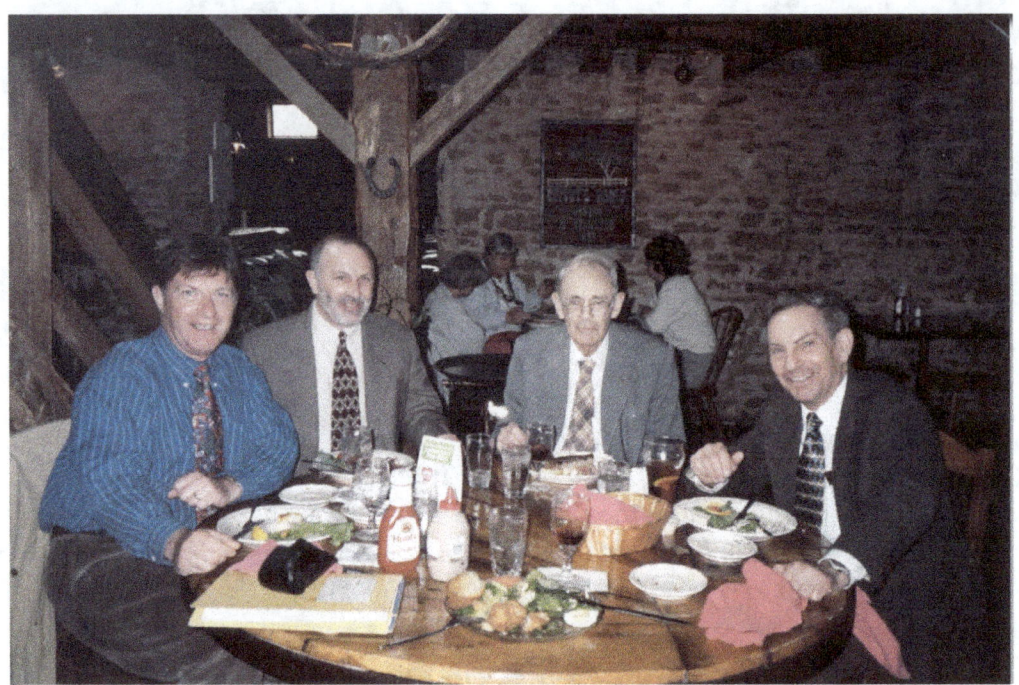

Figure 7. *Yves Delmotte, Jim DiOrio, John Ferry and me lunching in Madison.*

My group, the Madison contingent, and folks from Baxter Healthcare, met regularly to discuss work in progress, and Ferry almost always attended (Figure 7). At one of our meeting in 1996, that was held in the parlor room of a Madison bed and breakfast establishment, we presented our latest work involving longitudinal versus transverse fibrin cross-linking. That was followed by a stimulating discussion. A few days afterward I received a handwritten sketch (top of Figure 8) plus a letter (Addendum 4) explaining *"…what might happen…if the double-stranded fiber opened up to support tension only through a sequence of covalent-bond-linked units. This would increase the length by a factor of about 1.8."* That estimate was based upon X-ray scattering measurements of stretched fibrin films that he and Roska had made some twenty years earlier [25;26].

The subtilty behind Ferry's insights escaped me until several months later, while I was doing a pool lap swim, an activity that afforded me the opportunity to focus my thinking and reasoning. On that occasion, I was sifting evidence for and against transverse cross-linking, and suddenly Ferry's message became crystal clear. Why had it taken me so long to understand what he had been driving at? Until that day, I had been concerned mainly with structural details of the controversy, but I had not given much thought to the functional consequences of fibrin cross-link positioning. But at last I had made that connection! Transversely positioned cross-links would limit the extensibility of fibrin undergoing stretch, just as depicted by Ferry *(Figure 8)*. The alternative possibility, 'Longitudinal' cross-linking, would provide no limitations on the amount of fibril slippage (Figure 9). There was now a biomechanical corollary in favor of 'transverse' cross-linking.

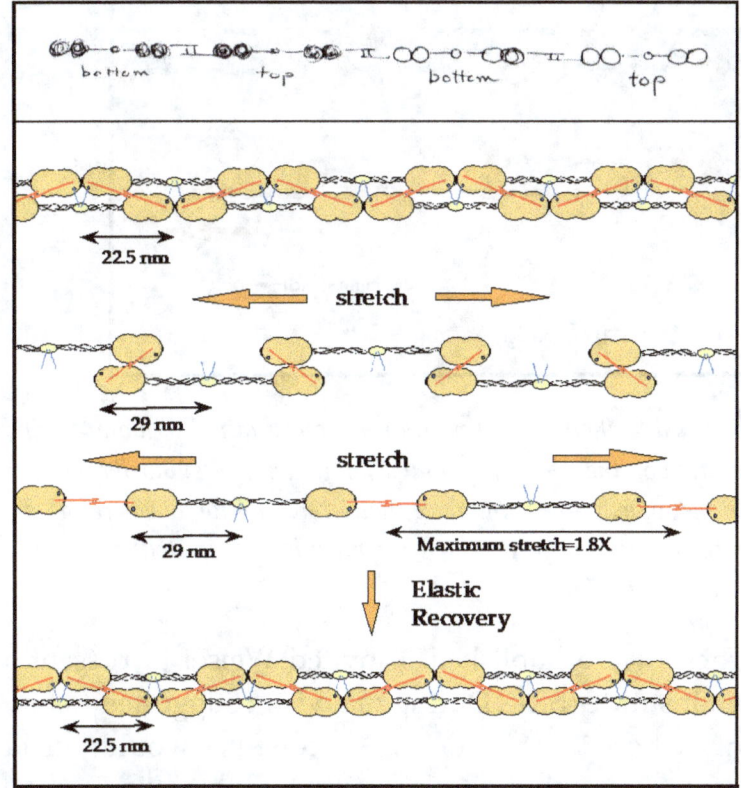

Figure 8. *The consequence of stretching 'transversely' cross-linked fibrin (cross-links in red) and then releasing the stress. John Ferry's pencil diagram is at the top. When cross-linked fibrin networks are stretched, the fibrils can extend up to 1.8 times their original length before breaking, a limitation imposed by transverse positioning of the γ chains. When the stress is released, the fibrils return to their original form. From [27].*

The Great Debate and a Failed Collaboration

In 2003, *Robert Ariens*, then an Associate Editor of The Journal of Thrombosis and Hemostasis (JTH), invited me and Weisel to a debate on the γ chain cross-linking issue. John Weisel would take one side and I the other. Ariens told me that he favored longitudinal cross-linking simply because "Nature is parsimonious." I could not understand such specious reasoning. Our articles were published side-by-side in 2004 and were soon followed by our rebuttals [27-30]. I doubt whether Russ Doolittle bothered to read any of them.

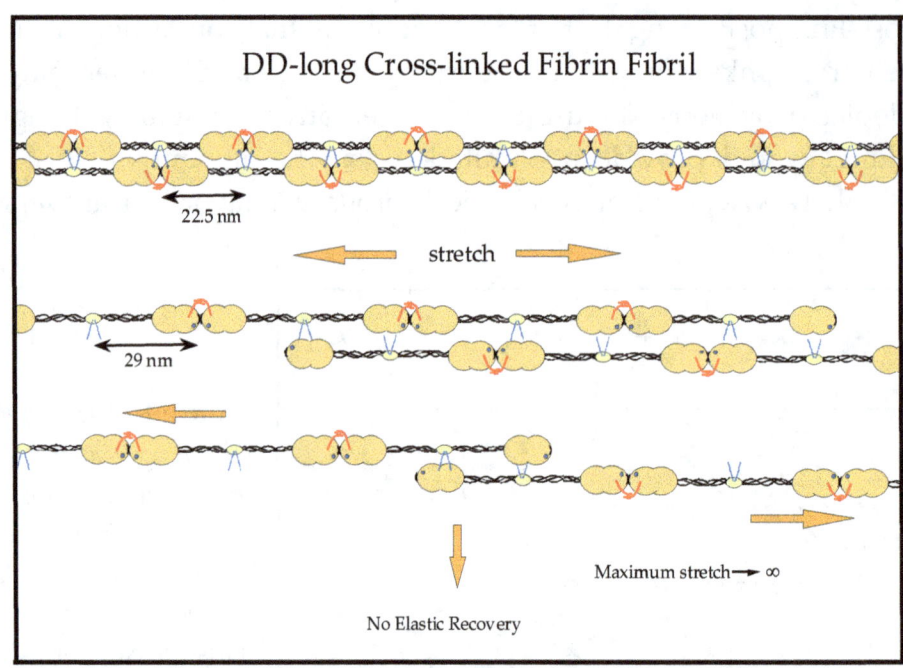

Figure 9. *If there were cross-linked γ chains (red) positioned 'longitudinally' along fibril strands, there would be no limitation on the amount of elongation under stress. Fibril strands would simply continue to slide past one another, and once that stretching force was released the network could not retract to its original form. Such behavior is inconsistent with the known elastic properties of fibrin. From [27].*

Shortly after those articles were published, I invited Weisel to present a seminar at the Blood Research Institute (BRI). During that visit I suggested to him a collaborative experiment whose outcome, if successful, would yield unambiguous results with respect to the two cross-linking hypotheses. The experiment had been suggested to me by *Paul Bishop*, a Factor XIII maven from a company called Zymogenetics. His idea was to orient the fibers of a cross-linked fibrin clot in a parallel plane by stretching, then fix the clot in that stretched position by snap freezing in liquid nitrogen, and finally, cryo-section the fiber-oriented polymer in the transverse plane at a calibrated section thickness. After collecting the frozen sections, we would then measure the lengths of the resulting cross-linked fibrin fragments by electron microscopy. The lengths of molecular fragments derived from a *transversely* cross-linked fibrin matrix would be longer by a factor of two than fragments that had been derived from a *longitudinally* cross-linked matrix. Bishop had proposed a great experiment!

It wasn't that I felt the need for additional evidence to bolster my transverse cross-linking argument. Rather, I was searching for an experiment that might possibly bring John Weisel into my camp. The one proposed by Paul Bishop was tailormade for that purpose. I wanted the fibrin fibers to be as uniformly oriented in a parallel direction as possible, like the noodles in a box of spaghetti, and that was where Weisel came in. He had a device in his laboratory for magnetically orienting fibrin fibers in a parallel plane. The equipment had remained in his possession from the days when *Jim Torbet* (France) had visited his laboratory to carry out some other types of experiments. I would provide the fibrinogen preparation, and Weisel would return the frozen, magnetically aligned, cross-linked fibrin specimens to me for cryo-sectioning and imaging by TEM, preferably using his own microscope (offering to make the measurements myself by STEM or TEM would have amounted to overkill and I did not suggest that particular route to him).

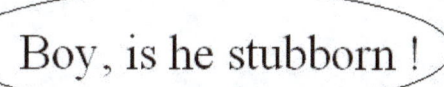

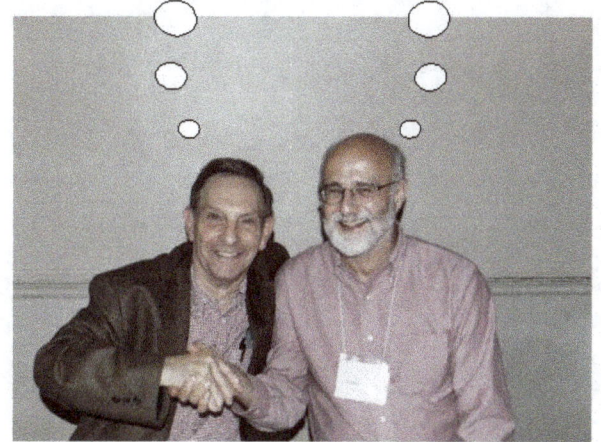

Figure 10. *Me and Weisel at a Fibrinogen Society Workshop in Chapel Hill, NC (2006). John's wife, Johanna, once confided to me that he was a 'very thoughtful person who took time to decide on any given issue.*

But once he had made up his mind, "Watch out -- he's stubborn!" She was unerringly correct.

I sent Weisel all necessary ingredients for the experiment, and together we worked out the exact conditions. To hasten the process along, I paid John a visit at the University of Pennsylvania in December 2006, and presented a seminar on a non-controversial subject, 'Antithrombin I'. During my visit John kept raising objections relating to potential 'preparation artefacts,' but he was never clear about what they might be and how they might affect the results adversely. Whatever his objections might have been, I suggested that we first do the experiment and deal afterward with its outcome.

By the spring of 2007, Weisel finally had sent me a magnetically oriented fibrin specimen. I promptly cryo-sectioned the specimen and returned all the slices to him for TEM analysis. That turned out to be the end of the collaboration. John did not share his results, if any, with me, and he continued to complain about 'artifacts' that might have interfered with image interpretation. Instead, I believe he was simply reluctant to share his observations. Exhausted by such a delaying tactic, I ended the collaboration, as I similarly end this narrative, confident that my ideas, bolstered by John Ferry's important inputs on fibrin polymer behavior, will prevail.[10+]

Michael Mosesson   *April 16, 2015*

---

[10] Clemens von Pirquet's statement *[February 25, 1907, Vienna]* reflects my own attitude regarding the cross-linking controversy, *"Professor Kraus in essence denies any scientific justification whatsoever of my theory. In fact, I am happy about this vigorous disagreement since it proves the great difference between my interpretation and that accepted hitherto. It protects me against the danger of having somebody say later, when my ideas have prevailed, "We have known that for a long time."* The quote was provided to me by Stanley Prusiner, the 1997 Nobel Laureate in Medicine for his discovery of 'Prions.' That discovery remained in dispute for many years after the prize had been awarded to him but is no longer in doubt today.

Afterword

In the months and years following the published 'Cross-linking Debate' (2004), further activity and interest in pursuing this controversy waned. For my part, I had published and summarized more than enough evidence than necessary to validate the *'transverse'* arrangement and invalidate the *'longitudinal'* cross-linking scheme. For his part, John Weisel probably had little more to offer in the way of new or revised protocols. In addition, as discussed, he had reneged on his part of a collaboration that could have brought new unambiguous evidence to bear on the issue. As far as Russ Doolittle was concerned, he was no doubt basking in the light shed by his X-ray crystallographic studies of cross-linked 'D-dimers', that he passionately believed had settled the matter.

As stated earlier in this discussion, Robert Ariens commented that "Nature is parsimonious", a phrase that I took to mean that the simpler of two competing hypotheses would be preferable for him, evidence notwithstanding, and not surprisingly, he chose the *'longitudinal'* cross-linking arrangement. He made this choice despite all the evidence to the contrary that he had had the opportunity to consider as the Editor of the cross-linking debate.

Six years after the furor had died down, Martin Guthold's group reported on the biomechanical properties of stretched cross-linked single fibrin fibers that had been analyzed by Atomic Force Microscopy [31]. To explain their findings, they proposed three possible mechanisms, but because they had assumed that cross-linked fibrin γ-chains were arranged *longitudinally*, they failed to consider a fourth possibility, namely that *transversely* positioned cross-linked γ-chains might also have been invoked to account for their results. When I recognized their error, I submitted a *Letter-to-the-Editor* detailing the problem [32]. That same year I exchanged a few emails with Guthold. He acknowledged his omission and promised to assess the evidence concerned with fibrin γ-chain cross-linking, but I never heard from him again about his re-assessments, if any.

Eight years after I had retired as Chairman of *The International Fibrinogen Research Society* (2003), I received an invitation to participate in a forthcoming Fibrinogen Workshop from its Chairman, Robert Ariens. I was flattered and responded enthusiastically that my participation would best be served by presenting a Plenary talk, or by organizing a Symposium focused on *'The Fibrin Cross-Linking Controversy.'* My goal was to revive the issue and hopefully, to stimulate new interest or even elicit new ideas. That proposal was not acceptable to Ariens and as a result I withdrew from participating in the conference.

Some months later, I was informed by John Weisel, who had been at the meeting, that when the notion of having a debate on 'fibrin cross-linking' was raised, it was met by derisive comments from a former close colleague, *Mattia Rocco*, who himself understood little about the nuances of fibrin cross-linking. In addition, there seemed to be no support among the conference participants for holding such an event, an outcome that was both hurtful and deeply disappointing. I let Rocco know about my displeasure and he apologized for his behavior. Since that episode I have assiduously avoided any further public engagement or statements on that subject, and I no longer believe that I can bring anything new to bear on the fibrin cross-linking issue. My belief in the correctness of the transverse γ-chain cross-linking arrangement remains strong and I feel certain that history will eventually vindicate that view.

Michael Mosesson *May 30, 2020*

Addendum 1

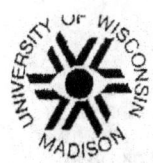

DEPARTMENT OF CHEMISTRY

1101 UNIVERSITY AVENUE
MADISON, WISCONSIN 53706
FAX # 608-262-0381

September 26, 1994

Michael W. Mosesson, M.D.
Sinai Samaritan Medical Center
945 North Twelfth Street
P.O. Box 342
Milwaukee, Wisconsin 53201-0342   FAX: 414/283-7477

Dear Mike:

Thank you for your letter and the two extremely interesting papers. (I just received the figures this morning.) The presence of double-stranded fibrils in cross-linked fibrinogen and the periodicity that goes with staggered overlapping is striking.

We did a few experiments on cross-linked fibrinogen (Shimizu and Ferry, Biopolymers, 27, 703 (1988)) and I think it is significant that the modulus of elasticity G is similar to that of fibrin under comparable conditions and moreover the gel is perfectly elastic with no irrecoverable deformation after holding stress for as long as one day.

It is confusing that John Weisel's observation of single-stranded fibrils under certain conditions favors "long" rather than transverse γ-γ cross-linking. I hope the meeting this week may resolve this question. Your new paper relieves a reservation I had about transverse, viz., whether the γ could stretch far enough to join; this is easier to see if the γ subdomain is proximal to the β.

The new trimolecular branch points are very interesting, especially the observation that they are more numerous in fine clots. I am now reviewing all our observations of irrecoverable deformation, scattered in various papers, to compare different types of clots. This may not be finished before I see you on Thursday, but I hope to have further comments soon.

After having been somewhat out of touch, I appreciate the opportunity of learning about these new and important developments.

Looking forward to the Thursday meeting,

Sincerely yours,

John D. Ferry

TOTAL P.01

Addendum 2

October 13, 1997

The location of crosslinked γ chains in fibrin

SIR — Spraggon, Everse, and Doolittle[1] recently reported on the crystal structure of crosslinked D dimer fragments that had been purified from proteolytic digests of crosslinked fibrin clots. They argued that these data had enabled them to address the question of the location of γ chain crosslinks in an assembled double-stranded fibrin fibril. That is, to be able to decide whether crosslinked γ chains in fibrin are positioned in an 'end-to-end' arrangement along each fibril strand bridging adjacent molecules, or whether they connect neighboring D domains by extending 'transversely' across the strands of each fibril fibril. Based upon the inescapable observation that both components in the D dimer crystals were joined end-to-end, and notwithstanding the fact that crosslinked γ chain segments were not located very near to these ends, nor were they even visualized, they opted for the 'end-to-end' fibrin γ chain crosslinking arrangement.

Because structural conclusions based upon crystallographic experiments often are readily acceptable as definitive, we wish to outline here the basis for our opinion that in this case, the crystallographic evidence does not warrant such an extrapolation: First, data derived from crystals of a D-dimer/GPRP complex should not be assumed *a priori* to be an accurate reflection of the position taken by crosslinked γ chains in assembled fibrin fibrils, because intermolecular associations that exist in fibrin create geometries that are not likely to be the same as they are in the isolated D-dimer fragment. The important effect of non-covalent D:E:D interactions among fibrin molecules is lacking in D-dimers, such interactions having been disrupted both by proteolytic degradation of the fibrin and the dissociative conditions that were used to separate D-dimer from the E domain.

Second, since neither the peptide structures containing the C-terminal crosslinking sequences, nor the crosslinked γ chain peptides themselves, were visualized, one must ask what structural feature of crosslinked D-dimer crystals could help decide in favor of one type of crosslinking arrangement? Regardless of whether crosslinking in fibrin is 'end-to-end' or 'transverse', crosslinked γ chains in the D-dimer fragment will nevertheless be covalently joined at their ends and be located somewhere between the adjacent D domains, as indeed they were.

Third, the D dimer crystal structure indicates that regions involving D domain intermolecular end-to-end association are aligned reciprocally, as are GPRP binding pockets and calcium binding sites, each pair of which appear to be catty-cornered. Further, C-terminal regions of the γ chains emerge from opposing sides of the fragment, rather than from its ends. Consider the geometry of an 'end-to-end' γ chain crosslinking process as it might occur in a fibrin fibril (diagram A). GPRP binding pockets in the D:E:D complex would be aligned on the same side of the opposing E domain to which they bind, and γ chain crosslinks would be formed at the ends or possibly be aligned end-to-end at or near the top of the two joined D fragments. That configuration would suggest that the ends of D domains are not aligned reciprocally, contrary to what is indicated by the D dimer crystal data.

On the other hand, consider the possible structure of D-dimer fragments that could result from a transverse fibrin crosslinking arrangement, in which the individual strands within each fibril twist around one another (as they are well known to do)(diagram B). In this structure, the ends of the D domains are aligned *reciprocally* and C-terminal γ chains emerge from *opposite* aspects of the D fragments, as would be anticipated if they had been positioned transversely in fibrin. The D dimer fragment derived from that configuration in fibrin would resemble the one found by Spraggon et al. for D dimer crystals.

October 13, 1997

The distinction between an 'end-to-end' and a 'transverse' crosslinking arrangement in fibrin is an important one to be made since it bears heavily on our ability to correctly interpret the physical behavior and physiological function or dysfunction of normal and abnormal fibrinogen molecules. We can suggest that better evidence for the γ chain crosslinking arrangement in fibrin might be obtained from crystals of fibrin or crosslinked fibrin, but that achievement has proven to be an elusive goal. Until that event or something equivalent comes about, most biochemical and ultrastructural evidence[2-5] still points toward transverse crosslinking in fibrin.

Michael W. Mosesson
Kevin R. Siebenlist
David A. Meh
University of Wisconsin Medical School
Milwaukee Clinical Campus
Sinai Samaritan Medical Center
Milwaukee, WI 53233

1. Spraggon, G., Everse, S.J., & Doolittle, R.F. Crystal structures of fragment D from human fibrinogen and its crosslinked counterpart from fibrin. *Nature* **389**: 455-462 (1997)
2. Selmayr, E., Thiel, W., & Müller-Berghause, G. Crosslinking of fibrinogen to immoblized des AA-fibrin. *Thromb. Res.* **39**:459-465 (1985)
3. Selmayr, E., Bachmann, L., Deffner, M., & Müller-Berghause, G. Chromatography and electron microscopy of crosslinked fibrin polymers-a new model describing the crosslinking at the DD-trans contact of the fibrin molecules. *Biopolymers* **27**:1733-1748 (1988)
4. Mosesson, M.W., Siebenlist, K.R., Hainfeld, J.F., & Wall, J.S. The covalent structure of factor XIIIa crosslinked fibrinogen fibrils. *J. Struct. Biol.* **115**:88-101 (1995)
5. Siebenlist, K.R., Meh, D.A., Wall, J.S., Hainfeld, J.S., & Mosesson, M.W. orientation of the carboxy-terminal regions of fibrin γ chain dimers determined from the crosslinked products formed in mixtures of fibrin, fragment D, and factor XIIIa. *Thromb. Haemostas.* **74**:1113-1119 (1995)

Addendum 3

GERMAN RESEARCHERS HOT ON TRAIL OF SAME DISCOVERY

I thought you might wish to see this. HHE

San Diego Team Racing to Wire in Scientific Quest

BY PAUL JACOBS
Times Staff Writer

LLA — An assault on Mt. Everest or an Olympic marathon may seem strange activities to choose for comparison to a scientific race.

But when Russell Doolittle, a professor of chemistry at UC San Diego, discusses the international scientific competition that has occupied several years of his life, he speaks of strategies and of endurance that seem more appropriate for an athletic feat.

Eight years ago, when he began his work on the molecule fibrinogen — with six chains and 3,000 pieces — he thought he was working alone in attempting to determine the exact chemical structure of one of the major blood-clotting factors.

Like Everest, fibrinogen was there, waiting to be conquered.

However, what Doolittle describes as a "cult of sequencers" — scientists who specialize in determining the exact order of the components of large molecules — has been growing, although most of the work had been on molecules of less Himalayan dimensions than fibrinogen.

One day, Doolittle found that his was not the only assault team on the mountain.

"You have to realize that the mountain was swathed in clouds," Doolittle said in a recent interview. "One morning the weather clears and it reveals another team, heading in the same direction you are but on a different ridge."

The unexpected competition was from a German group headed by Agnes Henschen of the prestigious Max Planck Institute for Biochemistry in Munich.

His competitor was no stranger. Both had worked together for a time in the Stockholm laboratory of Birger Blomback, a pioneer in the techniques used by sequencers.

The German effort is organized, Doolittle said, like a Panzer division, with the best equipment and an efficient staff capable of working in around-the-clock shifts if necessary to unlock the structure of a molecule.

Taken by surprise, Doolittle's lab lost one very important leg of the fibrinogen race.

He was determined — almost to the point of obsession, he admits — not to finish second in the final leg that would complete the structure of the molecule.

By June, the Doolittle lab was very close to filling in the last pieces of a giant chemical jigsaw puzzle that has more than 3,000 pieces.

The strategy was to finish the details in time to post a complete structure of the molecule at the International Congress of Hematology, meeting in Paris on July 28, and hope that the Henschen team would not be successful any sooner.

The fibrinogen competition is not unique in the annals of science, although few of the races are ever discussed outside the inner circles of scientific specialists.

One exception was the race to determine the general structure of the DNA molecule — the key to understanding heredity, multiplication and growth of all living things.

Among the losers in that race was

Please Turn to Page 10, Col. 1

Continued from First Page

Linus Pauling, who had already completed work in the basic structure of chemistry that would earn him a Nobel Prize.

The winners were Francis Crick, now at the Salk Institute, and James D. Watson, who showed in 1953 that DNA (short for deoxyribonucleic acid) was a double helix — two strands wrapped around one another that separated to form two duplicates of the original.

Watson, Crick and Maurice Wilkens won a Nobel Prize for their work on DNA, and Watson wrote "The Double Helix," a popular and human account of the stresses and joys of the competition.

The sometimes bitter competition between Roger Guillemin of Salk Institute and Andrew Schally has been chronicled in magazines like Science and New Scientist. The two scientists shared a Nobel Prize last year for their work in the discovery of brain hormones that control the release of other important body chemicals.

Like Henschen and Doolittle, other "sequencers" have been involved in races to complete the chemical analysis that can eventually lead to an exact three-dimensional model of molecules, put together like so many Tinker Toys.

Winning in such a race is not perfectly defined: The finish line is out of focus, the location of the summit ambiguous.

Fibrinogen is made up of 3,000 amino acids arranged in six chains. In Doolittle's two-dimensional representation of the molecule it looks something like a butterfly, impaled by two giant hatpins.

The problem of determining the order of pieces is made simpler because of the symmetry of the chains, since three chains are known to be the mirror image of the three others.

Doolittle credits Ms. Henschen with completing the structure of one of the chains and calls the race on a second chain a tie.

But because the third, remaining chain will complete the molecule, the competition to be first to determine its structure takes on special importance.

Doolittle went to the Paris conference last week with what he calls a "virtually completed" structure of the molecule.

For a few small sections, Doolittle knows the components but not the precise sequence.

However, the structure is complete enough so that he believes he can plant his flag on the summit and claim to have finished the job.

But he has not published his structure.

And among scientists, publication is the accepted way to establish accomplishments.

It is possible that Ms. Henschen's group could act quickly to confirm Doolittle's latest results, do the work on the remaining small areas of uncertainty and publish a totally completed structure first.

Strategy has been a constant consideration for Doolittle as he has faced the German challenge, which at times he compares to a battle between David (his lab) and Goliath (the Munich group).

Because the two teams have benefited from one another's results, there have been times when Doolittle chose to delay publication.

At a conference in New Hampshire in June, Ms. Henschen showed a slide that indicated she was only half way done with the final fibrinogen chain. "But later she said the slide was a

The bluffs are part of a strategy to keep the enemy off balance.

couple of months old," Doolittle said.

"I showed a slide, but it was very illegible. But I kept asking if it couldn't be focused a little better," he added.

The bluffs and tantalizing tidbits that the two sides have directed at one another are part of a strategy to keep the enemy off balance.

"A lot of it is childish," Doolittle said.

Ms. Henschen and her German colleagues are "honorable", he said, so honorable that Doolittle has decided to send his latest paper showing the essentially complete molecule to Nature, a British publication that is likely to send his paper to Ms. Henschen for review in deciding whether or not to accept it.

Other publications would be surer and faster.

Some journals are "unrefereed" — they publish results without submitting the work to the anonymous peer review that has been an important part of the establishment of high standards in modern science.

Although Doolittle describes most of his fibrinogen labors as "scut work" — as repetitious and demeaning and with little intellectual challenge — his colleagues see his approach to his work as imaginative and contributing to the techniques used by other sequencers working on other molecules. Ms. Henschen's approach "is to crank out the structure, amino acid by amino acid," said Dr. Robert Handin, an associate professor of medicine at Harvard Medical School.

Doolittle's approach is "more exciting, more interesting," said Handin, whose own research is on a separate but related area of blood chemistry.

And he cites Doolittle's willingness to use the data he has to speculate on the way fibrinogen works.

"His batting average has been very good," Handin said. "Most things he said have proved right."

But Doolittle, who will spend the next two months mopping up the areas of uncertainty in the long-chained molecule, believes he has given up opportunities to work on what has become an all-consuming goal.

But there have been pleasures along the way, in "seeing how the molecule reveals itself. I compare it to Balboa discovering the Pacific," Doolittle said.

Toward the end, several people in the lab, including Doolittle, were regularly contributing blood plasma — the source of fresh fibrinogen molecules — to speed up the effort.

The competition pushed Doolittle's relatively modest equipment budget to the limit. He became an expert tinkerer, a handyman of lab equipment.

He compares himself to Humphrey Bogart keeping the African Queen chugging up and down the river.

In contrast, the group in Munich had a professional staff of engineers to keep its equipment running efficiently.

"Pound for pound," Doolittle says, his crew was superior.

"I felt we could win on luck and smarts," he said, "more of the former than the latter."

If his structure is correct and he can sew up the details of establishing victory in the next two months, he will go on to other pursuits.

At the Paris conference, Ms. Henschen and Doolittle both agreed to loudly announce what they would be working on next to avoid an unnecessary duplication of effort, and another wearying race.

When Doolittle ran in the Mission Bay Marathon he was the 1,144th runner across the finish line. A certificate to that effect is proudly displayed in his office.

But fibrinogen has been a very different sort of race.

"I don't want to be second because second is bad in this business," Doolittle said. "It's like being Alydar to Affirmed."

The race is virtually over now, but those on the sidelines will be waiting for the official results and holding onto their betting tickets.

Addendum 4

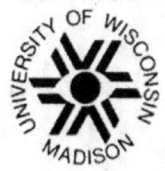

DEPARTMENT OF CHEMISTRY

1101 UNIVERSITY AVENUE
MADISON, WISCONSIN 53706
FAX # 608-262-0381

March 11, 1996

Michael W. Mosesson, M.D.
Sinai Samaritan Medical Center
945 North Twelfth Street
P.O. Box 342
Milwaukee, Wisconsin 53201-0342

Dear Mike:

I want to thank you again for inviting me to attend the hemostasis meeting last month. I enjoyed very much renewing associations with the research groups and hearing your review of your recent ingenious experiments, reprints of which you had sent me earlier.

The question came up in the discussion as to the implications of DD-long vs. DD-transverse on mechanical properties. We are hampered by lack of any real theory connecting elasticity with structure. However, it occurred to me that DD-transverse has the possibility of a large extension under tensile stress if the D:E non-covalent bonds (and the D:D interactions discussed in your paper on Tokyo II) can yield under tensile stress. The enclosed sketch indicates what might happen to the lower diagram of Fig. 1, p. 89 of your paper in *J. Struct. Biol.* if the double-stranded fiber opened up to support tension only through a sequence of covalent-bond-linked units. This would increase the length by a factor of about 1.8. Some lability of the D:E is indicated by the fact that unligated clots creep over long times even under low stresses and at large shearing stresses there are substantial modifications of structure, both of these effects being eliminated by ligation (cross-linking).

Although a clot can undergo a fairly large shearing strain it cannot be stretched in elongation much without breaking. Anyway, the relation between macroscopic stretch and fibril elongation is complicated by orientation of the fibers. Fibrin film is tougher and can be cut in strips and stretched, although the relation of macroscopic stretch to fibril extension again would not be simple. We found that stretching fibrin film caused an apparent increase in x-ray spacing by a factor of 1.28 independent of the macroscopic stretch (Table I of Paper II enclosed, p. 1841). This has never been explained – the evidence is a little fuzzy and it may be a red herring.

Cross-linked (ligated) fibrin film recovers its original length after a stretch by a factor of 1.82 (Fig. 6 of Paper I enclosed). This macroscopic stretch has been attributed to the bending and orientation of fibers. I am curious as to the extension and recovery of such a film after soaking it in a GPRP solution to dissociate the non-covalent bonding. The fibrils might open up as in the enclosed sketch and would be unlikely to recover, leaving a permanent deformation. Unfortunately, however, the interpretation of results of such an experiment would be far from definitive. I wish I could offer some better thoughts.

With very best regards,

Sincerely yours,

John D. Ferry

Enclosures

References

[1] Ferry JD. The mechanism of polymerization of fibrinogen. Proc Natl Acad Sci USA 1952;38:566-9.

[2] Ferry JD. The conversion of fibrinogen to fibrin: events and recollections from 1942 to 1982. Ann NY Acad Sci 1983;408:1-10.

[3] Doolittle RF. Structural aspects of the fibrinogen to fibrin conversion. Adv Protein Chem 1973;27:1-109.

[4] Chen R, Doolittle RF. γ-γ Cross-linking sites in human and bovine fibrin. Biochemistry 1971;10:4486-91.

[5] Fowler WE, Erickson HP, Hantgan RR, McDonagh J, Hermans J. Crosslinked fibrinogen dimers demonstrate a feature of the molecular packing in fibrin fibers. Science 1981;211:287-9.

[6] Selmayr E, Thiel W, Muller-Berghaus G. Crosslinking of fibrinogen to immobilized DesAA-fibrin. Thromb Res 1985;39:459-65.

[7] Selmayr E, Deffner M, Bachmann L, Muller-Berghaus G. Chromatography and electron microscopy of cross-linked fibrin polymers--a new model describing the cross-linking at the DD-trans contact of the fibrin molecules. Biopolymers 1988;27:1733-48.

[8] Mosesson MW, Siebenlist KR, Amrani DL, DiOrio JP. Identification of covalently linked trimeric and tetrameric D domains in crosslinked fibrin. Proc Natl Acad Sci USA 1989;86:1113-7.

[9] Weisel JW, Francis CW, Nagaswani C, Marder VJ. Determination of the topology of factor XIIIa-induced fibrin γ-chain cross-links by electron microscopy of ligated fragments. J Biol Chem 1993;268:26618-24.

[10] Siebenlist KR, Meh DA, Wall JS, Hainfeld JF, Mosesson MW. Orientation of the carboxy-terminal regions of fibrin γ chain dimers determined from the crosslinked products formed in mixtures of fibrin, fragment D, and factor XIIIa. Thromb Haemost 1995;74:1113-9.

[11] Wall JS, Hainfeld JF. Mass mapping with the scanning transmission microscope. Ann Rev Biophys Chem 1986;15:355-76.

[12] Kanaide H, Shainoff JR. Cross-linking of fibrinogen and fibrin by fibrin-stabilizing factor (factor XIIIa). J Lab Clin Med 1975;85:574-97.

[13] Mosesson MW, Siebenlist KR, Hainfeld JF, Wall JS. The covalent structure of factor XIIIa crosslinked fibrinogen fibrils. J Struct Biol 1995;115:88-101.

[14] Shimizu A, Ferry JD. Ligation of fibrinogen by factor XIIIa with dithiothreitol: mechanical properties of ligated fibrinogen gels. Biopolymers 1988;27:703-13.

[15] Doolittle RF. Fibrinogen and fibrin. Ann Rev Biochem 1984;53:195-229.

[16] Molecular Biology of Fibrinogen. 108 ed. New York Academy of Sciences; 1983.

[17] Spraggon G, Everse SJ, Doolittle RF. Crystal structures of fragment D from human fibrinogen and its crosslinked counterpart from fibrin. Nature 1997;389:455-62.

[18] Siebenlist KR, Meh DA, Mosesson MW. Position of γ chain carboxy-terminal regions in fibrinogen:fibrin crosslinking mixtures. Biochemistry 2000;39:14171-5.

[19] Doolittle RF. X-ray crystallographic studies on fibrinogen and fibrin. J Thromb Haemost 2003;1:1559-65.

[20] Veklich YI, Ang EK, Lorand L, Weisel JW. The complementary aggregation sites of fibrin investigated through examination of polymers of fibrinogen with fragment E. Proc Natl Acad Sci USA 1998;95:1438-42.

[21] Mosesson MW, Siebenlist KR, Hernandez I, Wall JS, Hainfeld JF. Fibrinogen assembly and crosslinking on a fibrin fragment E template. Thromb Haemost 2002;87:651-8.

[22] Mosesson MW, Siebenlist KR, Meh DA, Wall JS, Hainfeld JF. The location of the carboxy-terminal region of gamma chains in fibrinogen and fibrin D domains. Proc Natl Acad Sci U S A 1998;95:10511-6.

[23] Yakovlev S, Zhang L, Ugarova T, Medved L. Interaction of fibrin(ogen) with leukocyte receptor alpha M beta 2 (Mac-1): further characterization and identification of a novel binding region within the central domain of the fibrinogen gamma-module. Biochemistry 2005;44:617-26.

[24] Yakovlev S, Litvinovich S, Loukinov D, Medved L. Role of the beta-strand insert in the central domain of the fibrinogen gamma-module. Biochemistry 2000;39:15721-9.

[25] Roska FJ, Ferry JD, Lin JS, Anderegg JW. Studies of fibrin film. II. Small-angle x-ray scattering. Biopolymers 1982;21:1833-45.

[26] Roska FJ, Ferry JD. Studies of fibrin film. I. Stress relaxation and birefringence. Biopolymers 1982;21:1811-32.

[27] Mosesson MW. The fibrin cross-linking debate: cross-linked gamma-chains in fibrin fibrils bridge 'transversely' between strands: yes. J Thromb Haemost 2004;2:388-93.

[28] Weisel JW. Cross-linked gamma-chains in fibrin fibrils bridge transversely between strands: no. J Thromb Haemost 2004;2:394-9.

[29] Weisel JW. Cross-linked gamma-chains in a fibrin fibril are situated transversely between its strands. J Thromb Haemost 2004;2:1467-9.

[30] Mosesson MW. Cross-linked gamma-chains in a fibrin fibril are situated transversely between its strands. J Thromb Haemost 2004;2:1469-71.

[31] Liu W, Carlisle CR, Sparks EA, Guthold M. The mechanical properties of sing fibrin fibers. *J. Thromb Haemostas* 2010; 8:1030-6.

[32] Mosesson MW. [Letter to the Editor] Short by one mechanism. *J. Thromb Haemostas* 2010; 8:2089.

CHAPTER VII

MOLECULAR ARRANGEMENTS AT THE CORE OF FIBRIN BRANCHES

STEM

For more than 15 years I visited The Brookhaven Biotechnology Resource Facility on Long Island (BNL) on a regular basis to work at their Scanning Transmission Electron Microscopy (STEM) facility. Many of my studies involved fibrinogen and fibrin, including those described in the two chapters immediately preceding this one. Many of the conclusions we drew from experiments that were conducted at our home facility were substantially strengthened and often definitively proven by STEM analyses. Some studies required STEM for evidentiary support, and that was especially true for the studies of fibrin branch junctions described in this chapter.

Among the goals I set for visits to BNL were to investigate: 1) ultrastructural and functional aspects of fibrinogen molecules (chapter V), 2) cross-linked fibrinogen assemblies (chapter VI), and 3) fibrin network branch structure (this chapter). In addition to its inherent ability to yield high resolution images, another powerful feature of STEM is its capacity to accurately measure the *mass*[11] of objects in the microscope field under review. If mass analyses were carried out on fibrinogen molecules [●━●] that had been deposited on a microscope grid and then imaged by STEM, the mass value obtained for any given object in a field could be compared to the mass of a single fibrinogen molecule, 340,000 Da (340 kD), to compute how many fibrinogen molecules were present. For example, if two fibrinogen molecules were present in a field, the mass value returned would be twice that of a single molecule, 680 kD.

For mass analysis of STEM images of fibrils, we analyzed these structures using a 'fiber' program for determining the mass (kD) per unit length in nanometers (nm) (Figure 1). Thus, a two-stranded fibril comprised of a half-staggered arrangement of 340 kD molecules, each one 45 nm in length, would yield a value of 15 kD/nm. A four--stranded fibril would return twice that value, 30 kD/nm.

---

[11] *Protein Mass is expressed in Daltons (Da) or kiloDaltons (kD), Da ÷ 1000. Molecular Weight (MW) is expressed as g/mole and represents the mass of one Mole (6 X 10^{23} molecules) of a protein. Thus, given the MW of fibrinogen at 340,000 g/mole, the mass of a single molecule of fibrinogen would be 340 kD.*

Determining the Molecular Arrangements at Branch Junctions

It is useful to point out here that 'thick' fiber networks that had been imaged by Transmission Electron Microscopy (TEM) were the main source for assessing network branch structure. An example of such a network is shown on the book cover. This network formed under conditions favoring side-to-side fibril associations that resulted in thick fiber bundles. These structures presented an obstacle for precise determination of 'core' molecular arrangements.

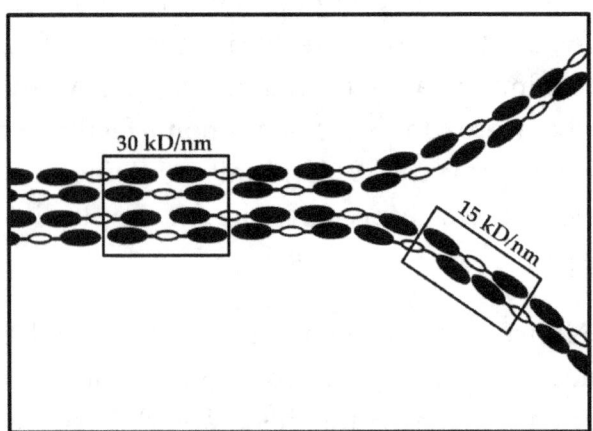

Figure 1. A *tetramolecular* branch junction forms when two double-stranded fibrils diverge. The rectangular field that encloses two fibril strands has a mass/unit length of 30 kD/nm, whereas the one enclosing a single fibril has a mass/unit length of 15 kD/nm.

Based upon examinations of these thick fiber networks, the prevailing view was that branches occurred predominantly, if not always, at *'tetramolecular'* junctions[12] (Figure 1). Please bear in mind, however, that the fibril structures depicted in Figure 1 are the *minimum* number of fibril strands required to form the *'core'* arrangement at a tetramolecular junction, and they are not revealed in networks containing thick fibers.

The evidence that any proposed molecular arrangement exists at the core of these branch points is obscured by the presence of the thick fiber bundles themselves. In examining thick fiber networks from other studies including ours, in addition to 'tetramolecular' type branching, we sometimes identified junctions composed of three arms that were equal in width.(1) These observations suggested that a second type of core molecular arrangement, a so-called *'trimolecular'* branch point, might exist.

That possibility had already been inferred in an earlier study of cross-linked fibrin degradation products (2). In that study, we identified *covalently 'cross-linked'* [13]

---

[12] Because the *'core'* of this type of fibril branch point is formed from four fibrin molecules it is called a *tetramolecular* junction. A second type of branch point whose arms are each the same in width is called a *'trimolecular'* junction. Its *core* is comprised of three fibrin molecules.

[13] In the presence of an enzyme called 'Factor XIII', fibrin fibrils become *covalently* linked intermolecularly through their D domains. Such covalent bonds are *not* dissociable in aqueous solutions. When cross-linked fibrin networks are degraded enzymically to their constituent core fragments, *cross-linked* D domains are

degradation products ('*D domains*') that had been derived from two, three, or four *cross-linked* fibrin molecules. We named them accordingly, '*D-dimers*', '*D-trimers*', and '*D-tetramers*'. It was clear that D-dimers were derived from cross-linking of two-stranded fibrils, but we were puzzled by the presence of D-trimers and D-tetramers. We suspected that these molecular fragments might have been derived from cross-linked trimolecular and tetramolecular branch junctions, but we needed better evidence to confirm that speculation.

Those studies prompted us to explore fibrin networks under conditions favoring thin fiber formation. Such conditions could lead to a clear understanding of the molecular arrangements at the core of branch points. Accordingly, we prepared thin fibrin networks, loaded them onto microscope grids, 'rotary shadow cast' them with heavy metal grains of platinum to enhance contrast, and then imaged them by TEM (Figure 2).

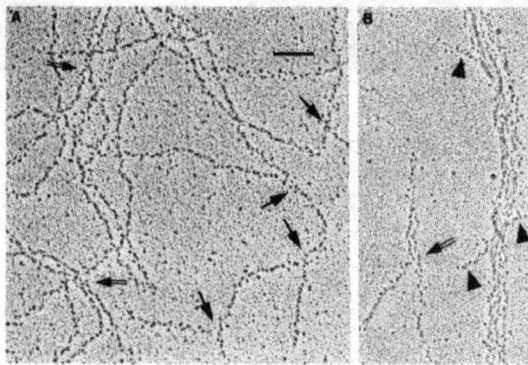

Figure 2. *TEM images of fine fibril networks.* **Arrows** *indicate trimolecular fibril junctions having three arms of equal width.* **Double-shafted arrows** *indicate tetramolecular junctions one arm of which is twice the width that of the other two.* **Arrowheads** *indicate thin fibrils protruding from a fiber bundle. Such branched structures are consistent with tetramolecular branch junctions. Bar = 100 nm. (Reproduced from Ref. 1 with permission.)*

Examination of these images revealed an extensive network of thin fibrils, fibril branch junctions, and thin fibers (panel B) that exhibited two types of branch junctions. The first type, the more common one, had three arms of equal width (arrows). We named them *trimolecular* junctions. The other type of junction had two arms of equal width, plus a third arm twice that width, a so-called *tetramolecular* junction (double arrows). Thus, these studies provided morphometric evidence for both types of branch junctions, but we wanted even more evidence to prove their existence.

---

released from the digest and are subsequently identifiable by their size and by their morphology. They were named *D-dimers*, *D-trimers*, or *D-tetramers*.

To accomplish this goal, we prepared thin fibril networks under the same solvent conditions used for the TEM studies and imaged them by STEM (Figure 3). The types of structures we found were like those we had previously observed by TEM.

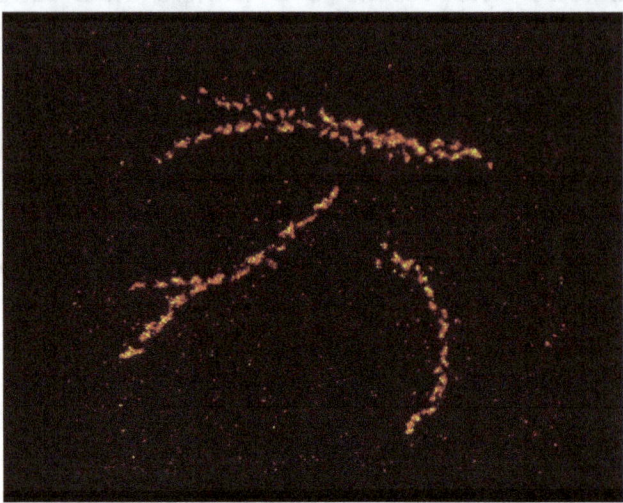

Figure 3. *An array of pseudo-colorized fibrils and fibril junctions selected from among the STEM images. The fibril junction at the top is a tetramolecular junction; the fibril branch in the middle is a trimolecular junction. Toward the right is an unbranched fibril strand.*

We subjected these fibrils to mass analysis and calculated their mass per unit length. As expected, *tetramolecular* junctions consisted of one four-stranded arm with a mass of 30 kD/nm, and two single-stranded arms, each having a mass of 15 kD/nm (see Fig. 1). *Trimolecular* junctions had three single stranded arms, each having a mass of 15 kD/nm. This finding confirmed its identity and permitted us to deduce the molecular arrangement at its core (Figure 4).

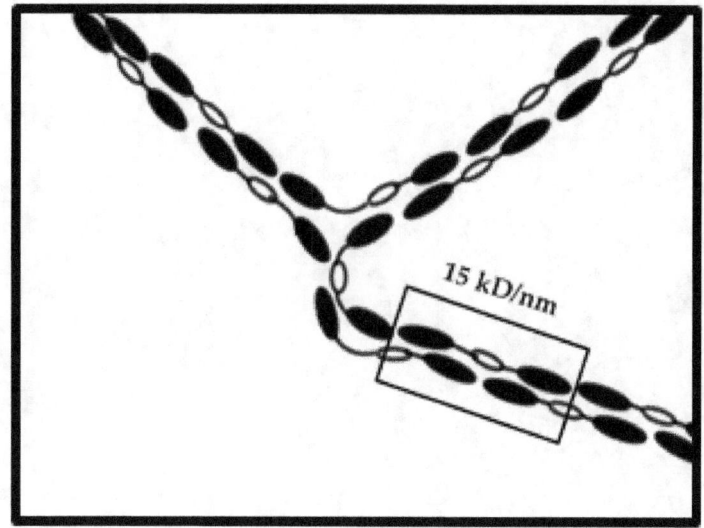

Figure 4. *A trimolecular fibril branch point. -Three fibrin molecules comprise its core structure.*

At the time these studies were conducted, and though we had identified and properly named the two types of branch junctions, I couldn't immediately figure out what the arrangement of the fibrin molecules comprising the core of a trimolecular junction would be. An answer was not long in coming. Shortly after I admitted my puzzlement to my colleagues at a group meeting. Without saying a word *Kevin Siebenlist* exited from our conference room and retreated to his office. A few hours later he gave me a hand-drawn diagram showing precisely what the trimolecular arrangement had to be. That arrangement is diagrammed in the above figure.

The discovery that *trimolecular* junctions predominate in fine fiber networks, has significant implications for its rheological properties. Fine fiber network polymers exhibit nearly perfect elasticity after deforming stress. Although the molecular composition of the core structures in thick fibrin networks cannot be precisely assessed, I strongly believe that *trimolecular* junctions play a leading role in conferring the elastic properties of both polymer types. In contrast, *tetramolecular* junctions in thick fibrin networks, if derived from tetramolecular core arrangements, would allow fiber slippage and structural realignments when stressed. The *trimolecular* core arrangements would resist such deformations.

Michael Mosesson   *May 14, 2020*

References

1. **EVIDENCE FOR A SECOND TYPE OF FIBRIL BRANCH POINT IN FIBRIN POLYMER NETWORKS, THE TRIMOLECULAR JUNCTION.** MW Mosesson, JP DiOrio, KR Siebenlist, JS Wall, JF Hainfeld. *Blood* 82:1517-1521, 1993
2. **IDENTIFICATION OF COVALENTLY LINKED TRIMERIC AND TETRAMERIC D DOMAINS IN CROSSLINKED FIBRIN.** MW Mosesson, KR Siebenlist, DL Amrani, JP DiOrio. *Proc Natl Acad Sci, USA* 86:1113-1117, 1989

CHAPTER VIII

ANTITHROMBIN I AND THE TRANSGENIC MOUSE THAT ROARED

Antithrombin I, '...in the right place at the right time.'
~ Walter Seegers, 1947

During blood clotting, thrombin[14] is generated from a circulating precursor called *prothrombin*. Thrombin cleaves and activates many proteins that participate in blood coagulation, but its most prominent activity is to cleave fibrinogen molecules and convert

---

[14] Glossary:
Allele: Any of the alternative forms of a gene that may occur at a given locus.
Allosteric: A long-range effect produced by ligand binding at a site on a protein that is remote from the site of the induced effect.
Antithrombin I: A property of fibrin attributable to its capacity to bind thrombin.
Antithrombin III: A protein in blood that binds to and inhibits thrombin using heparin as a cofactor (often referred to simply as 'Antithrombin').
Congenital Afibrinogenemia:- An inherited disorder characterized by absence of fibrinogen from the circulation.
Deep venous thrombosis (DVT): Formation of an intravascular blood clot in the venous system.
Embolus: A blood clot that breaks loose from its origin, migrates in the blood stream until it becomes lodged in a downstream vessel.
Enzyme: A protein having the ability to catalyze (speed up) a reaction such as cleavage of protein peptide bonds.
Fibrinolysis: Dissolution of a fibrin clot by a proteolytic enzyme such as plasmin.
Hemolytic Anemia: Lysis of red blood cells in the circulation resulting in anemia.
Intravascular thrombosis: Formation of blood clots within blood vessels.
Ischemia: reduced blood/oxygen supply to a tissue or organ.
Heterozygote: An individual with a defective, or mutant, gene at one locus while the other locus (allele) is normal.
Homozygote: Inheritance of a genetic defect or mutation on both alleles of a gene.
Microvascular surgeon: One who performs surgical procedures on small blood vessels.
Phenotype: The somatic product produced from a given gene.
Prothrombotic: A condition promoting intravascular thrombosis.
Thrombophilia: A tendency to form blood clots (thrombi) within the circulatory system.
Thrombin generation: When blood coagulation results in generation of thrombin from a precursor protein, *Prothrombin*.
Thrombin exosites 1 and 2: Domains in thrombin that bind to complementary sites on fibrinogen, fibrin, heparin, and other molecules.
Transgenic: Pertaining to an organism in which one or more genes have been altered, e.g., by deletion ('knock-out') or by insertion ('knock-in').

them to fibrin (Figure 1). Unlike soluble fibrinogen molecules, fibrin undergoes a self-assembly process that results in an insoluble fiber network called the *fibrin clot*. After clot formation occurs, thrombin remaining bound to fibrin becomes sequestered and its fibrinogen cleaving capacity becomes impaired. That activity is called *'Antithrombin I'*- one of several known mechanisms for inactivating or down-regulating thrombin activity. In this monograph I will discuss its discovery, analyze its inhibitory potential by defining its constituents, explain how they function synergistically, and explore its physiological importance in the context of other known inhibitors of thrombin.

Thrombin-induced clotting of blood (*thrombosis*) at sites of injury seals wounded

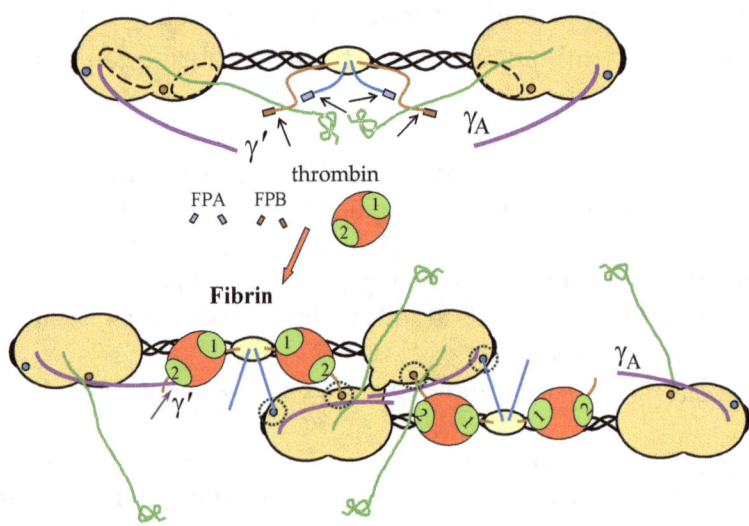

Figure 1. *A diagram illustrating fibrinogen conversion to fibrin by thrombin and the thrombin binding sites on fibrin that contribute to Antithrombin I activity. A symmetrical fibrinogen molecule (top) contains one central domain (◯) and two outer domains (⬭) that are connected through 'coiled' segments (⋙). The small arrows point to parts of the central domain that are cleaved by thrombin (🟢), releasing two small peptides termed FPA and FPB, respectively, a process that converts fibrinogen to fibrin. Below are two fibrin molecules that are linked by end-to-middle domain interactions (circled, ◌). Thrombin molecules bind via exosite '1' (green circled '1') to the central domain, whereas exosite '2' (green circled '2') binds to a fibrin γ' chain (→).*

blood vessels and limits blood loss, usually a beneficial effect. Adverse consequences occur when thrombosis in an artery occludes blood supply to a distal organ or tissue (*ischemia*). If that vessel supplies heart muscle occlusion results in cardiac muscle death, a myocardial infarction (MI). If the occlusion obstructs the blood supply to brain tissue, a 'stroke' results. Occlusive thrombi in veins impair the return of blood to the heart and commonly result in *'deep venous thrombosis'* (*DVT*). DVTs sometimes break loose from their moorings in a vein and migrate through the heart, becoming lodged in pulmonary arterial vessels; they are called *'pulmonary emboli.'*

Given the catastrophic consequences of intravascular thrombosis, it is not surprising that robust mechanisms are in place for regulating the extent of thrombin's activity. One of those mechanisms, *'Antithrombin I,'* is today's topic.

History and Terminology

More than sixty-five years ago *Walter Seegers* at Wayne State University reported that when thrombin became bound to fibrin, its capacity to induce more clotting was measurably reduced. Seegers termed the activity 'Antithrombin I' and he also defined other thrombin inhibitory activities he termed Antithrombins II, III, and IV [1]. Although at that time he could not know what their roles were, he asserted that Antithrombin I was important because it occurred "in the right place at the right time." I take his view to be farsighted and essentially correct. Nevertheless, for many years the relevance of Antithrombin I was disparaged in favor of Antithrombin III, another thrombin inhibitor that was touted as the most physiologically important.

To emphasize that disparagement, an expert 'Committee on Thrombin Inhibitors' sponsored by The International Society on Thrombosis and Hemostasis (ISTH) convened in the mid-1980's to evaluate the known circulating thrombin inhibitors. They concluded that 'Antithrombin III' (AT-III) was the only inhibitor worthy of a designation, and they recommended that AT-III be called simply *'Antithrombin,'* in effect repudiating the importance of other thrombin inhibitors, including 'Antithrombin I.'

Antithrombin I 'Deficiency' (Afibrinogenemia) and Thrombophilia

The belief that a single thrombin inhibitor, AT-III, accounted for all significant thrombin regulatory aspects continued to gain favor until shortly after the turn of this century when Norma de Bosch and I reported our findings on thrombin generation in plasmas from subjects with *Congenital Afibrinogenemia* [2]. This rare inherited disorder is characterized by the total absence of fibrinogen from the circulation. That deficiency provided us with an important tool for discovering what happens when fibrinogen is absent from blood.

We found that activation of clotting in afibrinogenemic plasma was associated with a marked increase in thrombin generation. Normalizing the fibrinogen level prior to initiation of clotting also normalized thrombin generation. When we added γ'-chain containing fibrinogen ['Peak 2 fibrinogen' ($\gamma'/\gamma A$)], thrombin generation was suppressed to a greater extent than with fibrinogen containing γA chains ['Peak 1 fibrinogen' ($\gamma A/\gamma A$)][2]. Clearly, the γ' sequence in fibrin contributed to Antithrombin I activity. More importantly, our experiments demonstrated that fibrin formation was important for down-regulating thrombin activity in blood. The absence of fibrinogen from the circulation (*Congenital Afibrinogenemia*) and Antithrombin I Deficiency were one and the same.

Prior to our report, every review article or book chapter that I had read portrayed Afibrinogenemia as a moderate to severe bleeding disorder. That there was bleeding tendency was true, of course, but it was an incomplete representation. Numerous reports of severe, sometimes fatal, intravascular thromboembolic disease in Afibrinogenemic subjects were in the literature but had been ignored. We emphasized all of those reports in our first Antithrombin I publication as well as in subsequent reviews and textbook chapters [3-6]. We also pointed out that a Murine model of Afibrinogenemia had displayed thrombophilic behavior [7]. Taken together, this left little doubt that Afibrinogenemia was a thrombotic as well as a hemorrhagic disorder.

A few months after our initial publication, *Klaus Preissner,* then Editor-in-Chief of Thrombosis and Haemostasis, requested that I write a review about fibrin-mediated thrombin inhibition. I was delighted to have been asked. Naturally, I entitled my manuscript 'Antithrombin I', a title that prompted a telephone call from the Preissner. He would gladly accept my article provided I remove 'Antithrombin I' from the title and from the text. "Mike, there is only one important 'Antithrombin.' It was called 'Antithrombin III' but now it is simply *'Antithrombin.'* "

"Calling it 'Antithrombin I' will confuse the readers," he added. I replied that I'd sooner withdraw the manuscript than change the title. Klaus demurred and the article was published exactly as I had written it [3].

Thrombin Binding Sites on Fibrin

The discovery of the γ chain variant, γ', began at DBS when John Finlayson and I subjected fibrinogen to gradient elution column chromatography. The fibrinogen eluted in two distinct chromatographic peaks that we termed 'Peak 1'and 'Peak 2' [8;9]. Peak 1 fibrinogen accounted for 15% of the total fibrinogen. A few years later John and I showed that Peak 1 γ chains were the platelet-binding variety termed γA. Peak 2 fibrinogen contained γA and a newly discovered variant chain, γ', in about equal amounts. The γ' chains had a higher negative charge that accounted for delayed chromatographic elution of Peak 2 fibrinogen [10].

A few years after that *Carlotta Wolfenstein-Todel* determined the unique amino acid sequence that accounted for the behavior of the γ' chains. Carlota was a biochemist from Argentina whose family had fled there from Europe to escape The Holocaust. After obtaining her PhD in Buenos Aires, she came to *Edwin Franklin's* laboratory at NYU in 1976 as a post-doctoral fellow to participate in his research on immunoglobulins. Ed knew that I had been searching for a protein chemist to join my group, and when he could no longer support Carlota's salary from his grants, he contacted me.

Shortly after that I hired her-she joined my group in 1978. Several months later she isolated a 20 residue peptide from a tryptic digest of γ' chains, determined its unique amino acid sequence, and that this peptide was situated at the carboxyl terminal end of the γ' chain [11;12]. After completing that stellar work, she returned to Argentina to be with her family. We met each other again in 1982 when she came to New York to attend the NY Academy of Sciences Symposium on Fibrinogen that I had organized [13]. That warm and cordial encounter turned out to be our last one.[15] I do not know if Carlotta, who was so modest and self-effacing, fully realized what a valuable contribution she had made.

During that same period, *Claude Legrêle* (University of Reims, France) came to my laboratory to study rat fibrinogen. We found that rats, like humans, had a 'Peak 2' fibrinogen that containing γ' chains [14]. Coupled with earlier reports on the chromatographic heterogeneity of several other animal fibrinogens [15] we suggested that γ' chains were a common constituent of Peak 2 vertebrate fibrinogen. It took several more years before we were able to figure out whether these chains contributed to Antithrombin I activity. In the years following our identification of the γ' chain sequence there were several reports concerning 'non-substrate' thrombin binding, most of them inferring that the site on fibrin was in the middle of the molecule near the substrate thrombin binding site. Pechik et al. subsequently determined the exact location of this site [16].

Other studies suggested that there were two thrombin binding sites on fibrin, one of 'low' affinity and the other 'high' [17;18]. We confirmed their existence and reported that 'low' affinity thrombin binding site was in the central domain of fibrin whereas the 'high' affinity site was on γ' chains [19;20] (Figure 2). An additional aspect of thrombin binding to fibrin concerned the 'long range' (allosteric) effect of Exosite 2 binding to thrombin on the catalytic site [22].

---

[15] Carlota and I had another very pleasant reunion in Buenos Aires in December 2019, 37 years later, during my visit to Chile and Argentina.

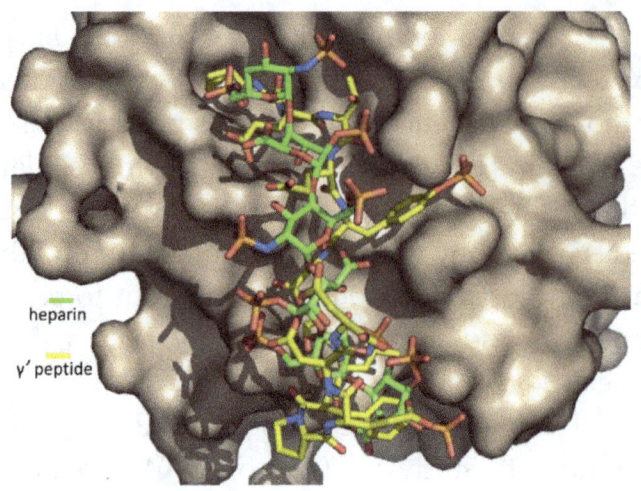

Figure 2. *Drawing of a thrombin molecule (brown) showing how heparin (green) or the γ' sequence (yellow) binds to its 'Exosite 2'. From Pineda et al.[21].*

Antithrombin I Deficiency and Thrombophilia

Ordinarily, low affinity thrombin binding sites on fibrin exceed by more than 20-fold the number of high affinity sites on γ' chains since these variant chains amount to less than 10% of the total γ chain population. Nevertheless, high affinity sites turned out to be important contributors to fibrin's thrombin binding function as dramatically illustrated by the 'Fibrinogen Naples I' dysfibrinogenemia [23-25].

Fibrinogen Naples I result from a mutation in the β chain gene of fibrinogen that eliminates low affinity thrombin binding at affected sites. Members of the kindred who were *homozygotic* for the defect (i.e., both β chain gene alleles were mutated) had severe and recurrent thromboembolism. Low affinity thrombin binding was absent from their fibrin and high affinity thrombin binding was significantly reduced. In contrast, *heterozygotic* members of the kindred, whose low affinity thrombin binding sites were reduced by 50%, were clinically unaffected, almost certainly because the residual low affinity binding fully supported normal bridge-binding between low and high affinity γ' chain sites [25]. The disparity between heterozygotes and homozygotes was due to diminished high affinity thrombin binding combined with absent low affinity binding in the fibrin of Naples I homozygotes, and had effectively eliminated Antithrombin I function, whereas heterozygotic fibrin retained normal Antithrombin I function.

Fibrinogen 'New York I' is an equally dramatic but less well studied example of Antithrombin I deficiency expressing severe thrombophilia. The dysfibrinogen is characterized by a mutation in the β chain gene that results in defective thrombin binding to fibrin at low affinity sites [26].

Human γ' Chain Antithrombin I Function in Transgenic Mice

In 1999, shortly after 'The Milwaukee Heart Project' had been dissolved for lack of funding, I resigned my position at SSMC and transferred my NIH Grants and some of my staff to the Blood Research Institute (BRI) of the BloodCenter of Wisconsin. *Irene Hernandez* joined me and continued as a highly valued associate. *David Meh* left after a few months for a position in industry and disappeared from my radar screen.

Moving to the BRI afforded me an opportunity to expand the scope of my inquiry on Antithrombin I by developing a transgenic mouse whose fibrinogen had been engineered to mimic a specific attribute of human fibrinogen. *Hartmut (Hardy) Weiler* was a key player for this project. He was Director of the BloodCenter Transgenic Mouse Facility. Hardy, a Molecular Biologist, was mainly interested in developmental aspects of hemostasis in animal models. It wasn't difficult to recruit him to collaborate in developing what we referred to as our 'gain-of-function Antithrombin I mouse.' I carried out preliminary experiments to illustrate the feasibility of the project and shortly afterward sent our grant proposal to NIH. The project was funded for four years.

Murine γ' chains arise through an alternative processing event similar to the process in humans and other mammals [27]. The murine γ chain gene codes for γ' sequences that terminate at position 418, whereas in humans the sequence ends at position 427. Both human and murine fibrinogen γ' chains have a binding site for plasma Factor XIII [28], but murine chains which lack the human γ' chain residues 419-427 do not exhibit high affinity thrombin binding [29], and possess only low affinity thrombin binding in its central domain. The absence of those residues meant we could create high affinity thrombin binding sites by replacing the murine γ' chain sequence with the human sequence. If successful, that would result in a 'gain-of-function' modification that would enable us to explore the *in vivo* role of γ' chains in Antithrombin I function. We called this creature the *hu-γ' fibrinogen mouse*.

Hardy knew exactly how to produce the hu-γ' mouse, but he needlessly delayed advancing the project for nearly three years. During year one we hired a post-doc named *Yi-He Guo* who was supposed to work on developing the hu-γ'mouse. I placed Yi-He under Hardy's supervision who then set him to work on an unrelated subject concerning an observation by *Berend Isermann* (a former post-doc) that fibrin degradation products caused cells to self-destruct, a process called 'apoptosis.' I had no interest in using my grant funds for that purpose, but I also knew little about the logistics of creating a hu-γ' mouse. My hands were effectively tied. Irene and I helped Yi-He prepare the fibrin degradation products that he needed for his experiments and we guided him in designing these experiments. I naïvely played along, relying on Hardy's promise that the hu-γ' mouse project would also move forward. It did not. These delays eventually torpedoed any hopes of renewing or extending the project.

By year three we finally had made the hu-γ' mouse and had its humanized fibrinogen in hand. At my end of the deal, I soon completed biochemical/functional characterization of hu-γ' fibrinogen as a necessary prelude for *in vivo* studies in the hu-γ' mouse. To improve our chances of success with this model, we crossed the hu-γ' mouse with transgenic mice having a known prothrombotic disorder called 'Factor V Leiden.' *Brian Cooley*, an animal experimentalist and gifted microvascular surgeon in the Orthopaedic Surgery Department at MCOW, examined the *in vivo* effects of hu-γ' fibrinogen on electrically induced femoral vein injury and thrombosis in the chimeric Factor V Leiden/ hu-γ' mice. He showed that the hu-γ' phenotype protected these mice against intravascular thrombosis. The gain-of-function hu-γ' mouse project had indeed been worth our efforts.

I was not at the BRI on the day that Cooley came over from MCOW to disclose his findings, but Hardy and Irene were there. Shortly after Brian presented the results Hardy Weiler (as retold by Irene) ran down the BRI hallway waving his arms and shouting, *"Mike was right! Mike was right!"*

While the hu-γ' fibrinogen mouse project was going on, *Uitte de Willige* reported that there was a direct association between low levels of γ'chains in human subjects and the risk of developing deep venous thrombosis (DVT) [30]. During that same period, I completed measuring the content of fibrinogen γ' chains in plasmas from human subjects with an often lethal syndrome called *Thrombotic Microangiopathy* (TMA). TMA is characterized by widespread microvascular thromboses, blood platelet consumption, and hemolytic anemia. The fibrinogen γ' chain levels in TMA subjects were significantly lower than those in normal controls, permitting the inference that reduced Antithrombin I potential in these subjects predisposed them to increased thrombin generation, platelet consumption, and microvascular thrombosis [31].

With all relevant data from the hu-γ' mouse study finally in hand I soon wrote a draft of the hu-γ' mouse manuscript. It did not meet Hardy's expectations. He wanted us to merge (or better still, *submerge*) our data from the murine model with data he had obtained from collaborators in Germany who had studied human γ' haplotype behavior in thrombophilic pediatric subjects. Although their data were interesting, they were, at best, tangential, and they did not belong in my paper. What was even worse, Hardy minimized the value of data I had generated for validating and characterizing the hu-γ' mouse phenotype. I had fully characterized hu-γ' murine fibrinogen and developed an immunoassay for measuring hu-γ 'epitope expression in murine plasma. He insisted that we include that information only as a footnote. I categorically refused to do that.

Our personal relationship deteriorated. Between July and September that year we had numerous contentious meetings. Hardy continued to insist that murine data be merged with the German pediatric group data. As to my choice of The Journal of

Thrombosis and Hemostasis (JTH) to publish our results, Hardy characterized JTH as a "throw-away" journal. He preferred a journal with a 'higher impact factor.' I rejected his suggestion immediately and submitted our paper to JTH (whose *impact factor*, by the way, was good enough for me). The paper (without including data from or attribution to Hardy's German colleagues) was published in JTH just as it had been written [29].

The Kaminski Effect-A Footnote

In 1974 Sinai Samaritan Medical Center established 'The Milwaukee Clinical Campus (MCC) of The University of Wisconsin Medical School in Madison (UW).' MCC The Milwaukee campus was founded and directed by *Dick Rieselbach* who served as the campus Dean and Chairman of The Department of Medicine. In 1981, he recruited me from SUNY-Downstate to become Vice-Chairman of The Department of Medicine and Director of The Research Division, a newly founded Division that was housed in a renovated 20,000 ft^2 office building called the 'Winter Family Research Institute.' I became a tenured Professor at UW, an appointment that afforded easy access to faculty, house staff, and students in Madison, about 90 miles west of Milwaukee. To cement our relationship, I frequently visited the Madison campus to participate in departmental meetings and on some occasions to orchestrate the discussion at a 'Medical Grand Rounds.' On one of those occasions I met *Marek Kaminski*.

The 'clinical case' for discussion and analysis that day was related to my recent work on fibrin and its role in thrombin inhibition. Kaminski was one of the medical residents in the audience, all six foot eight inches of him. He was called 'Marek the Great' by coworkers to differentiate him from another resident with the same name of considerably smaller stature. *Marek The Great* posed some interesting questions during and after my presentation that had gotten my attention.

A few weeks later Kaminski telephoned to ask whether he could come to Milwaukee for a Hematology Fellowship, and work in my laboratory as a 'Research Fellow.' That seemed like a good idea and I arranged a 'Clinical Fellowship' for him in *Hugh Davis'* Hematology Section. Although Marek wanted credit for the Hematology Fellowship, he was unwilling to earn it. He did not want to see 'cancer patients' who constituted much of our Hematology service and he did not want to be 'on call' for any reason. Neither Hugh Davis nor I could put up with that behavior, and we terminated the Hematology fellowship. I kept him on, however, as a Research Fellow because of my interest in his ideas on catalytically inactivated thrombin's effects on fibrin polymerization, a phenomenon that we began to call '*The Kaminski Effect*' (Figure 3).

Several years before he moved to Madison to become a Medical Resident, Kaminski had been a research fellow in *Jan McDonagh's* lab in Boston. He had obtained some interesting results on the non-catalytic effect of thrombin on fibrin polymerization.

Jan had given him little help or guidance with these experiments. In frustration Kaminski made copies of his experimental data, moved from Boston to Madison, and from there wound up in Milwaukee. It soon was obvious that my laboratory had been his intended target all along.

Marek showed me his results from Boston and asked me to help him publish them. I was now in the position of dealing with ideas that were not mine and experiments that had not been conducted in my laboratory. To alleviate that uncomfortable situation, I telephoned McDonagh and asked whether she wanted to collaborate in publishing Marek's data. Her response startled me; she declined. She had little or no appreciation of Kaminski's discovery and worse, little faith in his results, notwithstanding that five years earlier she had presented his observations at a Fibrinogen Workshop conference (*Enhancement of Fibrin Polymerization by Active Site Inhibited Thrombin*)[32]. Following our discussion, I felt more comfortable about my participation.

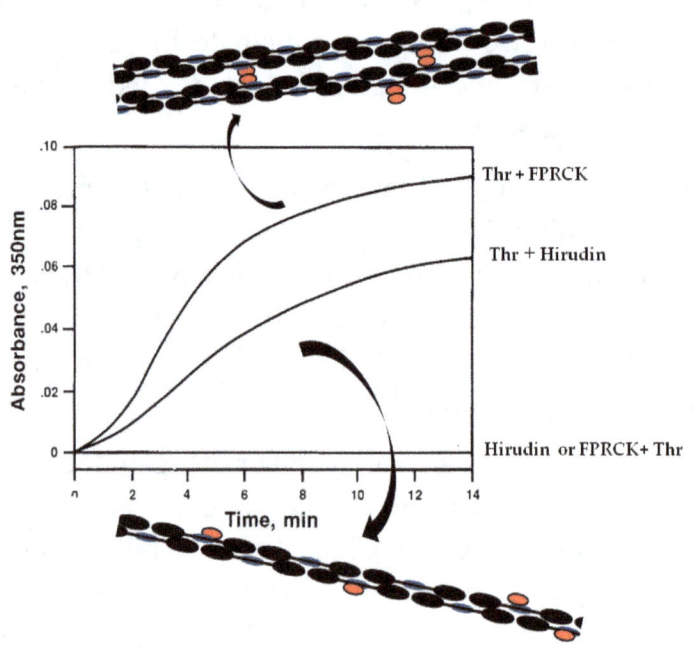

Figure 3. *The Kaminski Effect- Hirudin and FPRCK (D-phenylalanyl-L-propyl-L-arginine chloromethyl ketone) are both potent catalytic-site thrombin (Thr) inhibitors. In addition, hirudin binds to Exosite 2 and impairs thrombin dimer formation. When either inhibitor was added to a fibrinogen solution prior to thrombin, absorbance remained at baseline levels since no fibrin had formed. However, when thrombin was added at a measured interval before adding the inhibitor, fibrin formed, as reflected by the rise in absorbance (turbidity). The turbidity after FPRCK inhibition was consistently greater than after hirudin, as explained by the diagrams-the upper drawing shows two double-stranded fibrin fibrils (black) connected by FPRCK-inhibited thrombin dimers (red). Dimer-mediated bridging results in thicker fibers as reflected by higher turbidity. The lower drawing shows hirudin-inhibited thrombin monomers that do not form dimers and therefore cannot promote inter-fibril bridging, resulting in lower rise turbidity.*

During the next month or two we repeated key parts of Kaminski's Boston experiments. I confirmed that fibrin polymerization (turbidity rise) and fibrin-fibrinogen incorporation into clots were greater with FPRCK inhibited thrombin (FPR-thrombin) than with hirudin inhibited thrombin (HIR-thrombin) from which I could infer that FPR-thrombin was a cofactor for accelerated clot formation, whereas Hir-thrombin was not. We published those data in 1991 but we had gotten no further in our understanding, beyond what McDonagh and Kaminski had reported several years before [33]. Marek was probably satisfied with that achievement and wanted no more to do with this discovery, since shortly later he departed for a career as an Emergency Room physician somewhere in upstate Wisconsin. Never saw him again.

I did not think again about *The Kaminski Effect* until well after I had relocated from SSMC to the BloodCenter of Wisconsin. My renewed interest came during the hu-γ' mouse project. I chose Irene Hernandez, who had previously supervised my electron microscope facility at SSMC, to undertake those studies. She adapted admirably to this task and soon became as good a biochemical experimentalist as she had been as a microscopist. Once I clarified the design and goals of an experiment for her, she took charge. The protocols I had outlined were complex, involving multiple permutations of thrombin-interactive reagents, including exosite-binding nucleotides called DNA 'aptamers' (HD-1 and HD-22).

Irene handled these challenges with alacrity. It took several months for us to complete the experimental protocols and interpret them correctly but eventually we explained what 'The Kaminski Effect' was due to. Thrombin Exosite 1 accounted for FPR-thrombin fibrin binding and these inhibited thrombin molecules formed dimers via Exosite 2 interactions that could be blocked with an aptamer like HD-22 [34;35]. Thrombin dimerization surely increases thrombin binding to fibrin, thus increasing thrombin sequestration. Thrombin dimers also modify clot network structure and its inherent resistance to fibrinolysis. This amounts to a footnote to the Antithrombin I story.

Michael Mosesson   April 22, 2015

References

[1] Seegers WH. Multiple protein interactions as exhibited by the blood-clotting mechanism. J Phys Colloid Chem 1947;51:198-206.

[2] de Bosch NB, Mosesson MW, Ruiz-Sáez A, Echenagucia M, Rodriguez-Lemoin A. Inhibition of thrombin generation in plasma by fibrin formation (Antithrombin I). Thromb Haemost 2002;88:253-8.

[3] Mosesson MW. Antithrombin I. Inhibition of thrombin generation in plasma by fibrin formation. Thromb Haemost 2003;89:9-12.

[4] Mosesson MW. Update on antithrombin I (fibrin). Thromb Haemost 2007;98:105-8.

[5] Mosesson MW. Hereditary abnormalities of fibrinogen. In: Beutler E, Lichtman MA, Coller BS, Kipps TJ, Seligsohn U, editors. Williams Hematology. sixth ed. New York: McGraw-Hill; 2001. p. 1659-71.

[6] Mosesson MW. Hereditary Fibrinogen Abnormalities. In: Lichtman MA, Beutler E, Kipps TJ, Seligsohn U, Kaushansky K, Prchal JT, editors. Williams Hematology. 7 ed. New York: McGraw-Hill; 2006. p. 1909-27.

[7] Ni H, Denis CV, Subbarao S, Degen JL, Sato TN, Hynes RO, et al. Persistence of platelet thrombus formation in arterioles of mice lacking both von Willebrand factor and fibrinogen. J Clin Invest 2000;106:385-92.

[8] Finlayson JS, Mosesson MW. Heterogeneity of human fibrinogen. Biochemistry 1963;2:42-6.

[9] Mosesson MW, Finlayson JS. Biochemical and chromatographic studies of certain activities associated with human fibrinogen preparations. J Clin Invest 1963;42:747-55.

[10] Mosesson MW, Finlayson JS, Umfleet RA. Human fibrinogen heterogeneities. III. Identification of γ chain variants. J Biol Chem 1972;247:5223-7.

[11] Wolfenstein-Todel C, Mosesson MW. Carboxy-terminal amino acid sequence of a human fibrinogen γ chain variant (γ'). Biochemistry 1981;20:6146-9.

[12] Wolfenstein-Todel C, Mosesson MW. Human plasma fibrinogen heterogeneity: evidence for an extended carboxyl-terminal sequence in a normal gamma chain variant (γ'). Proc Natl Acad Sci USA 1980;77:5069-73.

[13] Molecular Biology of Fibrinogen. 108 ed. New York Academy of Sciences; 1983.

[14] Legrele CD, Wolfenstein-Todel C, Hurbourg Y, Mosesson MW. Evidence for two classes of rat plasma fibrinogen γ chains differing by their COOH-terminal amino acid sequence. Biochem Biophys Res Commun 1982;105:521-9.

[15] Finlayson JS, Mosesson MW. Chromatographic heterogeneity of animal fibrinogens. Biochim Biophys Acta 1964;82:415-7.

[16] Pechik I, Madrazo J, Mosesson MW, Hernandez I, Gilliland GL, Medved L. Crystal structure of the complex between thrombin and the central "E" region of fibrin. Proc Natl Acad Sci U S A 2004;101:2718-23.

[17] Liu CY, Nossel HY, Kaplan KL. The binding of thrombin by fibrin. J Biol Chem 1979;254:10421-5.

[18] Hogg PJ, Jackson CM. Heparin promotes the binding of thrombin to fibrin polymer. J Biol Chem 1990;265:241-7.

[19] Meh DA, Siebenlist KR, Mosesson MW. Identification and characterization of the thrombin binding sites on fibrin. J Biol Chem 1996;271:23121-5.

[20] Meh DA, Siebenlist KR, Brennan SO, Holyst T, Mosesson MW. The amino acid sequences in fibrin responsible for high affinity thrombin binding. Thromb Haemost 2001;85:470-4.

[21] Pineda AO, Chen ZW, Marino F, Mathews FS, Mosesson MW, Di Cera E. Crystal structure of thrombin in complex with fibrinogen gamma' peptide. Biophys Chem 2007;125:556-9.

[22] Siebenlist KR, Mosesson MW, Hernandez I, Bush LA, Di Cera E, Shainoff JR, et al. Studies on the basis for the properties of fibrin produced from fibrinogen containing γ' chains. Blood 2005;106:2730-6.

[23] Koopman J, Haverkate F, Lord ST, Grimbergen J, Mannucci PM. Molecular basis of fibrinogen Naples associated with defective thrombin binding and thrombophilia. Homozygous substitution of B beta 68 Ala-->Thr. J Clin Invest 1992;90:238-44.

[24] Di Minno G, Martinez J, Cirillo F, Cerbone AM, Silver MJ, Colucci M, et al. A role for platelets and thrombin in the juvenile stroke of two siblings with defective thrombin-absorbing capacity of fibrin(ogen). Arterioscl Thromb 1991;11:785-96.

[25] Meh DA, Mosesson MW, Siebenlist KR, Simpson-Haidaris PJ, Brennan SO, DiOrio JP, et al. Fibrinogen Naples I (Bβ A68T) non-substrate thrombin binding capacities. Thromb Res 2001;103:63-73.

[26] Liu CY, Nossel HL, Kaplan KL. Defective thrombin binding by abnormal fibrin associated with recurrent thrombosis. Thromb Haemost 1979;42:79abs.

[27] Holmback K, Danton MJ, Suh TT, Daugherty CC, Degen JL. Impaired platelet aggregation and sustained bleeding in mice lacking the fibrinogen motif bound by integrin alpha IIb beta 3. EMBO J 1996;15:5760-71.

[28] Siebenlist KR, Meh DA, Mosesson MW. Plasma factor XIII binds specifically to fibrinogen molecules containing γ' chains. Biochemistry 1996;35:10448-53.

[29] Mosesson MW, Cooley BC, Hernandez I, DiOrio JP, Weiler H. Thrombosis risk modification in transgenic mice containing the human fibrinogen thrombin-binding gamma' chain sequence. J Thromb Haemost 2009;7:102-10.

[30] Uitte de Willige S, de Visser MC, Houwing-Duistermaat JJ, Rosendaal FR, Vos HL, Bertina RM. Genetic variation in the fibrinogen gamma gene increases the risk of deep venous thrombosis by reducing plasma fibrinogen {gamma}' levels. Blood 2005;106:4176-83.

[31] Mosesson MW, Hernandez I, Raife TJ, Medved L, Yakovlev S, Simpson-Haidaris PJ, et al. Plasma fibrinogen gamma' chain content in the thrombotic microangiopathy syndrome. J Thromb Haemost 2007;5:62-9.

[32] Kaminski M, McDonagh J. Enhancement of fibrin polymerization by active site-inhibited thrombin. In: Henschen A, Hessel B, McDonagh J, Saldeen TG, editors. Fibrinogen. Structural variants and interactions.Berlin: Walter de Gruyter; 1985. p. 51-63.

[33] Kaminski M, Siebenlist KR, Mosesson MW. Evidence for thrombin enhancement of fibrin polymerization that is independent of its catalytic activity. J Lab Clin Med 1991;117:218-25.

[34] Mosesson MW, Hernandez I, Siebenlist KR. Evidence that catalytically-inactivated thrombin forms non-covalently linked dimers that bridge between fibrin/fibrinogen fibers and enhance fibrin polymerization. Biophys Chem 2004;110:93-100.

[35] Mosesson MW. The effect of a thrombin exosite 2-binding DNA aptamer (HD-22) on non-catalytic thrombin enhanced fibrin polymerization. Thromb Haemost 2007;97:327-8.

CHAPTER IX

THE FIBRINOLYTIC POTENTIAL OF BLOOD

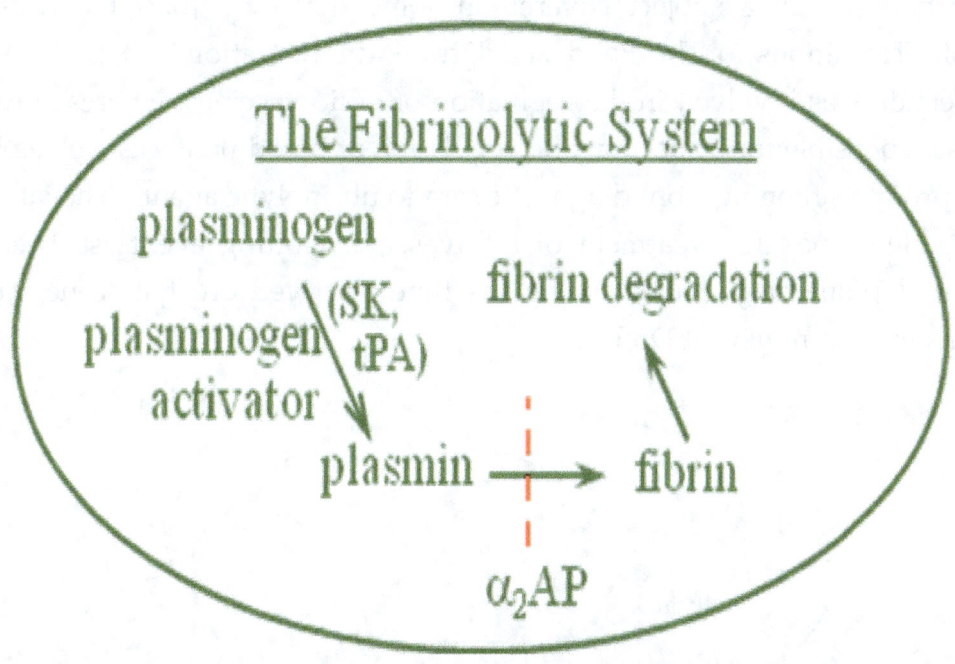

The Division of Biologics Standards

In 1961 I enlisted in The United States Public Health Service (USPHS), straight out of internship at Boston City Hospital (a story detailed elsewhere), received a commission as 'Senior Assistant Surgeon' (First Lieutenant), and then was assigned to serve in The Laboratory of Blood and Blood Products (LBBP) of The Division of Biologics Standards (DBS).

DBS, a Federal regulatory agency, was eventually folded into the Food Drug Administration (FDA), a subject covered in some detail by John Finlayson in his monograph 'Transitions to The Food and Drug Administration.' At that time DBS's virology section was involved in the regulation of polio vaccines, whereas my section, LBBP, was responsible for inspection and regulation of Blood Banks as well as licensing biological products ranging from diagnostic sera to fibrinolytic agents. The latter agents were being developed for treatment of intravascular clotting events such as venous thrombosis or pulmonary embolism. By the time I arrived on that scene, numerous applications were in review at DBS.

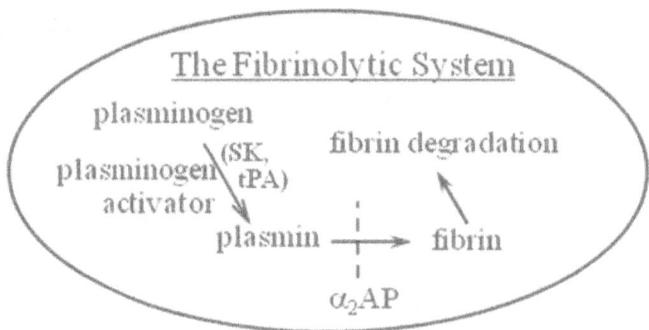

Figure 1. *The Fibrinolytic System. Precursor Plasminogen is converted to the enzyme plasmin by activators such as streptokinase (SK) or tissue plasminogen activator (tPA). Plasmin then degrades fibrin. The most potent plasmin inhibitor \ is α2-antiplasmin (α2AP).*

These products commonly contained an activator of plasminogen such as streptokinase (SK), either alone or in combination with a fibrinolytic enzyme like plasmin (Figure 1). My task was to develop and standardize methodologies for measuring and distinguishing each component. Existing methodologies suffered from the fact that the usual fibrin substrates for measuring clot lytic activity were heavily contaminated with plasminogen.

It took me nearly four months to develop a method for separating fibrinogen and plasminogen. I accomplished this simply by precipitating plasminogen-contaminated fibrinogen in the presence of the amino acid lysine. In the presence of lysine plasminogen and fibrinogen dissociated from one another, permitting the fibrinogen to be precipitated while plasminogen remained in solution. That discovery led to my first publication entitled *'The Preparation of Human Fibrinogen Free of Plasminogen'* [1], as described in Chapter II. More important than the contribution it had made toward evaluating fibrinolytic agents, these studies kindled a lifelong interest in this subject.

Discovering an Inhibitor of Fibrinolysis in Plasma Fibrinogen

Having learned how to prepare plasminogen-free fibrinogen, I turned my attention to determining whether removal of plasminogen had altered any of the properties of the fibrinogen. Except for the absence of plasminogen, I could find no changes. Among the procedures I used for comparing fibrinogens was gradient elution ion exchange chromatography, a technique that had been taught to me by John Finlayson. Unexpectedly, John and I found that instead of emerging from the chromatography column as a single peak, there were two distinct peaks (Figure 2) [2]. Those findings led to many more studies that kept me occupied for the next fifty years. One of them involved the discovery of an enzyme inhibitory activity associated with plasma fibrinogen, the subject of this present chapter.

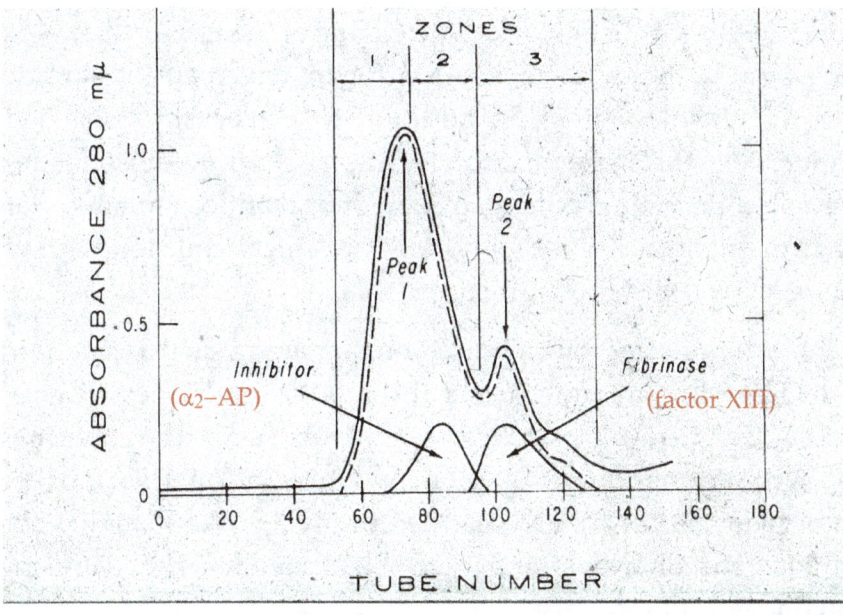

Figure 2. *Ion exchange chromatogram of fibrinogen reproduced from [3]. Current terminology has been added in red. The dashed line indicates the coagulability of the column fractions that had emerged. The 'inhibitor' activity, 'α2-AP', was located between peaks 1 and 2. Fibrinase is now called 'factor XIII.'*

I began investigating potential differences between the two fibrinogen peaks by collecting and analyzing the fractions that emerged from a chromatography column. In one experimental set I converted fibrinogen in the fractions to fibrin and then measured the lysis rates of clots to which plasmin or trypsin had been added. There was a region displaying slowed clot lysis rates that emerged between the two fibrinogen peaks. Although these findings didn't get me closer to understanding the differences between peaks 1 and 2 fibrinogen, we reported our findings on the inhibitory activity [3]. I then moved on to other subjects and did not return to the inhibitory activity for a long while.

Identification of α2-Antiplasmin

Thirteen years after my report (1976) *Desiré Collen* identified and characterized a potent plasma inhibitor of fibrinolysis, that is now known as α2-Antiplasmin [4]. It took several more years for me to connect Collen's inhibitor to the one I had found in fibrinogen. It came about in the following way.

In 1986 *John Hoak* (University of Iowa) asked me to investigate a family from Cedar Rapids, Iowa, several members of whom had exhibited a strong *thrombophilic* tendency (*a proclivity for forming blood clots in the circulation*) that occurred in the setting of a functional fibrinogen abnormality (*'dysfibrinogenemia'*). Thrombophilia in the family first surfaced when one member of the family died suddenly at age 19 of a massive pulmonary embolism a few days after giving birth to her first child. After that event, two of her sisters experienced recurring thrombotic disorders including mesenteric artery thrombosis, venous thrombosis and pulmonary embolism. The dysfibrinogenemia is now called 'Fibrinogen Cedar Rapids.'

While we were working on this problem Hoak referred one of the family members (Terry F) to my hospital, Sinai Samaritan Medical Center, for management of chronic active gall bladder inflammation (cholecystitis). In addition to cholecystitis she had previously experienced numerous thromboembolic events, including episodes of pulmonary embolism that resulted in chronic administration of oral anticoagulants. Her present situation called for urgent surgical intervention. My surgical colleagues were reluctant to undertake surgery while she was on anticoagulants.

To my knowledge, no one at that time had reported on managing such a situation. I felt that I had to devise a strategy that minimized her thrombotic tendencies without resorting to anticoagulants. I decided to use 'plasma exchange' to exchange the abnormal fibrinogen in her circulation with normal donor plasma containing normal fibrinogen. After this procedure she underwent successful gall bladder removal without significant bleeding or thrombotic complications. Shortly after surgery I restarted her anticoagulant medication and she made an uneventful recovery.

We found a mutation in the Cedar Rapids fibrinogen gene corresponding to amino acid 275 in the γ chain peptide sequence. Mutations affecting the γ275 site had already been reported in 18 other families, but only three of them had a thrombophilic clinical history. It thus appeared that the Cedar Rapids fibrinogen mutation might not be the main factor contributing to the thrombophilia. Indeed, in affected family members manifesting thrombophilia we also found a mutation in the coagulation factor V gene, *factor V Leiden* ('fV Leiden'); that mutation by itself is associated with an increased incidence of intravascular thrombosis. In our published report we concluded that coexistence of the 'fV Leiden-' and 'Cedar Rapids' fibrinogen gene mutation predisposed to *thrombophilia* [5].

In other experiments we found that Cedar Rapids fibrin(ogen) underwent fibrinolysis more slowly than our normal controls, an observation that called to mind my earlier investigations on the inhibitor of fibrinolysis in fibrinogen. Specific antibodies against α2AP were readily available by then and we soon identified α2AP and as a tightly bound constituent of both normal and Cedar Rapids fibrinogen. We included that information in the report [5]. The nature of the bond between α2AP and fibrinogen would remain unknown for several more years.

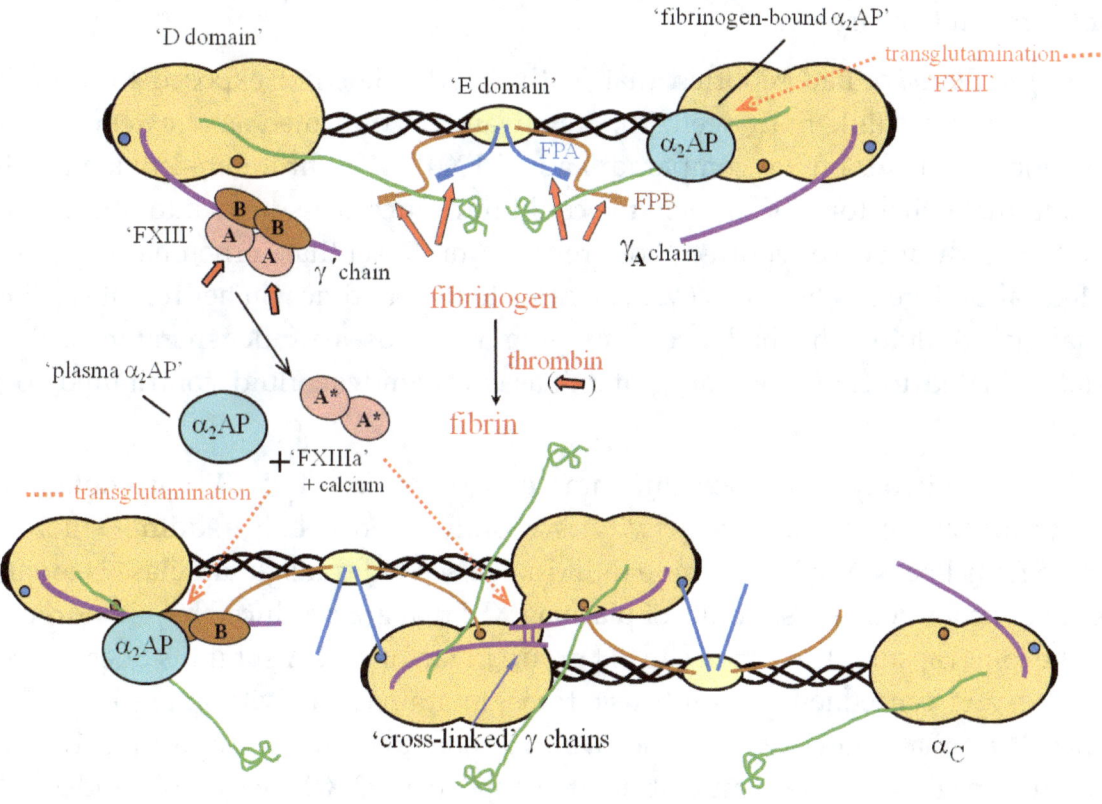

Figure 3. *Overview of Fibrinogen, α2AP, and Factor XIII. Upper-one molecule of fibrinogen molecule with Factor XIII [FXIII, A₂B₂] bound to its γ' chains. Some plasma α2AP is bound to fibrinogen αC domains (green); most is tightly (covalently) bound to form 'fibrinogen-bound α2-AP'. Middle, fibrinogen is converted to fibrin by thrombin cleavage of FPA (blue) and FPB (brown); the A subunits of FXIII are also cleaved to form FXIIIa [A*]. Lower-two molecules of fibrin are aligned end-to-middle by FPA and FPB*

contacts; extending this alignment process results in double-stranded fibrin fibrils. Aligned γ chains (purple) from two fibrin molecules are covalently cross-linked by FXIIIa; plasma α2AP molecules become cross-linked to fibrin's αC domains by FXIIIa.

Factor XIII, The Circulating Transglutaminase

I will digress at this point to discuss some relevant features of plasma Factor XIII. In the early 1960's *Ariel Loewy* (Haverford College), published his studies on a fibrin 'cross-linking' enzyme in plasma that he named 'Fibrinase.' Among these publications he described a fibrin-based method for measuring cross-linking activity. We still use this method [6]. Fibrinase is now termed *Factor XIII* (FXIII); it belongs to a class of enzymes called *transglutaminases* that catalyze the formation of covalent 'isopeptide' [ε-(γ-glutamyl) lysyl] bonds between aligned lysine and glutamine residues in substrates like fibrinogen and α2AP (Figure 3). Most transglutaminases are constitutively active, that is, they express activity in their native form. FXIII was believed to be an exception to that rule, in that it remained inactive until cleaved by thrombin to form 'FXIIIa'. That postulate did not turn out to be true.

Birger Blombäck had reported that 'native' FXIII (i.e., not exposed to thrombin) could readily cross-link fibrinogen [7]; Kevin and I confirmed and extended those observations [8]. Later on we compared 'native' FXIII with thrombin-activated FXIIIa, and found that either form of the enzyme could introduce cross-links into fibrinogen or fibrin [9]. Shortly after we reported those results Ann Rosenthal, a rheumatologist from The Medical College of Wisconsin (MCW), came to us for advice on her recent studies of synovial (joint) fluid. She had been studying the causes of degenerative arthritis, especially related to how the transglutaminases in synovial fluid contributed to the disorder.

There are two types of transglutaminase in joint fluid. 'Type II' transglutaminase is 'constitutively' active, and its activity is rapidly quenched by adding Thiol (SH) binding agents like N-ethyl maleimide (NEM). The second transglutaminase is identical to the catalytically active A subunits of plasma FXIII that are produced by 'chondrocytes' lining the joint capsule. The active site SH group in factor XIII A subunits does not react with NEM, and consequently its intrinsic transglutaminase activity is preserved in its presence. With that knowledge at hand, we were able to easily distinguish activity due to Type II transglutaminase from that due to chondrocyte FXIII-we simply added NEM to an assay mixture of joint fluid and only the chondrocyte FXIII remained active. These experiments provided another demonstration that FXIII is an active transglutaminase. For her part, Rosenthal used that discovery to extend her understanding of how chondrocyte FXIII synthesis is regulated and how transglutaminases contribute to the pathogenesis of degenerative arthritis [10].

A Covalent Bond Between α2AP and Fibrinogen

Following the Cedar Rapids fibrinogen studies, I turned my attention to the type of bond linking α2AP and fibrinogen. In the first set of experiments we showed that 'native' FXIII could cross-link α2AP to fibrinogen [11], thus inferring that α2AP bound to fibrinogen came from plasma α2AP, very likely through the cross-linking activity of FXIII. The next task was to show that the bond linking α2AP and plasma fibrinogen was covalent. I went after that proof with immune-blotting experiments (Western Blotting) as illustrated in Figure 4.

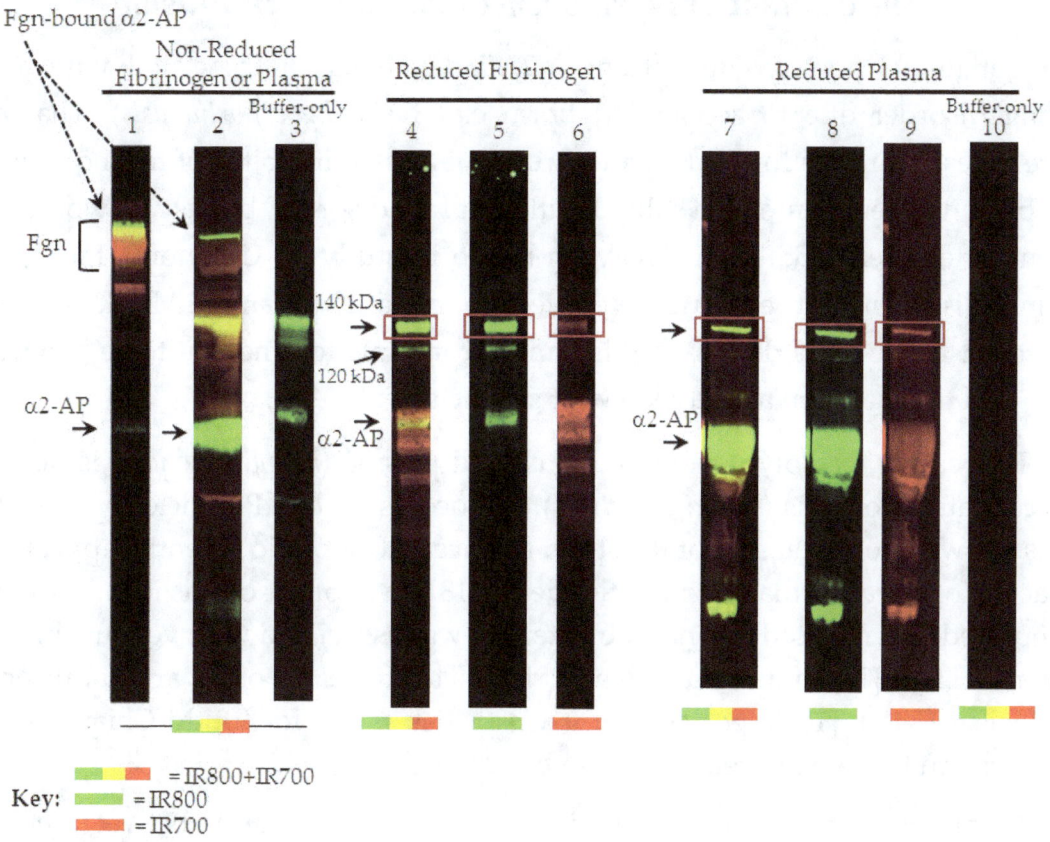

Figure 4. *An electrophoretic immune-blot ('Western Blot') using fluorescent antibodies to identify α2-antiplasmin or fibrinogen Aα chain epitopes [12]. In non-reduced fibrinogen or plasma specimens (lanes 1 and 2) α2-antiplasmin (green/yellow) migrated in the upper region of the broad ~340 KDa fibrinogen band (red). Disulfide-bond reduced fibrinogen (lanes 4-6) or plasma containing fibrinogen (lanes 7-9) showed a band of ~140 kDa that reacted with antibodies to both α2-antiplasmin and the fibrinogen Aα chain. The two proteins comprising that band were ~70 kDa each, thus proving that the two peptide chains were covalently linked to produce a 140 kDa 'heterodimer.'*

In non-reduced specimens (fibrinogen or whole plasma) tagged with fluorescent antibodies we found α2AP (green/yellow) migrating in the upper region of the red ~340 kDa fibrinogen band (lanes 1 and 2). Monomeric α2AP (~70 kDa) would not have occupied such a high molecular weight position had it not been covalently linked to the fibrinogen.

In the disulfide-reduced specimens (lanes 4-9), the ~340 kDa fibrinogen band was absent, and in its place were its constituent monomeric Aα, Bβ, and γ chains. The fibrinogen specimen (lanes 4- 6) or the fibrinogen-containing *plasma* specimen (lanes 7-9) possessed a prominent green (α2AP) and red (Aα chains) staining band of ~140 kDa. Its two components were each half the size of that band, thus providing unequivocal evidence that they were covalently linked to form a *'heterodimer.'*

The Content of Fibrinogen-Bound α2AP in Plasma

Congenital homozygous plasma α2AP deficiency is associated with a severe bleeding disorder due to accelerated fibrin clot lysis (*hyperfibrinolysis*). That clinical picture gives testimony to α2APs critical role as a potent inhibitor of fibrinolysis. I have never personally encountered a subject with that rare disorder, but as fate would have it, not long after I left DBS, John Finlayson began to study an Oklahoma family with a bleeding disorder that eventually proved to be due to an α2AP deficiency [see Addendum 1]. He and I discussed this family from time to time, but to be honest, I had little to add to what John already knew or suspected.

Decreased fibrinolytic potential of clotted plasma (*hypofibrinolysis*) is opposite to the accelerated clot lysis (*hyperfibrinolysis*) that occurs in α2AP deficiency, and there is far less known about that side of the story. Reduced fibrinolytic potential appears to be a risk factor for intravascular thrombotic events [13]. In support of this idea, Lisman et al. [14] reported that reduced fibrinolytic potential was associated with venous thrombosis, Guimaraes et al. [15] found that it was a risk factor for early onset arterial thrombosis, and Hoekstra et al. [16] reported that it was a risk factor for 'Budd-Chiari' syndrome (thrombosis in the hepatic veins or the inferior vena cava).

Numerous earlier studies had failed to show an association between the plasma level of α2AP and the lysis rate of a clot formed from that plasma, implying that there was an alternative explanation for α2AP's profound effects. Since α2AP is a better inhibitor after it binds to fibrin [17], I speculated that there should be a relationship between the amount of bound α2AP bound to plasma fibrinogen and the *fibrinolytic potential*. Expressed another way, 'fibrinogen-bound α2AP', rather than 'free α2AP', plays a decisive role in down-regulating the fibrinolytic rate of clotted blood. At that time there was no information concerning what the content of fibrinogen-bound α2AP might be in individual plasmas and that was where I would go next.

Reaching the Finish Line

I no longer had extramural funding, but I did retain my appointment at the BRI as an *Emeritus Investigator*. That enabled me to develop a collaborative project with the Diagnostics Laboratory at The BloodCenter to develop an ELISA for fibrinogen-bound α2AP, as a means for eventually studying its role in regulating the fibrinolytic potential of plasma. We agreed to split the expenses. Our modest budget permitted us to hire a part-time technologist, *Mary Ann Budish*.

She and I set out to develop the fibrinogen-bound α2AP ELISA. After nearly three years we finally had the assay we needed [see Addendum 2]. The principle behind this sensitive assay was first to capture plasma α2AP with an anti-α2AP, and then detect the fibrinogen that was bound to the captured α2AP using an anti-fibrinogen antibody.

While the immunoassays for measuring fibrinogen-bound α2AP (and plasma α2AP) were being developed, I collected 200 normal plasmas from the BloodCenter Donor population, and I also obtained more than 600 patient plasmas from the 'ATTAC' population that had been studied by Guimaraes et al. [15], courtesy of *Dick Rijken* (Erasmus University, The Netherlands). That study had involved determination of clot lysis times, CLTs, as a measure of the 'fibrinolytic potential' in subjects with 'early-onset' arterial thrombosis. My goal was to compare the Fgn-Bound α2AP levels with the CLTs that had been determined in that study, but just as light was appearing at the end of the tunnel, we exhausted our budget for this project. The Diagnostics folks were not anxious to extend the budget and I had insufficient funds to continue the project on my own. Consequently, we were able to measure only a small proportion of the 600+ ATTAC samples (Addendum 2, Figure 6). There were too few samples analyzed to determine whether there was any relationship between the CLT and Fgn-bound α2AP levels.

We also analyzed our collection of normal plasma samples for their content of fibrinogen-bound α2AP. The values were Gaussian in distribution, as was the distribution of fibrinogen and α2AP. There was no suggestion of a relationship between α2AP levels and Fgn-bound α2AP (Addendum, Figure 3). Other analyses did not get to the core of the problem. What remained was for me to determine the fibrinolytic potential (i.e., CLT by thromboelastography) of plasma samples to examine whether there might be a correlation between the CLT and the levels of Fgn-bound α2AP. I am currently carrying out these thromboelastographic measurements myself in the hope that I might re-energize the original enthusiasm for the project. (PS, they did not work.)

It is disappointing to have come so far over such a long period of time without achieving the goal, to define the role of Fgn-bound α2AP in the fibrinolytic process. Toward that end, I leave this essay as a guide for future investigators.

Michael Mosesson   June 24, 2015

References

[1] Mosesson MW. The preparation of human fibrinogen free of plasminogen. Biochim Biophys Acta 1962;57:204-13.

[2] Finlayson JS, Mosesson MW. Heterogeneity of human fibrinogen. Biochemistry 1963;2:42-6.

[3] Mosesson MW, Finlayson JS. Biochemical and chromatographic studies of certain activities associated with human fibrinogen preparations. J Clin Invest 1963;42:747-55.

[4] Collen D. Identification and some properties of a new fast reacting plasmin inhibitor in human plasma. Eur J Biochem 1976;69:209-16.

[5] Siebenlist KR, Mosesson MW, Meh DA, DiOrio JP, Albrecht RM, Olson JD. Coexisting dysfibrinogenemia (gammaR275C) and factor V Leiden deficiency associated with thromboembolic disease (fibrinogen Cedar Rapids). Blood Coagul Fibrinolysis 2000;11:293-304.

[6] Loewy AG, Dunathan K, Kriel R, Wolfinger HL. Fibrinase I. Purification of substrate and enzyme. J Biol Chem 1961;236:2625-33.

[7] Blomback B, Procyk R, Adamson L, Hessel B. FXIII induced gelation of human fibrinogen--an alternative thiol enhanced, thrombin independent pathway. Thromb Res 1985;37:613-27.

[8] Siebenlist KR, Meh DA, Mosesson MW. Plasma factor XIII binds specifically to fibrinogen molecules containing γ' chains. Biochemistry 1996;35:10448-53.

[9] Siebenlist KR, Meh D, Mosesson MW. Protransglutaminase (factor XIII) mediated crosslinking of fibrinogen and fibrin. Thromb Haemost 2001;86:1221-8.

[10] Rosenthal AK, Mosesson MW, Gohr CM, Masuda I, Heinkel D, Siebenlist KR. Regulation of transglutaminase activity in articular chondrocytes through

thrombin receptor-mediated factor XIII synthesis. Thromb Haemost 2004;91:558-68.

[11] Mosesson MW, Siebenlist KR, Hernandez I, Lee KN, Christiansen VJ, McKee PA. Evidence that alpha2-antiplasmin becomes covalently ligated to plasma fibrinogen in the circulation: a new role for plasma factor XIII in fibrinolysis regulation. J Thromb Haemost 2008;6:1565-70.

[12] Mosesson MW, Holyst T, Hernandez I, Siebenlist KR. Evidence for covalent linkage between some plasma alpha2-antiplasmin molecules and A alpha chains of circulating fibrinogen

1. J Thromb Haemost 2013;11:995-8.

[13] Catena C, Novello M, Lapenna R, Baroselli S, Colussi G, Nadalini E, et al. New risk factors for atherosclerosis in hypertension: focus on the prothrombotic state and lipoprotein(a). J Hypertens 2005;23:1617-31.

[14] Lisman T, de Groot PG, Meijers JC, Rosendaal FR. Reduced plasma fibrinolytic potential is a risk factor for venous thrombosis. Blood 2005;105:1102-5.

[15] Guimaraes AH, de Bruijne EL, Lisman T, Dippel DW, Deckers JW, Poldermans D, et al. Hypofibrinolysis is a risk factor for arterial thrombosis at young age 3. Br J Haematol 2009;145:115-20.

[16] Hoekstra J, Guimaraes AH, Leebeek FW, Darwish MS, Malfliet JJ, Plessier A, et al. Impaired fibrinolysis as a risk factor for Budd-Chiari syndrome. Blood 2010;115:388-95.

[17] Sakata Y, Aoki H. Significance of cross-linking of α_2–plasmin inhibitor to fibrin in inhibition of fibrinolysis and in hemostasis. J Clin Invest 1982;69:536-42.

ADDENDUM 1

[Abridged and modified from John Finlayson's chapter, 'Transitions to The Food and Drug Administration']

This narrative is about a familial bleeding disorder discovered by James Hampton of the University of Oklahoma Medical Center who then contacted John for help. Affected family members "did not bleed spontaneously, yet they did bleed after trauma." Hampton believed that there was deficiency in Factor XIII because "the blood of such people clots at a normal rate, but the clots tend to be unstable." As more experiments were performed, inconsistencies arose in that hypothesis, and Hampton began to suspect that the problem "might lie in the fibrinogen itself." Such so-called "congenital Dysfibrinogenemias" (i.e., inborn abnormalities of fibrinogen) were often named after the place where they had been discovered. Hampton called this one 'Fibrinogen Oklahoma.'

'To advance the study of *Fibrinogen Oklahoma*,' Jim sent his prize student, Bob Morton, to work with Finlayson. Since he was quite keen to learn what his prize student was up to, Jim telephoned John every week to inquire about progress on their joint project. John would dutifully answer the telephone (with Bob standing by, absorbing every word) and describe the previous week's observations. In reality, numerous observations were made, but no salient conclusions emerged. Nevertheless, each week Jim became more eager to publish the results that had accumulated. Consequently, each week John had to stand more firmly, insisting that there could be no meaningful publication until there was a story to be told. In doing so, he had to walk a fine line. On the one hand, he was very appreciative of Jim's willingness to send additional plasma samples. On the other, he felt that with two previous misdiagnoses of this bleeding condition, no one would be served by rushing into print.'

'Eventually, fall came, and Bob returned to finish medical school. He then went to Massachusetts General Hospital for a residency and subsequently migrated to the NIH Clinical Center for additional training. During the latter stint, he and John were able to get together on several occasions. Afterward, Bob returned to the South. Exquisitely trained and credentialed, he became a full-time clinician.'

'John continued to spend part of his time wrestling with the business of Jim's bleeding patients, and Hampton continued to send him plasma samples. Among the techniques John used was that simple one that he had taught to Bob Morton years previously, namely, clotting diluted plasma and winding up the clot. When cross-linking was prevented, the peptide chains of the patients' fibrin sometimes resembled those of the high-solubility fibrinogen or the plasmin-digested fibrinogen that Mike and John had studied.'

'This gave John the idea that maybe something *was* missing from the patient's fibrinogen after all. However, the true situation became clear after a few simple experiments. (Almost all experiments are simple—after you know the answer.) If the clots were wound up and allowed to incubate in their own serum, they underwent digestion. They continued to undergo digestion if the incubation was prolonged. By contrast, if both the cross-linking and the digestion were prevented by using appropriate inhibitors, the fibrin clots were stable, and the peptide chains looked perfectly normal. In other words, there was (just as all the previous experiments had indicated) nothing abnormal about the fibrinogen. The apparent abnormality was being *created* during the incubation.'

'This suggested two things. Either there was too much of the digesting enzyme (plasmin) or its precursor (plasminogen), or there was not enough of a plasmin inhibitor. The first possibility was ruled out by some straightforward assays. The latter issue required help from Franco Carmassi, a postdoctoral fellow in Jack Folk's laboratory.' (Located nearby on the NIH campus).

'Franco was setting up an immunological analysis for another plasmin inhibitor and agreed to run some samples for John. As the results accumulated, the situation became somewhat like that in the old days when stock market quotations were received on tickertape. One felt the excitement rising but tried not to become too excited by the news. But, in this case, the news was genuinely exciting.'

'Finally, some 11 years after Bob had arrived in John's lab, it was possible for John to report (in a conference co-organized and co-chaired by Mike, of all things) that this long-studied 'Fibrinogen Oklahoma' family had a partial deficiency of the inhibitor that Franco was studying. This meant that the blood of the afflicted family members clotted in normal fashion but that the clots were being digested away before they had completed their job, that is, not only to stop bleeding but also to prevent its recurrence.'

'Remarkably, we now know, thanks to much additional work carried out in Mike's lab, that this inhibitor was the same one that Mike and John had discovered in the course of investigating normal fibrinogen 20 years earlier (α2-antiplasmin).'

ADDENDUM 2

Report and Analysis of a 'Plasma Fibrinogen-Bound α2AP ELISA'

(Presented at a BRI conference, March 2013)

Background, Rationale, and Goals

Dissolution of intravascular fibrin-rich thrombi by fibrinolysis is an important physiological mechanism for resolving occlusive or ischemic events that often accompany *intravascular thrombosis*. The rate at which fibrinolysis occurs after clotting has taken place is commonly estimated by determining the *fibrinolytic potential*, which is measured by quantitative assessment of the Clot Lysis Time (CLT). CLTs vary from one individual to another, and there is insufficient evidence to explain the basis for the variability.

There is, however, some evidence indicating that reduced fibrinolytic potential (i.e., prolonged CLT) is associated with an increased risk for arterial thrombosis [1]. In addition, Hoekstra et al. [2] implicated impaired fibrinolysis as a risk factor in the Budd-Chiari syndrome (spontaneous thrombosis in hepatic veins or the inferior vena cava). Several other recent studies showing that hypofibrinolysis is associated with an increased occurrence of intravascular thrombosis are not listed.

There are two α2-antiplasmin (α2AP) compartments in blood, a well characterized freely circulating monomolecular component ('free α2AP') accounting for most of the circulating α2AP, plus a recently characterized component that is covalently linked to circulating plasma fibrinogen ('fibrinogen-bound α2AP') [3]. Although α2AP, per se, is the most important inhibitor of plasmin-mediated fibrinolysis, there is no information that distinguishes the roles played by 'fibrinogen-bound α2AP' compared with 'free α2AP' in regulating *in vivo* fibrinolysis.

Alpha2-AP is an effective inhibitor of fibrinolysis after having been incorporated into fibrin. We infer from this that α2AP that has been incorporated into circulating fibrinogen, namely 'fibrinogen-bound α2AP', plays a definitive role in regulating fibrinolysis *in vivo*. The hypothesis behind this statement is that increased levels of 'fibrinogen-bound α2AP' serve to slow fibrin clot dissolution (hypofibrinolysis). It follows that hypofibrinolysis increases the risk of incurring an occlusive intravascular event. Having a quantitative method (i.e., an ELISA) for measuring this component of plasma could provide a new way of predicting and assessing thrombotic risk.

Our goal is to determine whether 'fibrinogen-bound α2AP' is a thrombosis risk modifier, by first developing an immunoassay (ELISA) to determine the normal range and distribution of values for this plasma constituent. We will then determine the fibrinolytic potential of each plasma sample. To add breadth to the study we will also develop an ELISA for estimating 'free α2AP' plasma levels.

Once that is accomplished, we will measure the levels of fibrinogen-bound α2AP in patient populations with clinically proven thrombophilic states that are associated with hypofibrinolysis (i.e., a prolonged CLT). For this purpose, we have obtained 600+ plasma samples from the population reported by Guimaraes et al. [1].

References

[1] Guimaraes AH, de Bruijne EL, Lisman T, Dippel DW, Deckers JW, Poldermans D, et al. Hypofibrinolysis is a risk factor for arterial thrombosis at young age. Br J Haematol 2009;145:115-20.

[2] Hoekstra J, Guimaraes AH, Leebeek FW, Darwish MS, Malfliet JJ, Plessier A, et al. Impaired fibrinolysis as a risk factor for Budd-Chiari syndrome. Blood 2010;115:388-95.

[3] Mosesson MW, Siebenlist KR, Hernandez I, Lee KN, Christiansen VJ, McKee PA. Evidence that alpha2-antiplasmin becomes covalently ligated to plasma fibrinogen in the circulation: a new role for plasma factor XIII in fibrinolysis regulation. J Thromb Haemost 2008;6:1565-70.

'The Plasma Fibrinogen-Bound α2AP ELISA'

Principle of The Assay- Capture plasma α2AP with anti-α2AP, and subsequently detect the fibrinogen bound to the α2AP with a second antibody against fibrinogen.

Assay Calibration- Employ a standard fibrinogen ELISA to determine the amount of fibrinogen that was captured by the anti-alpha2 AP antibody. [*Note:* the plasma dilution required for detection of fibrinogen in the *Fibrinogen-Bound α2AP ELISA procedure* is 50X lower than that for the fibrinogen assay.]

- *Plasma Fibrinogen Standard,* 'Cryocheck' Normal Reference Plasma (Precision Biologics) (Fgn concentration, 2.96 mg/ml).

- Diluted fibrinogen concentrations range from 0.296 μg/ml to 0.009 μg/ml. (1:1000 to 1:32,000).

ELISA Procedures

1. Dilute plasma samples or other standards with PBS; incubate for 2 hr at RT.

2. Coat each plate well for 2 hr at RT with 100 μl anti-alpha2 AP antibody (Everest Biotech, EB08777) (diluted 1:4000 in carbonate buffer, pH 9.6).

3. Wash 2x with PBS/Tween (0.05%).

4. Add 100 μl per plate well of diluted plasma samples or known standards; incubate for 1 hr at RT.

5. Wash plate 4x with PBS/Tween (0.05%).

6. Add 100 μl per plate well of biotinylated Rabbit anti-Fibrinogen (DAKO; diluted 1:3333 in PBS).

7. Wash plate 4x with PBS/Tween (0.05%).

8. Add 100 μl per plate well of ALKP-Streptavidin to plate (Jackson, 1:5000 in PBS).
9. Wash plate 4x with PBS/Tween (0.05%).

10. Add 100 μl per plate well of PNPP.

11. Stop reaction with 1 N NaOH.

12. Read plate-"endpoint read" at 405 nm.

'The Plasma α2AP ELISA'
Assay Principle-

Capture plasma α2AP with anti-α2AP, and subsequently detect bound α2AP with a second anti-α2AP antibody (Sandwich ELISA).

Establishing Plasma α2AP Standard-

An *in-house* α2AP plasma standard was prepared from a commercial α2AP-depleted plasma to which had been added a known amount of purified α2AP (1 μMol per ml) [databook ref., MWM 5-11). The plasma used for standard preparation was 'Cryocheck' Normal Reference Plasma (CCNRP). [CCNRP is commonly used at BCW for preparation of standard plasma protein curves, but had no previously assigned value for the plasma α2AP concentration.]

The *in-house* standard was run 5 consecutive times against CCNRP and an average result of 94% was obtained. The α2AP-depleted plasma was also run against CCNRP and yielded an average value of 15%. Since the *in-house* standard was equivalent to 79% of the CCNRP value (94%-15%), the absolute α2AP concentration in CCNRP was calculated as 1.27 μM.

ELISA Procedures-

1. Coat plate wells with 100 μl per well of diluted anti-α2 AP (Everest Biotech EB08777, diluted 1:1000 in carbonate buffer, pH 9.6). Incubate for 2 hrs at RT. Wash 2x with PBS/tween (0.05%)

2. Dilute Standards and other samples in 1.0% Milk Casein in PBS. Add 100 μl per plate well of diluted standards and samples to wells.

3. Wash 2x with PBS/Tween (0.05%); incubate plate for 1 hr at RT.
4. Wash plate 4x with PBS/0.05% Tween.

5. Add 100 μl per plate well of biotinylated Rabbit anti-α2AP (ABCAM, diluted 1:1500 in 1% Milk Casein).

6. Wash plate 4x with PBS/0.05% Tween.

7. Add 100 μl per well of ALKP-Streptavidin to plate (Jackson, 1:5000 in 1% Milk Casein); incubate fir 30 minutes at RT.

8. Wash plate 4x with PBS/0.05% Tween.

9. Add 100 μl per well of PNPP.

10. Stop reaction with 1 N NaOH.

11. Read plate-"endpoint read" at 405 nm.

RESULTS
Normal Plasmas

After many iterations, we developed a reproducible and reliably accurate Fgn-Bound α2AP assay. The standard for calibrating this assay was unique, the Plasma Fibrinogen assay itself. Developing an absolute fgn-bound standard proved to be difficult and we instead opted for fibrinogen ELISA itself. To summarize this procedure, we used the standard fibrinogen assay values (at ~1:50 higher dilution) to estimate the amount of fibrinogen that had become bound to the analysis plate using anti-α2AP capture. I believe that this is a unique standardization procedure since we used an antibody to α2AP for capture and an antibody to fibrinogen for tagging the fibrinogen that was bound to α2AP [and it is the main basis for patenting this ELISA procedure].

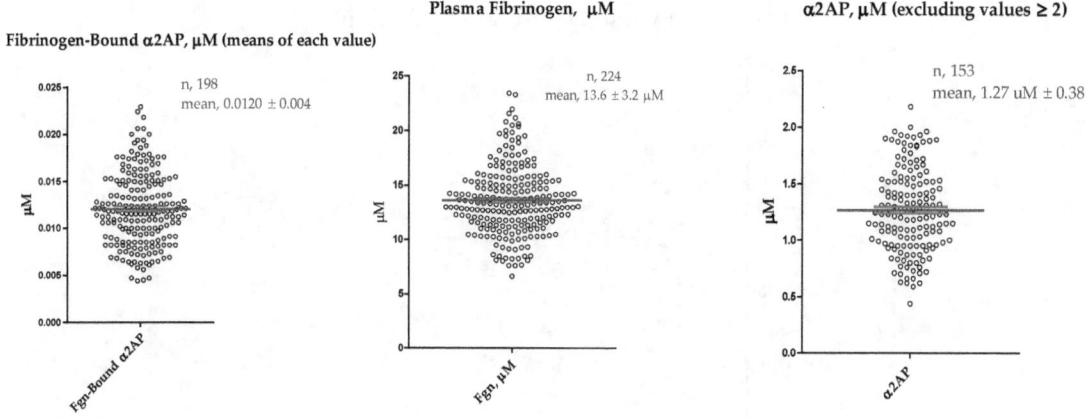

Figure 1. Distribution plots of Fgn-bound α2AP, Fibrinogen, and α2AP

Interpretations

The values for each measurement are Gaussian in distribution. We encountered some difficulties with the α2AP ELISA in that some values suggested that α2AP was self-associating or aggregating. This behavior resulted in apparent values for α2AP that were unrealistically high. For that reason, for this presentation, I excluded values for α2AP ≥ 2. [*We will need to revisit this assay to eliminate this problem.*]

We have compared the concentration dependence of Fgn-bound α2AP with fibrinogen levels (Fig. 2). The slope of the regression line for the absolute levels (in μM) of plasma fibrinogen versus Fgn-bound a2AP [panel A] is not significantly different from zero (p, 0.9), suggesting that there is no correlation between the fibrinogen level and the Fgn-Bound α2AP levels.

When the same plasma fibrinogen data were plotted against the relative level of Fgn-bound a2AP (i.e., % Fgn-bound a2AP) [panel B], the slope of the regression line was negative (p, 0.0001), indicating an inverse relationship between the absolute fibrinogen level (μM) and the relative level of Fgn-bound

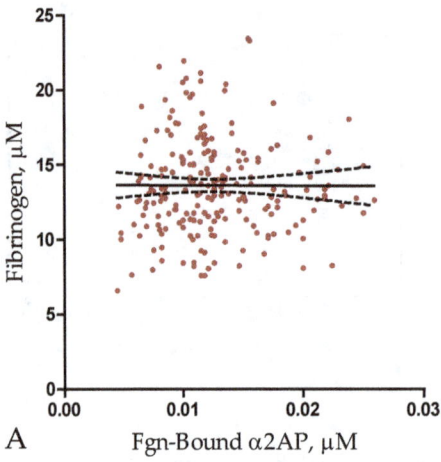

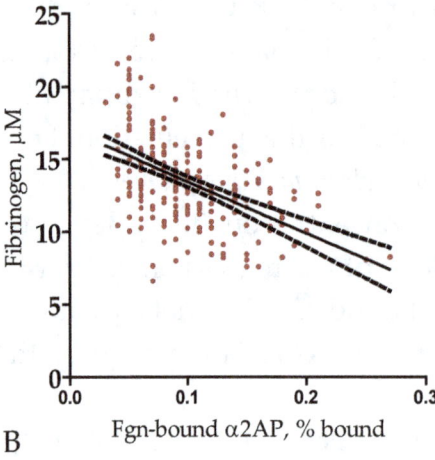

Figure 2. Fibrinogen levels (μM) plotted against Fgn-Bound α2AP levels in μM [panel A] or as a % of the total fibrinogen [panel B].

Taken together, we conclude that within this range of plasma concentrations, fibrinogen itself does not play a significant role in affecting the process of α2AP incorporation into fibrinogen.

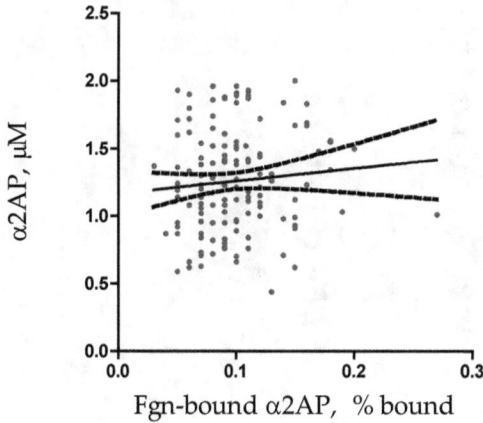

Figure 3. α2AP, μM, versus % Fgn-bound α2AP

We plotted the level of α2AP (μM) against % Fgn-bound α2AP. The slope of the regression line was not significantly different from zero (p, 0.3). This implies that there is no correlation between α2AP levels and the relative levels of Fgn-bound α2AP, an anticipated result.

The Haplotypes of the Val/Leu Factor XIII Polymorphism

Factor XIII or a related transglutaminase is the enzyme responsible for catalyzing the incorporation of α2AP into fibrinogen in the circulation to form Fibrinogen-Bound α2AP [3]. There is a polymorphism in the Factor XIII that results in Val or Leu at positon 34 of the A subunit. Several groups reported that the Leu variant has a significantly higher enzyme activity than the Val form. For that reason we posited that the Leu variant might be more active in incorporating α2AP into plasma fibrinogen.

We determined the normal subject donor DNA haplotypes (LL, VL, and LL) and plotted them versus the Fibrinogen-Bound α2AP levels (Figure 4).

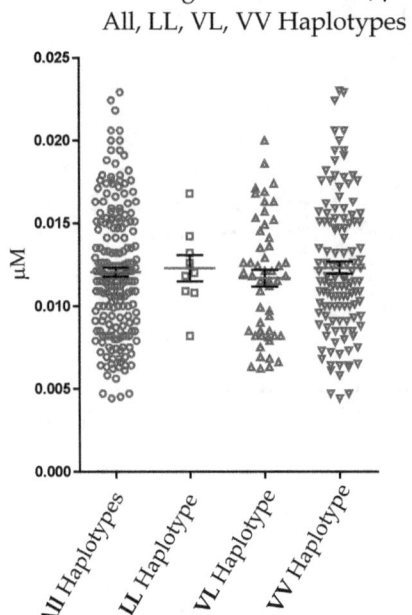

Figure 4. Factor XIII Haplotypes versus Fgn-Bound α2AP

There were no statistical differences between the mean or median Fgn-bound α2AP values for 'All' haplotype samples versus each of the individual haplotypes (LL, VL, VV) [p, >>0.05], and more particularly between the LL and VV haplotypes. The number of samples of the LL haplotype was relatively small (9 of 199 total plasmas) and we may want to augment that number with additional determinations. However, we infer from these results that there is no evidence suggesting that one Factor XIII Val/Leu haplotype is more active than the other one with regard to incorporation of α2AP into circulating fibrinogen.

Plasma Samples from the 'ATTAC Study' Published in Guimaraes et al. [1]

We obtained plasma samples from the 'ATTAC' population studied by Guimaraes et al. [1] (provided to us by D. Rijken, Erasmus University, The Netherlands). That study involved determination of the clot lysis time, CLT, as an inverse measure of the 'fibrinolytic potential' in a cohort of subjects with clinically proven 'early-onset' thrombophilic states, compared with an age and sex matched cohort of normal subjects. Our goal was to measure the Fgn-Bound α2AP levels in each sample and analyze their distribution with respect to the CLT. For further breadth we also included measurements of plasma fibrinogen- and plasma α2AP levels.

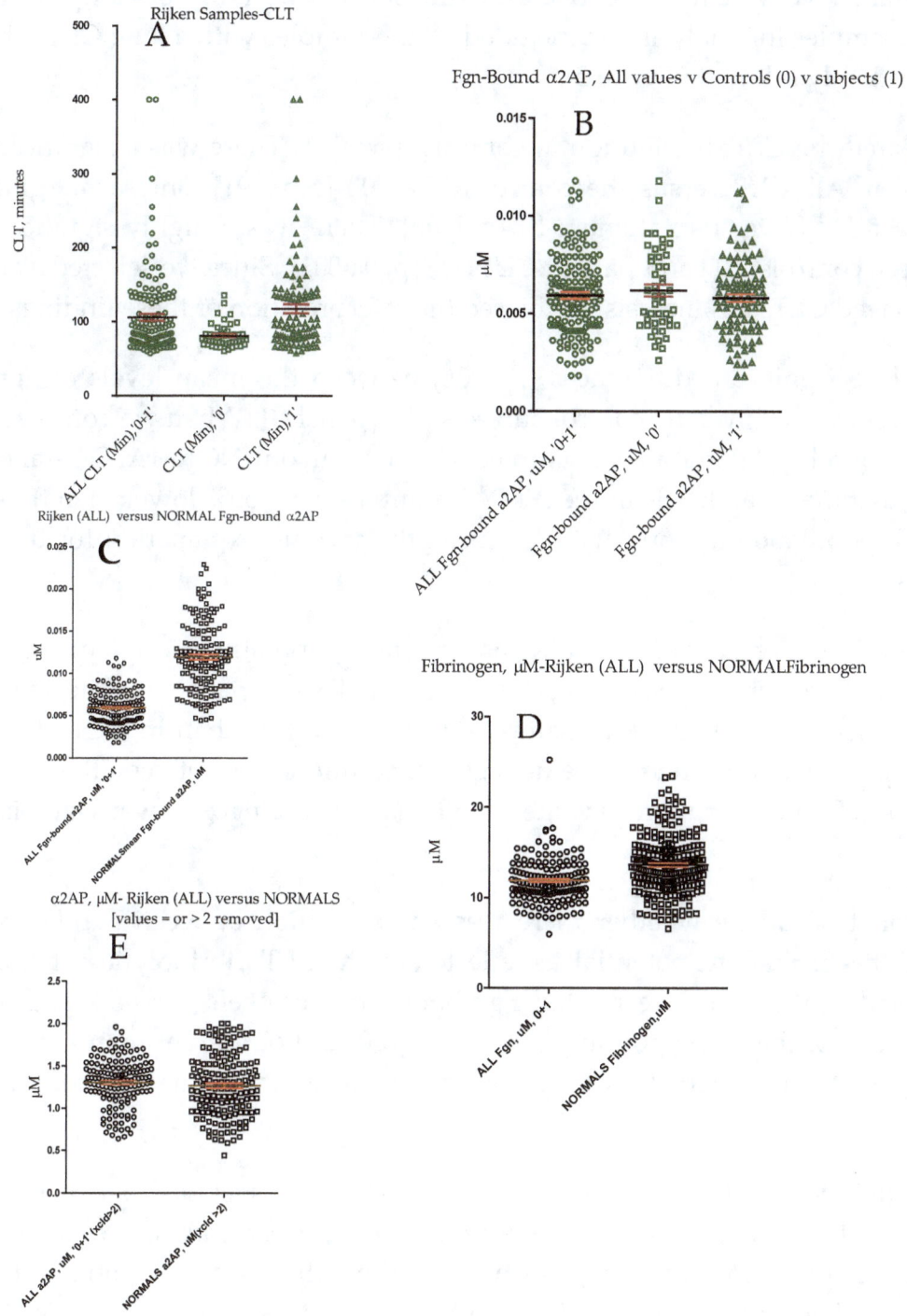

Figure 5. The ATTAC study samples (Rijken). A. CLT, 'All' v control v pts; B. Fgn-bound α2AP, uM; 'All' v Controls (0) v Pts (1); C. Fgn-bound α2AP-Normal subjects v ATTAC subjects; D. Fibrinogen, 'ATTAC subjects v 'Normal subjects', uM. E. α2AP, ATTAC subjects v Normals, μM.

About one-third of the ATTAC samples that we analyzed were from control subjects (n, 47) and the others were from patients with thrombosis (n, 100). Because of budgetary constraints we were not able to analyze the entire cohort of ~600 samples. In selecting patient samples for analysis, we included all the samples with a long CLT. The controls were randomly selected (Figure 5).

We compared the CLT distribution in controls (panel A. There was a significant difference between 'All' CLT versus the control CLTs ('0') [p, 0.001], only a marginal difference between 'ALL' versus patients ('1') [p, 0.05]. There was a highly significant difference between controls ('0') and patient CLTs (1) [p, 0.0001]. Since we selected *all* of the patient prolonged CLTs for analysis, we biased the interpretation of these findings.

We found no significant differences (p, 0.36) between the mean levels of Fgn-bound α2AP in controls ('0') versus control subjects ('1') [panel B]. When we compared the levels of Fgn-bound α2AP in ATTAC samples with those in our NORMALS (2-tailed t test) we found that the mean levels in the ATTAC samples were 50% lower than those in our NORMAL population ((p, <0.001). We currently have no explanation for these large differences.

This large difference between ATTAC and normal populations was not found when we compared the fibrinogen- (panel D) or α2AP levels (panel E). The mean fibrinogen levels mean levels in ATTAC samples were 13% *higher* than in NORMALS (13.6 v 11.9 μM; p, <0.001), and there were no significant differences between the mean α2AP levels (p, 0.2). The distribution of values in all analytical categories was Gaussian in all cases.

In an effort to examine whether there was an association between Fgn-bound α2AP levels and the 'fibrinolytic potential' as reflected by the CLT (fibrinolytic potential is inversely related to the CLT), we plotted Fgn-bound α2AP levels versus the CLTs (Figure 6). The slope of the regression line was not significantly different than zero (p, 0.4), and consequently the higher CLT values were not associated with higher values for Fgn-Bound α2AP.

This finding does not provide evidence that there is an association between the amount of a2AP that is bound to fibrinogen and the *fibrinolytic potential (CLT)*. There is insufficient evidence to warrant drawing a firm conclusion. The assay is sound and the concept behind its development is sound. The subject deserves more study. We do, however, have enough information to warrant submitting a patent application dealing with the new assay.

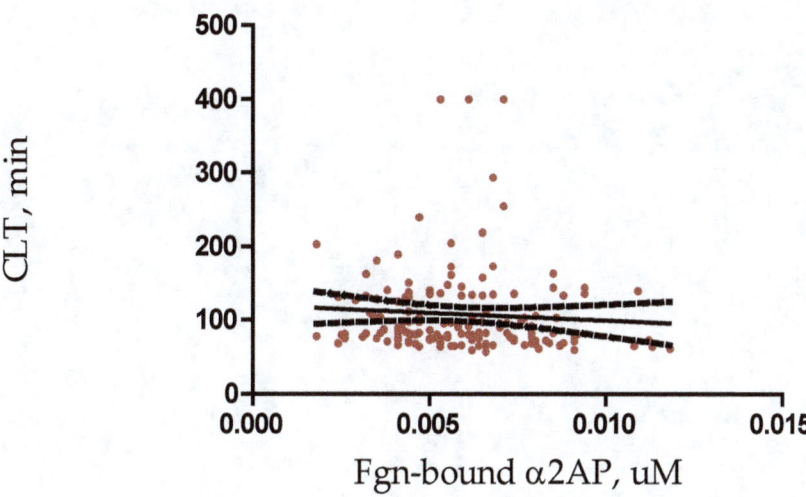

Figure 6. Fgn-Bound α2AP versus CLT

Respectfully Submitted,
Michael W. Mosesson, MD

CHAPTER X

SWEET CLOVER DISEASE OF CATTLE AND THE PRODUCTION OF TRANSGENIC FIBRINOGEN IN COWS' MILK

The year was 2012. Two people from a company named *Pharming* paid me an impromptu visit one afternoon at my office in the Blood Research Institute on Watertown Plank Road. One of them was a Veterinarian and the other a Project Manager. *Pharming's* home office was in Utrecht, The Netherlands, but my visitors had come from a farm located in DeForest, Wisconsin, not far from UWM-Madison. They were interested in my expertise on Fibrinogen and, as it turned out, they had come to the right person. The subject we discussed that day related to an active project at their farm, namely the production of Human Fibrinogen in cows.

To understand *Pharming's* basis for deciding to produce human fibrinogen in cows I digress with an abbreviated history of the development of human blood banking and plasma fractionation. The first 'Blood Bank' in the United States was established in Chicago more than 80 years ago and was designed to facilitate the collection of whole blood and to provide a convenient and relatively stable source of blood and blood products for intravenous transfusion. In those days drawn blood that had been properly refrigerated was stable for only a few days at most and therefore the product had limited usefulness outside of a hospital perimeter. By the onset of World War II, it was clear that whole blood transfusions could be life-saving assets under battlefield conditions, but their limited stability and other shortcomings (e.g., blood typing required) blunted that pathway. However, a byproduct of whole blood, *blood plasma*, could readily be separated from cellular elements by centrifugation. The resulting liquid plasma was more stable than whole blood and could be freeze-dried to produce a product that after reconstitution, was useful as a blood volume expander to treat, for example, battlefield casualties. But that was not enough.

It was clear at that time that stable and more highly purified by-products of plasma would significantly extend their clinical usefulness. Because it was wartime, a top-secret project was launched by the Federal government that was staged at 'The Protein Foundation' in Boston under the direction of EJ Cohn of Harvard University. The goal was to develop methods for separating plasma constituents into stable components that might be used on the battlefield or elsewhere as blood protein replacements and/or blood volume expanders. The participants in this project included Harvard faculty members and doctoral level people who had been conscripted or had enlisted in the armed forces and then assigned to work at The Protein Foundation. Many of them continued their work in this field after the war and became famous for their wartime efforts and their other subsequent achievements. Names like John D. Ferry, DJ Mulford, JN Ashworth, K Morrison come readily to mind.

The various fractionation processes that were developed were known as 'Cohn Fractionation Methods' and were eventually assigned numbers such as Method VI or Method X. Details concerning the developed schemes were not published or made public until after World War II had ended. Among the useful plasma products that emerged from the project were Albumin ('Fraction V'), The Immunoglobulin Fraction ('Fraction II+III'), and Fibrinogen ('Fraction I'). Fractionation was carried out in large vessels (2000+ liters) containing pooled plasmas that had been collected from hundreds of individual donors. Successful applications of Cohn subfractions obtained in this way were achieved during the war, some of which are still in use. For example, Albumin ('Fraction V') could be heated to inactivate infectious agents without changing its essential properties and as a result, has been in continuous use as a plasma volume expander since its introduction. On the other hand, the fibrinogen-rich subfraction ('Fraction I'), could not be 'sterilized' by heating or by any other procedure without becoming denatured, a feature that resulted in an appreciable incidence of transfusion-transmitted viral hepatitis. Consequently, although the therapeutic usefulness of fibrinogen subfractions was evident, the risk of transfusion-related infections led to abandonment of the original large volume fractionation procedure. In the years that followed, many alternative fractionation procedures have been developed that resulted in safer products and that assured continued utilization of fibrinogen-rich plasma fractions.

Fibrinogen-rich blood fractions were used clinically during World War II in several forms, e.g., 1) as a freeze-dried reconstituted liquid solution for intravenous infusion in individuals whose circulating fibrinogen levels had been depleted; 2) as *Fibrin Film*, a fibrin clot that originally had been freeze-dried and packaged under vacuum in large ampules and rehydrated for field use. Reconstituted fibrin film like that shown at the right was used to cover and contain gaping wounds suffered on the battlefield.

Concerns about preventing transmission of infectious diseases as well as economic considerations provided a compelling rationale for *Pharming's* attempt to develop a method for producing large amounts of virus-free Human Fibrinogen (rhFgn) in the milk glands of lactating cows. During their visit to my office they explained that the company had already been successful at their home base in The Netherlands in producing a human gene product termed 'rhC1-INH' in lactating cows' milk, a product that was intended as a treatment for Hereditary Angioedema (HAE), a congenital abnormality characterized by a deficiency of C1esterase inhibitor (C1-INH). They had achieved this by selectively inserting the human C1-INH gene into the milk glands of cows. When lactation was induced in these cows, they produced their expected milk product, but the milk also contained substantial amounts of rhC1-INH. This protein could subsequently be purified to homogeneity for use in human subjects with HAE.

More recently, they had purchased a farm in Wisconsin for the purpose of producing recombinant human fibrinogen (rhFgn) in cows' milk. At the time they contacted me they had already succeeded in producing rhFgn milk. They'd come to invite me to help them resolve several problems. After listening to their presentation, I gladly accepted their invitation and immediately began to investigate the issues they had related to me. These included the following: 1) Although they could readily identify human fibrinogen in their transgenic cows' milk, the yield of fibrinogen was significantly lower than anticipated; 2) milk production often became progressively reduced with successive milking; 3) the milk often contained visible 'clots'; 4) lactating cows often developed mastitis (an inflammatory condition involving the milk glands and their conduit channels), further reducing milk production. These problems were a serious impediment to their success and the Pharming people evidently had no useful ideas about what was going on and therefore no means of solving these serious problems.

To begin my involvement in their *human fibrinogen milk* project, I made several visits to the farm to see and examine the lactating cows and to investigate the problems they were encountering. I took several samples of fibrinogen-containing milk to my laboratory to retrieve and analyze the human fibrinogen/fibrin in the milk. I was able to show that the 'clots' we had observed in the milk were due to formation of *fibrin clots*. At the same time, I examined the histological sections of the mastitis biopsies. It was immediately clear that the milk channels were filled with and often obstructed by fibrin clots that must had been generated from the fibrinogen secreted into the milk. I also noted small but significant amounts of blood in the milk ducts in biopsy specimens. Obstruction to milk flow by these clots readily accounted for the occurrence of inflammatory mastitis. It did not take long for me to understand exactly what was going on. The next step in this investigation would be to explain my findings and conclusions to the Pharming people. I arranged a group meeting at the DeForest farm with all involved Pharming personnel including the CEO. My goal was to explicate the existing problems and place the presentation in historical perspective to offer a unique solution to the problems.

I started the conference with the following remarks (paraphrased): '*Fibrinogen is a soluble circulating clotting protein in blood. It is converted to an insoluble polymer, the* **Fibrin Clot***, by* **Thrombin***, a biological catalyst (enzyme) which is generated from its precursor,* **Prothrombin***, as the final product in the blood clotting cascade. Blood clotting can be triggered by many events including contact with underlying tissues that are encountered when blood* *escapes from a blood vessel. Because thrombin is an enzyme, only small amounts are required to produce extensive fibrinogen conversion to fibrin.'*

*'That's precisely what I believe happens when fibrinogen is secreted in cows' milk. **Remember**, fibrinogen is never found in milk from normal lactating cows. Even a small degree of tissue trauma (due to the milking process or to other minor events) will result in some blood escaping into the milk, as evidenced by the red blood cells that we've observed in the ducts. Ordinarily, such escape of blood would have no noticeable adverse consequences, **but** when the clotting protein **fibrinogen** is also present in the milk, as in rhFgn cows, the thrombin activity generated from the escaped blood is enough to catalyze fibrin clot formation. And when fibrin does form in those ducts it often obstructs milk flow, resulting in the mastitis that we see commonly in rhFgn cows. Fibrin clot formation in the milk and the consequent milk duct obstruction account for progressively reduced fibrinogen content. Furthermore, as you can imagine, the existence of substantial amounts of fibrin in the milk will limit the usefulness and the marketability of the human fibrinogen that is recovered.'*

*'So, what can be done to solve these problems? To understand what can be done I will start with the story of a hemorrhagic disease of cattle that was first recognized in the 1920s in Northern USA and Canadian cattle. Bleeding occurred only in cattle that had been fed moldy silage made from a sweet clover plant and the often-fatal affliction came to be known as **'Sweet Clover Disease.'** After eight years had passed a Canadian veterinarian named LM Roderick reported that the affected animals lacked the blood clotting factor **Prothrombin**, the precursor to the clotting enzyme **Thrombin**. The substance in the moldy silage that led to reduction of prothrombin levels remained unknown until Karl P. Link of the University of Wisconsin started his own investigations. Finally, in 1939 one of his students, Harold Campbell, isolated the anticoagulant, **Dicoumarol**, from these plants and showed that it inhibits prothrombin formation in cattle and in rabbits. A more potent version of dicoumarol, **Coumadin**, that had been synthesized from the coumarin-based anticoagulant, was patented by the **W**isconsin **A**lumni **R**esearch **F**oundation and became known as 'WARFarin.' As everyone now knows, **warfarin** became the most used anticoagulant for thrombotic disorders and remains in wide usage today. I want to extend this story concerning one of the greatest medical breakthroughs of the 20th century to a discussion of how we can take the story of sweet clover disease in cattle and turn it around to learn how to safely anti-coagulate our rhFgn cows.'*

My ideas took root immediately and we set about learning what was known about Coumadin anti-coagulation of cattle. Although there was a wealth of information about Coumadin use in humans, there was little known about its use in cows. We began by determining what an appropriate dose of Warfarin would be to effectively anti-coagulate cows while minimizing their hemorrhagic risk. That took us several weeks to accomplish but eventually we arrived at a dosage level (like that used in humans) that effectively reduced the prothrombin level without inducing significant hemorrhage and that also prevented clot formation and mastitis in the rhFgn cows. I believe that this simple intervention saved the rhFgn project. Shortly thereafter I withdrew from my involvement with Pharming and returned to my own more circumscribed interests at the BloodCenter of Wisconsin.

Michael Mosesson   *March 15, 2020*

CHAPTER XI

ORIGINS OF THE INTERNATIONAL FIBRINOGEN RESEARCH SOCIETY

A Personal Account

The first Workshop conference on Fibrinogen was conceived by Pehr Edman and organized in his honor by his wife, Agnes Henschen. The conference was entitled *'The Shape and Structure of Fibrinogen'* and was held in 1977 at Edman's Proteinchemie Department at The Max-Planck Institut für Biochemie in Martensried bei München. Edman was a renowned biochemist who had developed a new method for protein amino acid sequence analysis. The method came to be known as the 'Edman Procedure' and was a revolutionary improvement of existing methodologies. At the time of the conference Edman's procedure was being used by Henschen for sequencing Fibrinogen.

Many notable scientists contributed to that conference including Klaus Lederer, L. Bachmann, Gérard Marguerie, Dieter Heene, Helmut Hörmann, Friedrich Lottspeich, Edda Töpfer-Peterson, Preben Kok, and Micha Furlan, among others. The proceedings were published in a special issue of *Thrombosis and Haemostasis*.

That first meeting was succeeded by other Workshops that were held in different European cities. The composition of each Workshop Organizing Committee depended on its venue, but usually included Agnes Henschen on the roster, probably to acknowledge her primary role in starting them. I did not attend those early conferences and therefore my knowledge of them is limited, but I did participate actively in the 1986 Workshop organized by Gert Müller-Berghaus in Giessen, West Germany, that was held at Schloss Rauischholzhausen.

As a sidelight to that Workshop, I had been serving for three years prior to that conference as a member of Müller-Berghaus' *'Scientific Advisory Board'* (*Fachbeirat*) for the newly created *'Research Unit for Blood Coagulation and Thrombosis'* under the auspices of The Max-Planck Institut at Justus-Liebig Universität. During my tenure on the Fachbeirat I had been assigned to review the studies being carried out by Eberhard Selmayr, a Veterinary School Student who was spending his senior undergraduate year in that department. Selmayr had chosen to investigate the structural arrangement of cross-linked γ-chains in assembled fibrin polymers, a subject that was not controversial at the time, at least as far as I knew. After reviewing his experimental results and listening to his presentation at a Fachbeirat meeting, I realized that he had developed significant evidence that refuted existing dogma concerning the arrangement of cross-linked γ-chains in an assembled fibrin polymer. His experimental design was simple but clever and decisive, his findings unambiguous, and his conclusions definitive and unassailable, or so I believed.

After further discussions I was confident that once Selmayr's results had been published, existing dogma would fall by the wayside. I could n<u>o</u>t have been more wrong about that! In subsequent meetings, I encouraged Selmayr to continue his research studies, but he had already decided that what he wanted most was a career as a Clinical Veterinarian. Despite my urgings, he eventually left Müller-Berghaus' group to pursue his career goal. Although he was listed as a member of the 1986 Workshop Organizing Committee, and I was looking forward to seeing him again, he did not attend the Workshop meetings.

Following Selmayr's seminal publication, several new reports from other laboratories ignored his findings and conclusions, and instead presented their experiments that they believed had extended the prevailing hypothesis. I was surprised by their outright rejection of Semayr's report, and their unfailing support for a cross-linking scheme that I now believed to be incorrect. Given Selmayr's withdrawal, I decided to take up the cudgel on my own, a decision that led to a long series of experiments designed to critically examine the fibrin cross-linking question. The consequences of my decision were covered in detail in Chapter VI. Those investigations corroborated Selmayr's original conclusions and turned out to be one of the most rewarding 'quests for truth' of my career.

The following year, 1987, the boundaries of the Europe-bound Workshops were extended to Renfrew, Scotland for a meeting that was organized by Gordon Lowe (Glasgow), Patrick Gaffney (London), David Lane (London), and Agnes Henschen (Munich). During that conference I met with the Organizing Committee and with prior Workshop organizers and proposed Milwaukee, Wisconsin as the site for the 1988 Workshop. My offer met with enthusiastic approval. The conference would be the first Fibrinogen Workshop to be held on the other side of the Atlantic Ocean.

The following year the global reach of the conference was further extended to Kyoto, Japan, hosted by Michio Matsuda. Following that successful 1989 meeting, it was on to Rouen, France in 1990, a Workshop that had been organized by Nanette and Claudine Soria.

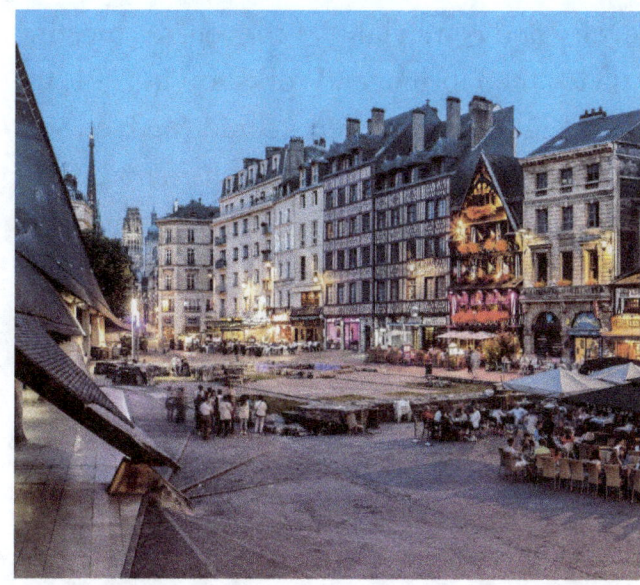

(Photo: Place du Vieux Marché with the eaves of the Église Jeanne d'Arc at the left).

During the two preceding Workshops, a working Committee composed of former organizers and participants, met to discuss the future of the Fibrinogen Workshops, to determine whether a more formal organization, namely *The International Fibrinogen Research Society (IFRS)*, should replace them, as well as to develop details of its ultimate organization, and the drafting of a Constitution to codify governance structure. Formal inauguration of the IFRS took place at Rouen, where Workshop members met one evening for dinner and other festivities at Place du Vieux Marché (Old Market Place). That Market Place is best known as the site where Joan of Arc was burned at the stake in 1431. In her memory, a modern church, Église Jeanne d'Arc, borders the Square.

That evening, Welsh-born John Owen from Bowman Gray School of Medicine whose weekend hobby was 'Church bell ringing' and who would become the IFRS Secretary-Treasurer, held forth eloquently. He mesmerized the audience with his Welsh accent and controlled and amused them for about fifteen minutes. When he had concluded his opening remarks, he announced the genesis of the IFRS and asked for approval by the 'soon-to-be members.' The response was explosively unanimous amid shouts, applause, and clicking of wine glasses. Owen announced that the Advisory Committee had selected me to be its CEO. I, of course, was aware of that decision, but nevertheless I was humbly appreciative, and accepted this honor in a brief acceptance speech.

The IFRS was subsequently registered in Wisconsin as a non-profit Corporation. Its first Board of Directors comprised: *President*, Agnes Henschen (Germany); *Chairman and CEO*, Michael Mosesson (USA); *Secretary-Treasurer*, John Owen (USA); *Counselors*: Frank Brosstad (Norway), Jessie T. Douglas (UK), Michio Matsuda (Japan), Leonid Medved (USSR), Gert Müller-Berghaus (Germany), Willem Nieuwenhuizen (Netherlands), John R Shainoff (USA), and Claudine & Nanette Soria (France).

The day following our evening of revelry and conviviality, I convened a meeting of The Board of Directors to choose a venue for the Fibrinogen Workshop in 1991, the first under the aegis of the IFRS. We selected Kiev, Ukraine, and Leonid Medved was chosen as its Chairman. The Soviet Union at that time was undergoing '*Perestroika*' that would eventually lead to its dissolution. In the months following the Rouen meeting, there was increasing turmoil and disruption throughout the USSR. Early the next year John Owen sounded the alarm concerning the potential hazards of holding the Workshop in Ukraine, and in addition, only a small number of participants had registered for the conference. After consulting at length with members of the Board, I reluctantly decided to cancel the meeting. Understandably, Leonid Medved was disappointed at that decision and so were we all, but at least the Kiev meeting had the distinction of being the only scheduled IFRS Fibrinogen Workshop that did not take place.

Michael Mosesson   *May 28, 2020*

CHAPTER XII

TRANSITIONS TO THE FOOD AND DRUG ADMINISTRATION

By John S. Finlayson, PhD

<u>Preface, Michael Mosesson</u>

In 2008 I telephoned my friend and long-time colleague John Finlayson to say hello—it had been quite some time since we last had spoken and I especially wanted to discuss my latest work on α2-antiplasmin (α2AP) bound to fibrinogen and ask him to read the manuscript. That subject had its origins at The Division of Biologics Standards (DBS) in the early 1960's with our discovery of a plasmin/trypsin inhibitory activity in purified fibrinogen specimens. In the narrative that follows John relates something of this early work as well as many other things that took place during those times.

The source of the inhibitory activity that we had uncovered in 1963 was obscure then but is now known to be due to α2-AP that is covalently bound to fibrinogen in the circulation. It was natural for me to want to share this latest development with John, not just because of his perspicacity, but more importantly because I could think of very few other people, world-wide or local, who could grasp its potential significance. He agreed to review my manuscript, and he did this promptly with his usual thoroughness and insightfulness. His comments, as always, were helpful, and led to my citing his contribution in the acknowledgement section.

During the course of our telephone conversation, I mentioned that I'd been writing some scientific/personal memoirs centering about my fibrinogen career, and I asked him whether he would be willing to contribute an essay or two concerning the early days of DBS, and how it evolved to become a branch of the Food and Drug Administration (FDA). It did not take much coaxing, and the results of this request appear in the essays that follow. John presents a detailed and personal portrait of early phases in the regulation of biologicals by the Federal Government and the Science that came with it. From my standpoint, his essays afford a pleasant journey into the past and a delightful reprise of some of the happiest and most productive days I ever spent. Many of the discoveries and observations described in his narrative eventually became major subjects that occupied me for the remainder of my career. Editing John's contribution was minor-after all, it was he who taught me how to write. Any comments or significant additions to the text are in italics. I have also inserted a picture or two to liven things up.

I gratefully admit that John was the most influential person in teaching me how to write and convey proper science, and how to critically assess one's own data—thank goodness I met him early enough in my career to make a long and permanent difference. My education did not occur soon enough for me to avoid the straight C's (or less) in English that I had regularly achieved in college. Other people portrayed and stories described in his essays attest to his self-effacing devotion to teaching and education. The narrative reveals his own skills as a writer, master teacher, scientist, collaborator, analytical thinker, and learner, to say nothing of the administrative and investigative abilities he perfected while at the evolving FDA.

Michael Mosesson   November 17, 2009

Part 1

The Early Days of the Division of Biologics Standards

It was David Aronson who said it. This was the only laboratory in the world that was studying blood clotting but did not arise by "budding off" from some other, preexisting laboratory studying the same subject. It arose, as Dave said, as a "sport," not in the sense of athletics, but rather in the meaning of the word as your botany teacher tried to explain it. In short, it was as close to spontaneous generation as one dares come in biology.

Who knows why it was formed? No one really—at least, no one now alive. Those of us in the original Coagulation Section always surmised that Dr. JT Tripp (John Theodore Tripp, who signed his name "J.T. Tripp" and was called "Ted" by his compatriots) thought that it would lend some class to his operation. That operation was called the Laboratory of Blood and Blood Products (LBBP). It was one of the units of the Division of Biologics Standards (DBS), which, in turn, was part of the National Institutes of Health (NIH).

DBS was, for all practical purposes, one of the institutes of the NIH—without achieving quite the level of prestige that went with being an institute. It didn't matter. In the pecking order at NIH, Institutes had not been created equal. The National Institute of Arthritis and Metabolic Diseases was considered more prestigious than the National Heart Institute which, in turn, was more prestigious than the National Cancer Institute. DBS must have been at the bottom of the food chain. After all, it was charged not only with doing research (as were all the institutes), but also with regulating all the biologic products—vaccines, allergenic extracts, blood products, antitoxins, etc.—manufactured or marketed in America *[originating as a result of the Public Health Service Act of 1944 that created the Laboratory of Biologics Control that eventually became DBS, and ultimately a major branch of FDA]*. Obviously, an organization that had double duties, one of which was completely practical, couldn't carry much academic cachet.

Nonetheless, there it was, *The Coagulation Section*, and it was a small part of the operation. Moreover, from the standpoint of truth-in-labeling, "small" was about as accurate as one could get. For nearly the first four months of its existence, the Coagulation Section had a staff of one—Sandy Shapiro (Sandor S. Shapiro). Sandy had come aboard in July 1958. He had been faced with the need to set up a lab from scratch, so he spent most of his early days ordering chemicals and equipment, and then reading scientific articles while waiting for the orders to be delivered. As the lab began to take shape, he decided that, rather than working on factors in blood that promoted clotting, he would concentrate on those that could ultimately dissolve clots—the so-called thrombolytic or fibrinolytic substances. That was still firmly within the "mission" of the section since it was responsible for regulating that type of product.

With the arrival of John Finlayson in October its size doubled, and when Dave Aronson showed up three weeks later, it increased by another 50 percent. Nonetheless, "small" was still an accurate description. In fact, the Section was so small that it had no "Chief", so we borrowed the Chief of the Blood Derivatives Section, Dick (Richard T.) Suchinsky. Like Sandy and Dave, he was a medical doctor, but at the University of Buffalo he had spent considerable time in the laboratory of Sidney Shulman, learning a variety of biophysical techniques. (When he left DBS in 1960, he did a residency and became a psychiatrist, but that's another story for another day.) Finlayson was the outlier. In addition to not having "M.D." after his name, he had no Ivy League connection, and he was the one and only biochemist in the Laboratory of Blood and Blood Products. He compensated for this shortcoming in some measure by regaling the group with stories from his days in graduate school at the University of Wisconsin. And, having spent a fair amount of time prowling around the UW's Medical School, he could leaven these monologues with a few of what Dave called "ward stories."

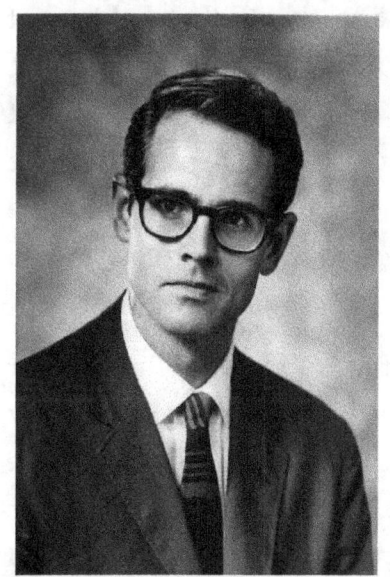

Photo: John Finlayson

Moreover, he seemed to intrigue Suchinsky. Months later Dick confessed, "When he came into the lab, I took one look at his CV and saw that he had just come from Sweden, and another look at his normal length hair, and I didn't know if I'd be able to talk to him!" (Remember, this was the '50s, when super-short hair was the American norm.) In any event, Dick rattled off a list of techniques that were then state-of-the-art in protein biochemistry. He seemed pleased that John had had hands-on experience with all of them.

Then the topic turned to chromatography. For readers who have not frittered away their lives in chemistry labs, suffice it to say that it is a process similar to water-softening. A solution of things that one is trying to separate is pumped through a tube filled with a solid material called an adsorbent, followed by one or more fluids such as salt solutions. As those things are repeatedly adsorbed to and desorbed from the adsorbent, one of them begins to get ahead of the others. If the process works, by the time they emerge from the other end of the tube, they will be coming out one at a time, in more-or-less pure form. That's the theory. In practice, chromatography proved to be a powerful technique for separating many different substances—plant pigments, vitamins, minerals, etc. But if the things one was trying to separate from each other were proteins, the outlook was quite different. There had been a few successes, and the failure rate was enormous.

It turned out that about two years previously, two scientists at NIH (Herbert Sober and Elbert Peterson) had invented a whole new class of adsorbents that held great promise for protein chromatography. They had done this by chemically modifying cellulose powder, which looks about like cornstarch but unlike cornstarch, doesn't dissolve in water. (Your cotton shirt, which is made of cellulose, also doesn't dissolve when you wash it—it just gets wet.) There was only one problem: one could buy cellulose powder, but no commercial firm sold the modified cellulose. If you wanted to use it, you had to make it yourself.

Suchinsky had already begun synthesizing one type of the modified cellulose. For simplicity, we called it by its initials: DEAE—and do to this day! (For the terminally curious, that stands for diethylaminoethyl, which is a very explicit descriptor if you have taken chemistry, but which you may ignore if you haven't.) John took over the process and saw it through to the end. He then poured a slurry of this newly synthesized adsorbent into a glass tube in preparation for performing a trial chromatographic run. Since we are now in the terminology business, we might as well say that chromatographers refer to the tube as a "column." That has a nice architectural ring to it, but it serves mainly to distinguish column chromatography from other variants of the process that involve different equipment and configurations.

Up to that point, things had gone well. The column looked good. There were no obvious bubbles, channels, air pockets, or other discontinuities that would disturb the flow and thereby decrease the column's separating ability. Now the next step was to hook the column up to a pump that was connected to a reservoir of salt solution and to pump away. This preliminary experiment would serve to check out the physical system and, equally important, let us find out which pump settings corresponded to what flow rates through the column. The results of the latter proved to be distressingly simple. No matter what setting was used, the flow rate was zero. It was like trying to pump water through a tube of concrete.

When informed of this sad event, Dick unceremoniously dumped the DEAE cellulose into the waste receptacle and announced that we had to start over. There was no disputing that, but Finlayson feared that repeating the same futile process would merely lead to the same frustrating conclusion. What to do?

The answer arrived by a most unexpected path, which was ultimately provided by the wise administrators of NIH. These visionaries had created a thing called "surplus." Simply put, it meant that if a lab, office, or other facility at NIH had something (a desk, a chair, a scientific instrument, etc.) that was serviceable but no longer needed, it could be placed in a central location and made available, free of charge, to another group. Thus, through "surplus," our lab had recently acquired a high-speed centrifuge (called a 'preparative ultracentrifuge'). We did not have a specific use for it in mind; it just seemed that no well-appointed biochemistry lab should be without one. In fact, many research scientists had reported that it was invaluable for separating proteins or other big molecules based upon different rates of sedimenting when spun at high speed.

Of course, our newly obtained pride and joy had to be installed, connected to the proper high-voltage line, and calibrated to assure that it attained the speeds that were claimed. Accordingly, an engineer from the firm that manufactured it was summoned to check it out. He arrived promptly and, after ascertaining that all the paperwork was in order so that his firm would be paid for the service, he set to work.

By now, John stood in awe of the volume of paper needed to accomplish even the simplest tasks in government. How, he wondered, had the NIH buildings ever been constructed? The mountain of paper needed for each must have exceeded the dimensions of the building! Nonetheless, others (including our visiting engineer) seemed to accept it all as a fact of life. He quickly disassembled the ultracentrifuge, replaced a few minor parts, reassembled it, poured the appropriate oils into the correct chambers, and revved it up. During acceleration it emitted a very satisfying whine, one that John recalled hearing in the corridors of the UW biochemistry department. It was vaguely reminiscent of the soundtrack from the movie, "Breaking the Sound Barrier."

After a few accelerations and decelerations, the engineer announced, "I've checked it out with your low-speed rotor and your intermediate-speed rotor." Then he continued, "Where do you keep your high-speed rotor?" We had to confess that we didn't own one. The generous scientist who had put the centrifuge and two rotors into surplus must have either kept it or decommissioned it because of metal fatigue. "Never mind," said our engineer, who was nothing if not resourceful, "I know where to borrow one." And so he did. An hour or so later he pronounced the centrifuge ready for operation at all indicated speeds, obtained the proper signatures (more paper, more awe), and departed. We proceeded about our business. It was great to have a functional preparative ultracentrifuge, but we had other things to do. There were Nobel Prizes to be won! However, even that would have to wait. First, we had to figure out what to do to make useful DEAE cellulose. At about this point, we noticed that the engineer had left the borrowed high-speed rotor behind. Perhaps, for a fleeting instant, we thought of keeping it. Immediately though, reality took over, and we set about discovering who the rightful owner was. That proved to be ridiculously simple—and very auspicious. There, inscribed on the bottom of the rotor, was the word, SOBER (as in less than 0.8% blood content).

More naïve scientists might have taken this as an admonishment not to operate the centrifuge at high speed while under the influence. But we knew better. This rotor came from the lab of Herb Sober, one of the co-inventors of the modified celluloses. It had to be returned at once. That would afford an opportunity to see what this cutting-edge biochemist looked like. And maybe, just maybe, to get some insight into the reason for our spectacular failure. Because Herb Sober had received his degree from the biochemistry department at UW (albeit several years previous), Finlayson was dispatched to return the rotor. Sober's lab was in a building not far from ours—about a four-minute walk. Rotor in hand, John found the great man seated at his desk, hard at work.

Sober had huge, bushy, black eyebrows, which gave him a somewhat fearsome mien. Nonetheless, he was quite cordial, considering that he had been interrupted by an unexpected visitor who was at least 20 years his junior. (Or perhaps he was just glad to get his rotor back.) After a few Wisconsin pleasantries, John recited his sad story.

"Hmm," was the response, "maybe Peterson has some ideas." John managed not to say, "Wow," or any other adolescent interjection, but he was certainly thinking it. "Peterson" was Elbert Peterson, the other co-inventor of the modified celluloses—the chemist who figured out how to turn the basic concepts of protein chromatography into chemical reality.

Peterson, all six feet four of him, stepped into the room and immediately began quizzing Finlayson. "Did you remember to …?" "Yes." Did you forget to …?" "No." "After the synthesis, did you suspend the cellulose and decant the fine particles?" "Yes, numerous times." "Before the synthesis, did you sift the cellulose powder?" "What?" "Oh, did we forget to put that in the paper?" Upon re-reading the now classic paper by Peterson and Sober, one could see that the concept of using cellulose with particles of a certain size was alluded to in several places. Unfortunately, there was no sentence intoning, "Thou shalt sift thy cellulose powder."

Whatever the etiology, the prognosis was clear. We were going to have to buy a set of so-called U. S. Standard Sieves, which have screens with precisely measured openings. And then, to have cellulose particles that were neither too coarse nor too fine, we would have to sift. And sift. And sift some more. The portent was that the weeks to come would be terminally boring.

The reality was just the opposite. Our little Coagulation Section had grown by the addition of a technician, Lou Leonard, a superb athlete who was assigned to work for David and Sandy. Then, just about the time that the Standard Sieves arrived, so did a technician who was assigned to John's lab, Nelson Roberts, who had just returned from duty in the Navy.

As one might imagine, there were many jokes about "Mr. Roberts" from the Navy. (Apparently, no one had enough sense of history to conjure up witticisms about "Admiral Nelson.") When these subsided, however, several happy discoveries were made. In addition to being a well-trained (former medical corpsman) and enthusiastic worker with an outgoing personality, Nelson had a glorious singing voice.

Thus the days (and the lab) were filled with song. Impromptu songs with a Calypso beat to accompany the shaking of the sieves. Irish airs or college fight songs during the preparation of various salt solutions. Arias from Handel's Messiah when the DEAE cellulose was being washed ("regenerated") between experiments. It was such a great time that the temptation is to describe every step—and every small triumph—blow-by-blow. Suffice it to say that DEAE cellulose was finally prepared successfully, the columns filled and packed evenly, and the flow rates were satisfactory. After a few fits and starts, it was possible to repeat some of the chromatographic experiments of Sober and Peterson and to reproduce their results.

Furthermore, as Sober and Peterson had reported new and improved salt solutions, these were incorporated into our program. When they invented an apparatus for automatically varying the composition of the salt solution being pumped onto the column, thereby permitting subtle separations of very similar proteins, we had the NIH instrument shop make one for our lab (below). And, along with this, we continued to upgrade our equipment and to become more sophisticated about handling—and analyzing—the proteins that we did separate.

Nevertheless, insofar as the Coagulation Section was concerned, Finlayson was still the outlier. Dave had initiated a program to purify prothrombin from human blood plasma, and Sandy joined him in this endeavor. The importance of prothrombin in blood clotting had been recognized for some 55 years, but there was considerable controversy about the purity of the "prothrombin" being studied in various laboratories. Clearly, Dave and Sandy were in the mainstream of blood coagulation.

Finlayson, meanwhile, at the suggestion of Dick Suchinsky, had undertaken the chromatography of albumin. Albumin made from bovine blood plasma, albumin made from human blood plasma, albumin that had been heated in the presence of "good" stabilizers, albumin that had been heated in the presence of questionable stabilizers, albumin that had been heated in the absence of stabilizers, albumin that had never been heated. All these, and several other variations on the theme (as Sandy, who was a truly virtuoso violinist, might have said), were fair game for Finlayson's columns.

Moreover, John had taught himself how to separate proteins of human blood plasma by the methods used by commercial manufacturers of therapeutic plasma products. These methods that had been carefully worked out during World War II by Edwin Cohn and his group at Harvard University, involved stepwise precipitation of the proteins, or groups of proteins, at low temperature. (The overall process is called "protein fractionation" by those who practice it.) John had carried them out in what Suchinsky called "our spacious laboratory out in the hall."

Eventually, JT Tripp decided that maybe Finlayson's chromatography was good for something after all. At the same time, he seemed to be terrified that John might leave in a year or so, and the Laboratory of Blood and Blood Products (read "J. T. Tripp") would have nothing to show for his efforts. When these two thought paths intersected in Tripp's mind, he called John into his office and encouraged him to undertake a "bread and butter" research project. All the projects offered seemed to have something to do with albumin. John therefore selected one that Dr. Tripp had initiated to evaluate albumin analogous to that which was being stored in the Department of Defense or the Civil Defense Stockpile. (Recall that this was the time of the Space Race, the Cold War, etc., etc. Thus, the thinking went, there would surely be a nuclear holocaust, attended by the need for huge volumes of resuscitation fluids.)

So, John delved deeper into the chromatography of albumin. What did this have to do with blood coagulation? Little or nothing. However, as the words chiseled in stone over the entrance to the National Archives predict: "What is past is prologue." Explanation of how chromatography of albumin (which Dave insisted, almost daily, was a "dead" protein) was prologue to anything will require not only a bit more time and space, but also the introduction of new characters in this human drama. The first two are, in order of appearance onstage, Mitsuo Yokoyama and Mike Mosesson himself. But each deserves his own act (or, at least, his own scene).

Part 2

Mitsuo Yokoyama To the Rescue

"Kuudjuu?" Mitsuo used the term so frequently that, at first, we thought it was a Japanese word. Eventually, it dawned on us that he was simply asking, "Could you?" Each person in the entirety of the Laboratory of Blood and Blood Products eventually became the recipient of that question. Often repeatedly. Yes, Mitsuo Yokoyama had come into our lives. To say that he was a unique personality would be the understatement of the century. Mitsuo was unique by any criterion one could muster—Eastern or Western, scientific or otherwise. He seemed to embody the deferential Asian diplomat, the slapstick comedian, and everything in between.

Tripp had met Mitsuo in Japan, shortly after World War II. Mitsuo was working with a U. S. Army medical unit. He was a medical doctor, and his specialty was blood grouping and typing. Tripp had invited him to America and now, years later, he had arrived on our doorstep.

For all his idiosyncrasies, Mitsuo was a prodigious worker. And he was certainly not shy. He seemed to know, or at least to have corresponded with, everyone in the blood typing field. As far as our little laboratory group was concerned, he was a phenomenon. Not only was he appropriately exotic, he was over 30! (None of us, except Tripp, was yet out of our 20's.)

"Kuudjuu?" This time he was addressing the question to Dick and John. It was the beginning of the question, "Kuudjuu make me some gamma globulin?" Inasmuch as the Japanese language does not distinguish between the "l" and the "r" sound, the entire sentence was a little problematic for Mitsuo, but we understood at once. Gamma globulin was the term that was used at that time to designate the class of blood plasma proteins that includes antibodies. "Of course," said Dick, always happy to volunteer John's services. "How would you like us to make it?" "What ways are there?" replied Mitsuo, whose grasp of biochemistry, to say the least, lagged far behind his knowledge of blood group serology. "Well, we can make it by salt precipitation, by Cohn fractionation, and probably by DEAE cellulose chromatography."

Mitsuo opted for the last of these, for reasons known only to him. Perhaps it sounded modern and cutting-edge (which, indeed, it was). Or perhaps he was simply intrigued because pronouncing it presented even more of a challenge than "gamma globulin." In any event, John began to outline the experimental approach. He would obtain blood serum from various donors (including many of us in the lab), prepare it for chromatography, use his experience to date for separating the various proteins on the column, and use test tubes to collect the protein-containing salt solutions that emerged.

"I'll measure the protein content of each tube," John explained, "and I'll give you the tubes that contain most of the gamma globulin. There will probably be five, six, or seven tubes for each donor." "How many tubes are there altogether?" Mitsuo asked. "You mean for the entire chromatographic experiment on each donor's serum? About 165." "OK," Mitsuo persisted, completely undaunted, "I test all."

Well, so he did, eventually. First, however, John unintentionally created a major diversion by asking what he thought was a simple, obvious question. "You realize," he said, "that the salt concentration and the acidity of the solutions are continuously changing throughout the experiment. What effect does this have on the reaction between the blood group antibodies and the red blood cells?" "I don't know." "Well, who does?" "I don't think anyone knows." John was incredulous. "How can that be? It seems like the first thing you would study when you are working out a test method!" "Maybe we ask Joel." And so we must now migrate down the hall and meet Joel Solomon, who was in neither the Coagulation Section nor the Blood Derivatives Section. If memory serves, he was in the Diagnostic Reagents Section, which was responsible for controlling the quality of all the blood grouping and typing reagents sold in America.

Joel had two master's degrees, one in Parasitology and one in Blood Banking, but he had not yet received a Ph.D. That was to come later, as were many other adventures during his service in the regulation of blood products. At the moment however, the most impressive thing about Joel stemmed from his room. Three walls of his office/lab were covered with shelves, literally from floor to ceiling. Every inch of these shelves was filled with those gray, cardboard boxes that used to hold medium-sized magazines, papers, etc. In scientific settings, they served to hold reprints of scientific articles. Such was the case in Joel's room. Every one of those boxes was stuffed full of reprints about one or another aspect of blood grouping, blood typing, and/or blood banking. Seemingly, Joel could tell you at least the summary of every article therein.

Surely, then, this was the man to answer John's simple question. Probably Mitsuo and John awaited the answer with bated breath, inasmuch as that was the going cliché at the time. "I don't know," Joel said slowly, taking a book off his desk, "I think Boyd has a sentence or two about it in his textbook of immunology." Joel's recollection, as usual, was correct. The concept was addressed in a rather vaguely worded sentence or two. Needless to say, John was not satisfied. This could not possibly be the extent of the world's knowledge about this mini-subject! And so, for the next three days, John was holed up in the NIH Library, combing every possible source of information. Eventually, he had to admit that Mitsuo and Joel were right. There was vanishingly little information in the scientific literature. In fact, the most useful paper that even mentioned the topic had been published in 1910 by Karl Landsteiner, the discoverer of blood groups. In German no less. Since then, apparently, the whole matter of whether (or how) salt concentration and acidity influenced the action of blood group antibodies had seldom appeared on anyone's radar screen.

There was only one thing to do. John and Mitsuo were going to have to investigate this area themselves. Only then could they be confident that the results obtained by testing all the tubes from the chromatographic experiments would be reliable. And so, an entirely new set of experiments was designed, executed, and written up for publication. Once again, there were so many twists and turns before the final version of the paper emerged that there is great temptation to describe every bend in the road. Suffice it to say, however, that most of the salts studied had similar effects on the reaction between red blood cells and their corresponding antibodies. Moreover, the reaction was relatively tolerant to changes in salt concentration and acidity. The "translation," then, was that the original study could proceed as planned. There was, though, an interesting historical wrinkle.

Mitsuo was approached by one of his many acquaintances, Dr. Tibor ("Tibi") Greenwalt. Greenwalt, who was already a grand old man of Blood Banking, albeit he lived and worked for nearly another half century. (*Among his accomplishments Tibi organized and became the first President of what is now The BloodCenter of Wisconsin. In the setting of The BloodCenter he intersected years later with Mike Mosesson after he had moved to Milwaukee.*) Tibi was planning a new scientific journal. It was to be the official journal of the American Association of Blood Banks and Greenwalt would be the first editor-in-chief. The journal would be called "Transfusion."

To assure that this new addition to the scientific literature did not die in infancy, Tibi was soliciting manuscripts, preferably enough to fill a year's worth of issues. The timing was perfect, so Mitsuo and John published in Volume 1 of Transfusion. Evidently, the fundamental questions addressed in the paper were not viewed as particularly fundamental—or even particularly interesting—by the scientific world because neither of the authors ever received any comments or inquiries about it. Nor, as far as they knew, was it ever cited by any other scientists.

So what came out of the original study, in which John was going to chromatograph sera from various donors and Mitsuo was going to test all the tubes containing effluent to see whether blood group antibodies were present? Each performed his tasks as planned, only more so. Mitsuo not only tested all 165 tubes per donor, he tested the contents of each tube against a whole series of different red blood cells. As Joel said at a meeting, "Every time one saw Yokoyama, he was standing behind rows and rows of tiny test tubes, so it's pretty certain that no one is going to repeat this work." Meanwhile, John was performing physical and chemical tests on the proteins that came off the column, and he enlisted Dick Suchinsky and Nelson Roberts in the endeavor. By virtue of Mitsuo's heroic testing, it became clear that the column could separate two classes of antibodies. This finding agreed with those made by a few other scientists.

The antibodies that emerged from the column first were very pure, so John and Dave Aronson used one of the new instruments—"toys" as they called them—purchased by JT Tripp to determine their molecular weight. (Again, for the benefit of the chemically challenged, we can say simply that molecular weight is a number indicating the relative size of a molecule. If a carbon atom "weighs" 12, a water molecule "weighs" 18 and an albumin molecule "weighs" about 66,500.) Their results agreed with those reported in many scientific papers—an outcome that was comforting but not very exciting.

On the other hand, the other antibodies—those that emerged much later in the chromatographic experiments—were mixed with many other serum proteins. It was clear from the analyses performed by Dick and John that they were "macroglobulins," but a precise molecular weight was not known. Most workers in the field just said that macroglobulins had a molecular weight of "about a million" and let it go at that. In view of the fact that our macroglobulin antibodies were decidedly impure and might never be purified by the methods then available, a more definitive molecular weight seemed out of the question. Then Dave rode to the rescue. The "MD" after his name notwithstanding, Dave was a physicist at heart. In fact, he had received the first bachelor's degree in biophysics that Yale University had ever conferred. And he had many colleagues in the world of physics.

One of these colleagues was Dr. John ("Buster") Preiss, a "real" physicist (no "bio") who was ensconced in an NIH building that was literally only a few steps away. Real or not, Buster knew where the action was. He often said, "Biochemists are the luckiest people in the world because they get to work on globular proteins." ("Globular" just means twisted and/or folded up in a glob, as opposed to being stretched out in a fiber.) The other John (Finlayson) enthusiastically agreed with him.

Buster, in addition to being a first-rate physicist, was a superb mechanician. In the basement of his uncle, who lived in the Washington, DC area, he had built an apparatus for target-volume irradiation, a technique that most scientists had never heard of—let alone used. In brief, the idea of this method is that if you prepare a series of identical samples of your dried, biologically-active protein, irradiate each sample with a different (and progressively increasing) dose of precisely known energy, then re-dissolve the samples and analyze them to see how much of the biological activity of each has been "killed," you can calculate back to determine the size of the molecule that has that activity. Inasmuch as a big molecular "target" (hence the name of the method) is easier to hit with radiation than a small one, the biological activity of a big molecule will be killed off with lower doses than will that of a small molecule.

The beauty of the technique is twofold. First, one obtains the molecular weight of the actual biologically-active entity, not some aggregated form of it. Second, it doesn't have to be pure. In addition to a well-calibrated "flux" of radiation, all one needs is a specific assay for the biological activity. Buster had the radiation. He had chosen low-energy electrons, which seemed ideal for irradiating macromolecules. Mitsuo had the biological assay. All that was needed to make it specific was to use the right red blood cells—group A cells to measure the amount of anti-A antibodies, group B cells to measure the anti-B.

The experiments were done, Dave pitched in to take the lead in doing the calculations, and voila! The molecular weight came out between 700 000 and 750 000. Because it implied less precision, the former value was published, along with a plethora of other data about blood group antibodies. In retrospect, this entire activity was laced with irony. The report of the molecular weight elicited no interest whatsoever. Mitsuo, who probably couldn't spell "target-volume irradiation," was the lead author on what must have been the only publication in history to report the molecular weight of blood group antibodies determined by this method.

Nevertheless, what was past was indeed prologue. What John had learned (often the hard way) about protein chromatography, including that of albumin, and about Cohn fractionation of plasma proved to be of genuine value in the study of antibodies. A technique that Dave had learned at Yale was clearly applicable to a wide range of proteins. And, at the risk of sounding unpardonably redundant, we can now say that this prologue was just the beginning.

Part 3

Changing of the Guard

As Sandy Shapiro said, the medical world, especially the academic medical world, moves on July 1. That meant that June 30, 1960 would be the last day for Sandy and for Dick Suchinsky as commissioned officers in the U. S. Public Health Service. Sandy, after two years at NIH, would head for Cambridge (Massachusetts) to begin a post-doctoral fellowship at MIT. Dick, pulling up stakes after four years in Bethesda, would begin a residency in psychiatry. His new home would be Cornell Medical School in New York City.

Two of our other PHS officers were not moving anywhere. John (always the outlier) was not bound by the annual rhythms of the medical world. Besides, he had come in October, so he had not yet completed his two years of obligatory service time. Dave, on the other hand, was passing the three-year mark; he was planning to make a career in the PHS. His first year had been spent in the tuberculosis epidemiology branch in Washington, DC. As testimony to his versatility, he served as the statistician for the group.

That June 30th, however, was an historic date for still another reason. When the Division of Biologics Standards was created in 1955, it had no building to call its own. Its members continued to labor in the same NIH buildings (of which there were at least three) they had occupied before the creation. Nonetheless, plans were afoot to bring them all together under one roof. A location had been surveyed, ground had been broken, and construction had begun. The building was not yet completed, but it was far enough along that a dedication ceremony could take place. And this was the day!

An appropriate reviewing stand had been set up in front of the building. August personages from Congress had been invited. After some behind-the-scenes scuffling between Dr. Roderick Murray, the director of DBS (who was said to be very anti-cleric), and Dr. James Shannon, the Director of NIH (who was reportably a devout Catholic), a clergyman had been invited to offer the invocation. But who would be the primary dedicator?

The answer was Prince Bhumibol of Thailand. If, upon reading this, you wonder what the good prince had to do with biological standards or the regulation of biological products, or the research underlying any of these, be assured that these thoughts were universal. The incisive minds in the Coagulation Section decided that he was selected because (1) he was available, (2) he was non-controversial, and (3) being a Harvard graduate, albeit in musicology, he spoke excellent English.

Now, of course, the prince and the other worthies who would sit on the reviewing stand would have to be given a tour of the building—or at least the ground floor of the building. Moreover, this tour would have to impress them not only with the architectural magnificence of the structure but also with the earth-shattering importance of the work that would be conducted therein. Accordingly, there had to be exhibits.

Therefore, early in the morning of the great day, John and Nelson arrived in their usual laboratory, prepared a column of DEAE cellulose, let a sample of human blood serum flow into the top of the column, and followed that with a suitable salt solution. After the serum proteins had progressed some distance down the column, they stopped the flow, placed the entire setup on a cart, and began the quarter-mile journey from the old building to the new.

The irony was not lost on Dave Aronson. For over a year, we had observed that whenever we asked Dr. Tripp if a particular piece of equipment could be discarded or sent to surplus, he would equivocate by saying, "Put it on a cart." As John and Nelson were gingerly rolling the cart into the elevator, Dave was chanting, "Put it on a cart." (*see photo below*). The quivering of that ancient elevator notwithstanding, the descent was relatively benign. Exiting the building was a little more challenging, crossing the roadway was even more so, and pushing the cart uphill got to be a bit arduous. The two lab denizens were discovering that the sidewalks at NIH were somewhat less smooth than they appeared at first glance.

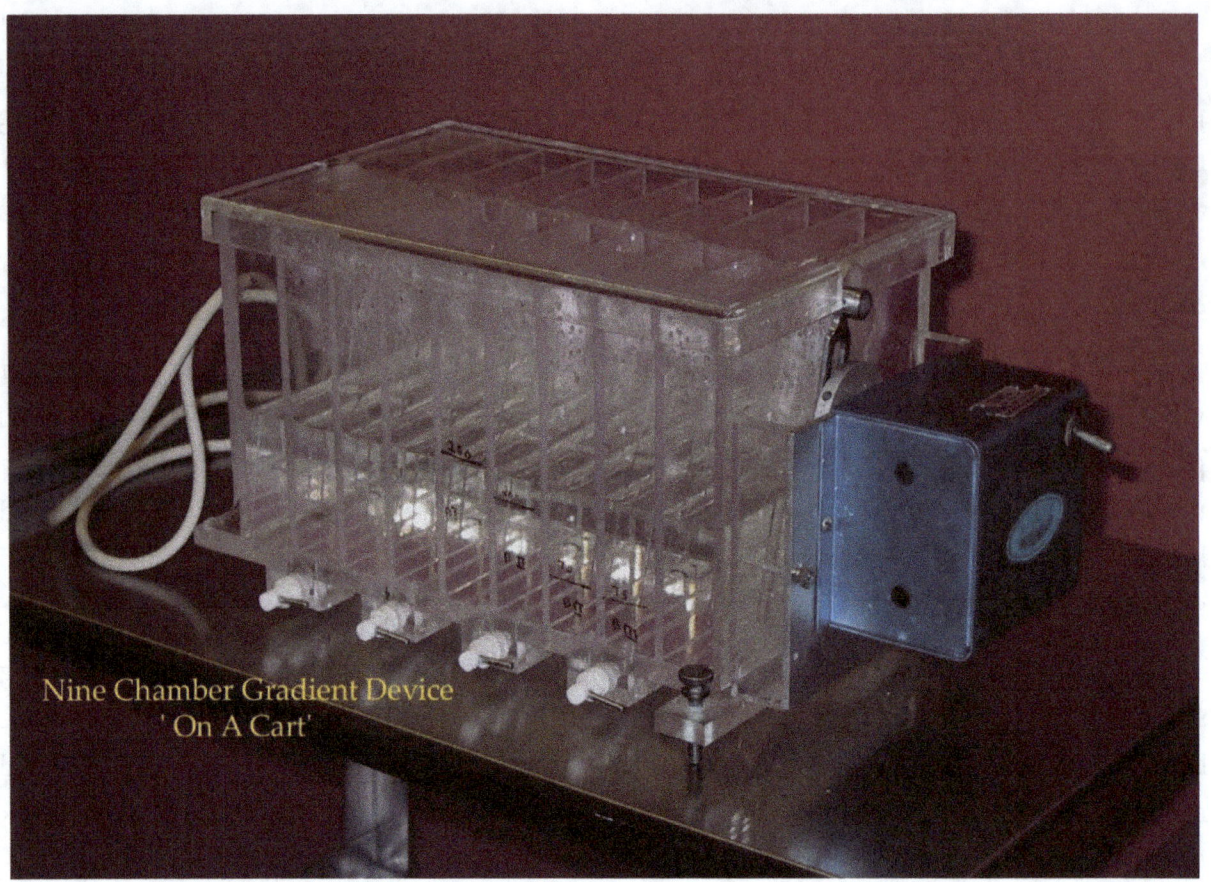

A nine-chamber device for imposing a salt-buffer gradient on an ion exchange column packed with a resin like DEAE-cellulose.

Just as great concern seemed to be transitioning into borderline anxiety, a Volkswagen, packed to the gills, hove into view. As it came nearer, John and Nelson could see that the driver was waving in salutation. It was Dick Suchinsky, taking his final voyage through NIH! Their spirits somehow renewed, the two carters pushed on and reached their destination with the column, the reservoir of salt solution, and the other equipment (all of which, did we mention, was made of glass) intact.

The setup was quickly transferred to a lab bench in the first room encountered, the flow was re-started, and soon it was dripping away, looking for all the world like a *bona fide* chromatographic experiment. In fact, the colorful proteins in the serum (most proteins in solution are colorless) were separating and showing up nicely against the white DEAE cellulose.

Emboldened by this transfer, John and Nelson returned to the old building and decided to set up another exhibit. For this, they would have to make the journey with the freeze-drying apparatus. There was no need to "put it on a cart" inasmuch as the apparatus had been fabricated that way, so as to facilitate moving it from one lab to another. The inventors, however, had probably not envisioned that those labs would be a quarter mile of uneven sidewalk apart.

Because the essence of freeze drying is the removal of water under a near-total vacuum, an essential part of the apparatus was a vacuum gauge. The type built into our freeze dryer was a McLeod gauge. One need not know the admittedly ingenious principle of its operation—only that it is made of glass and filled with mercury. Have you ever tried to tell mercury to hold still while its container is being jostled about? But this, too, would pass. The freeze dryer survived the journey, and the electrical outlets in the new building were operational. Thus the dripping of the chromatographic exhibit would be accompanied by the chugging of the vacuum pump on the freeze dryer.

There was never any mention of whether the distinguished visitors enjoyed, or even saw, the exhibits. No matter. John and Nelson took pride in the fact that they had performed the first chromatographic separation ever carried out in Building 29, even if it all happened some two months before we moved into the new quarters.

The dedication ceremony went off without the proverbial hitch. It was a pleasant day, the weather was good, and the speeches were long. The prince looked elegant in a sharkskin suit. The princess was absolutely stunning. Senator Lister Hill (after whom an NIH building would later be named) even managed to find a medical link, though admittedly a tenuous one, with the prince. "Mah fah-thah," he intoned, speaking to the prince in his marvelous southern accent, "lahk yoah fah-thah, was a fuh-sician!"

Otherwise, most of the speeches were of little note. It was interesting that, as we listened to them, we were looking at the speakers and, in the background, the building that we had obviously gathered to dedicate. Yet, with one exception, none of them called it a building. It was always "this magnificent facility." The one exception was the taciturn Dr. Murray. He said, simply, "We thank you for the building." He then went on to make a point that has often been overlooked in the years of its occupancy. He noted that it is not only the cutting-edge research in biology, but also the less glitzy investigation of previously-plowed ground (often the re-investigation of well-known biological products from a new point of view) that is both necessary and important.

Significant as they were, the new building and our new labs within it were not the only developments in the Laboratory of Blood and Blood Products. Personnel changes were underway. In keeping with the new month on the medical calendar, Sandy's replacement arrived in the person of a newly-commissioned PHS officer. This was Michael W. Mosesson, M.D., fresh from an internship in Boston. To say that Mike had little research experience would be a vast understatement, but whatever was lacking he more than made up for in enthusiasm.

In this connection, another prevalent cliché of that era was, "He rolled up his sleeves and got right to work." To apply this to Mike, one would have to say that he rolled up his sleeves past the shoulder blades. He quickly envisioned an important (and challenging) research project and then launched into it. In principle, it was very simple: allow pure plasmin to react with pure fibrinogen and analyze the resulting products. Of course, in principle, the project, "Climb Mount Everest," is also very simple. The complexity lies in the transition from principle to performance.

For one thing, neither pure plasmin nor pure fibrinogen existed at that time. In time, Mike was to learn—as were we all—that purity is an elusive, and sometimes relative, concept. (When asked about the purity of a particular reagent, Dick Suchinsky used to smile and say, "Pure as American womanhood.") Among the problems was that all preparations of human fibrinogen, regardless of the number of purification steps they had undergone, were contaminated with plasminogen, the precursor of plasmin. Furthermore, because of the similarity of plasmin to the pancreatic enzyme, trypsin, it was believed that plasmin could act on plasminogen to convert the latter to more of the active enzyme, plasmin. Clearly, this would complicate the interpretation of any results obtained from experiments with plasminogen-contaminated fibrinogen.

We learned later (much later) that plasmin does indeed act on plasminogen, but not in such a way as to produce additional active plasmin. That information, however, became apparent too late to help Mike. Nevertheless, getting rid of the plasminogen that contaminated fibrinogen preparations was challenge enough. And when that challenge was met another, even greater one, rose up in its place. But that story will have to wait a bit. For the moment, Mike was eagerly learning, and adapting, technique after technique. Moreover, his learning was not limited to the lab. He began studying all sorts of subjects so as to build up an infrastructure supporting his research. In fact, that fall he and John enrolled in a year-long class of differential equations.

Meanwhile, there was much activity in the Coagulation Section. John pointed out that we were probably the only NIH section with doctorate personnel whose names all rhymed (Aronson, Finlayson, Mosesson). Elaborating on this fact, Mike suggested that we should call ourselves "The Three Sons," a takeoff on the name of "The Three Suns," a popular musical group of the day. Soon we moved into our new building. Actually, we moved ourselves, despite the hindrance by the transportation personnel and the security staff. Dave and Mike occupied one room, and John was just across the hall. Then, in

October, John got a roommate. This was Bud (Edward H.) Mealey. In fact, John and Bud not only shared a room, they shared a single desk.

Bud had a fascinating history. He had grown up in a blue-collar family in Boston and never expected to attend college. After high school, however, he had gone to work in Edwin Cohn's group and thus became familiar with protein fractionation, literally from the ground up. As World War II progressed, he entered the Navy and was sent to college (Tufts) under the V-12 program, a concentrated educational approach to producing naval officers. After receipt of his bachelor's degree, he was commissioned and placed in command of a ship—one of the so-called Landing Ships that were widely used in invasions.

After the war, he entered graduate school at the University of Kansas and completed both an M.S. and a Ph.D. under the direction of Professor Dwight Mulford, one of Professor Cohn's former colleagues. In the course of his research for the latter degree, Bud had explored more variations of plasma protein fractionation than those of us in the Coagulation Section would encounter in a lifetime.

In contrast to the sometimes frenetic activity of the rest of us, Bud's research was characterized by its utter tranquility. He never seemed to be hurrying. Yes, he would be adding a reagent here, stirring a solution there, filtering and/or centrifuging something, but he would still have time for an occasional puff on a cigar. (Laboratories were indeed different in those days.) Nonetheless, at the end of the day, a remarkable array of precipitates (fractions, or "pastes," as they are called in the industry) would appear.

Bud was a wonderful addition to the lab. He was an endless font of information, a stabilizing influence, and a continuing source of wise counsel. Unfortunately for us, his many talents were soon identified by Tripp, with the result that Bud's research activities became progressively diluted by other duties. This, in turn, resulted in a meteoric rise in his position. By the time he left Bethesda, seven years after his arrival, he had become Acting Chief of the Laboratory of Blood and Blood Products.

In retrospect, he was one of the best leaders of Blood and Blood Products in its 35-year history. That same tranquil, unhurried approach, combined with a firm dedication to factual information, seemed to inspire confidence and cooperation among all his coworkers.

Part 4

Transition from Science and Biologics Regulation to Biologics Regulation and Science-Migration to the G59FDA

What follows will cover events that are undoubtedly described elsewhere, probably in much greater detail. It is tempting to say that this will be only the mortar that goes between the building blocks of these memoirs. In fact, it is a good deal less. If we pursue the analogy, it is more like the grout between tiles or paving-stones, simply providing background that may smooth the path.

As we saw in the previous part, Mike arrived and began to work with full vigor. He and Dave occupied a single lab in our new building, and their combined endeavors made that lab a virtual beehive of activity. Meanwhile, John and Bud continued just across the hall. It is fair to say that we were aware of, and reasonably well informed about, each other's work. However, except for the target volume irradiation experiments described previously, most of our work was not collaborative. We each, to use an expression that did not come into common usage for another decade, "did our own thing."

Mike, in particular, pursued the goal of preparing plasminogen-free human fibrinogen. And, remarkably, he succeeded. With an eye to publishing a paper describing this work, he began to explore ways to determine whether the fibrinogen had been altered by the steps he used to remove the contaminating plasminogen. Each potential approach that Dave or John suggested, Mike dutifully followed, and each yielded the same result: the removal process had introduced no detectable change in the protein.

Realizing that such a conclusion would be more readily accepted if the methods for detecting change were more powerful, Mike asked John if there were a method that could detect truly subtle changes in proteins. John, as noted previously, had performed numerous chromatographic experiments on DEAE cellulose and had found that the effects of heating albumin could be readily observed. Moreover, he found that changes in albumin occurring as a result of something as benign as storing the protein could be detected and, to some extent, quantified by means of chromatography.

John therefore suggested this approach and offered to carry out some chromatographic experiments on Mike's plasminogen-free fibrinogen. Thus began a collaboration that spread over the better part of two decades. Before considering these experiments, however, we should fast-forward about four years to include a vignette that is too delicious to ignore. It seems that John's work on the chromatography of albumin had attracted a bit of attention at NIH, as a result of which Drs. Peterson and Sober had invited him to give a seminar for their research group. This honor afforded John the opportunity to meet with the respected doctors and to have some individual discussions with their postdoctoral fellows. One of these fellows had recently published a paper about the chromatography of bovine albumin, but he had previously worked on fibrinogen. After noting the similarities of their findings on bovine and human albumins, John suggested that this fellow's earlier studies on fibrinogen might be expanded by using chromatography. "Oh," responded the fellow emphatically, "you can't chromatograph fibrinogen; it's too big and too insoluble!"

Obviously, four years previously, Mike and John did not have the benefit of this wisdom, so they went ahead and chromatographed fibrinogen. Evidently the fibrinogen was also unaware of this insurmountable obstacle because, during chromatography, it behaved just as well as the albumin. In this case it was John's turn to pontificate, with equally erroneous results. "You see," John told Mike, "if you haven't changed the fibrinogen during the process of removing plasminogen, the elution pattern should show one more-or-less symmetrical peak. If more than one peak appears, that means you've changed something."

Well, soon the first experiment was completed. The elution pattern consisted of a nice, large, generally symmetrical peak (representing about three-fourths of the protein that emerged from the column), followed by another peak, followed by a tiny "bumple," to use Mike's newly-invented terminology. "There," John said, "is the result. Clearly, about a fourth of the fibrinogen has been changed. When you test the chromatographic fractions for clottability, you will find that the first peak is the clottable protein and the second peak is non-clottable."

In view of the fact that the major biological role of fibrinogen is to form clots, this sounded like a rather dire indictment of Mike's purification process. To make matters more complicated, the nature of the salt solutions used to elute the protein from the column appeared to require some manipulation of the fractions before clottability measurements could be made. This led to a series of interesting, albeit not terribly productive, experiments. Nonetheless, ultimately some relatively simple, relatively straightforward methods were worked out, and Mike was able to obtain clottability results for every fraction that contained any detectable protein. (Does this sound like a re-run of Mitsuo and the blood group antibodies in chromatographic fractions of human serum? It should because the experimental design was virtually the same.)

Once again, fibrinogen demonstrated its ability to withstand dire predictions. Virtually all of the protein in the first two peaks of the elution pattern was clottable. That meant that it was indeed fibrinogen and, furthermore, its biochemical structure was so little changed (possibly not changed at all) that its functional activity remained intact. Even the tiny third "bumple" contained clottable protein.

After some serious head scratching and the passage of time, Mike and John actually ran the control experiment—that is, chromatographing the same quantity of fibrinogen that had undergone all of the purification procedures *except* those that were used to remove plasminogen. The result? The elution patterns—total protein, clottable protein, everything—were identical.

At about this time, Mike's success in preparing plasminogen-free fibrinogen had attracted sufficient attention that he had been invited to present it at the meeting of the Protein Foundation in Boston. (Actually, at that time, the meetings took place in Cambridge, just off Harvard Square.) Of course he accepted; this was a small but very prestigious meeting in the world of blood proteins. Mike and John began to wonder, however, if this latest chromatographic result should be included. It wasn't really directed toward fibrinogen's plasminogen-freeness, but it was interesting. So, they decided to let an older, presumably wiser head make the call. They asked Newt Ashworth. "Definitely include it," Newt said, "it'll be a bombshell!" Actually, it turned out to be more like a bomb—as in "the play bombed in Bridgeport." People were greatly excited by the prospect of having plasminogen-free fibrinogen available as a reagent, but the chromatographic heterogeneity barely raised a whisper.

Back at NIH after the meeting, John was undaunted and sought the advice of another older (and definitely wiser) head, namely, that of Dr. William Carroll. Years previously, Dr. Tripp had noted that when other NIH scientists found the work of the Division of Biologics Standards too practical (read "prosaic") for their tastes, Bill had always provided helpful advice and assistance. This occasion was no exception. After patiently listening to John's saga, he concluded that all the results were legitimate, but he suggested that re-chromatographing the individual peaks would be a good idea. It was a case of "no sooner said than done." Re-chromatography of the first peak (in the same chromatographic system) produced a single symmetrical peak. Re-chromatography of the second peak yielded two peaks. One was eluted at the same position as the former, and the second (almost exactly twice as large), at the position of the original second peak. This set of results allowed Mike and John to speak of "peak 1 fibrinogen" and "peak 2 fibrinogen" and to calculate that the latter amounted to about 15% of the total fibrinogen in Mike's preparations.

As is the usual case in science, however, these findings also raised additional questions. One was the obvious matter of what the chemical difference between these two types of fibrinogen might be. The other was even more worrisome. Clearly, this heterogeneity—this peak 1-ness and peak 2-ness—was not due to Mike's plasminogen-removal process or to John's chromatographic procedure. But could it be due to some kind of processing that the protein underwent before it was ever subjected to either of these steps? Thus began a series of experiments that today would probably be described as "retro." That is, instead of striving for more and more purification, Mike began to make (and, of course, John continued to chromatograph) progressively cruder fibrinogen preparations.

In each case, the distribution of *clottable* protein remained the same, leading to the inevitable conclusion that this retro pathway would have to embrace its ultimate beginning, namely, whole blood plasma that had undergone no purification whatsoever. The trick here was not in the chromatography but rather in the measurement of clottable protein. (Fibrinogen amounts to less than 5% of the total protein of plasma.) Fortunately, the way to accomplish this had already been worked out. Even though the elution pattern of plasma looked very much like that of serum (which John had chromatographed dozens of times during his collaboration with Mitsuo), with many peaks and valleys, the distribution of clottable protein was the same as in all the purified preparations. This finding provided enormous comfort. The heterogeneity was not a product of any purification procedure. It was real. Plasma that circulated in human beings really did contain these two—or maybe three, if you counted the "bumple"—kinds of fibrinogen. (A few years later, Mike worked out a method for chromatographing the plasma of individual blood donors; everyone tested had the same two kinds of fibrinogen and had them in about the same proportions.)

Now "all" we had to do was to find out the chemical basis for the difference. And so another trek began. Every analysis that John or Mike (or both) could think of was performed. And almost everyone yielded the same result: no detectable difference. The only positive findings were that (1) peak 1 always emerged before peak 2 during chromatography and (2) the two kinds of fibrinogen migrated at different rates in an electrical field. This was strong evidence of a difference in electrical charge. It explained some of the results that other workers had reported previously, but it defied all efforts to explain the reason for the charge difference itself.

Not necessarily in desperation, but certainly lacking any better approach, Mike and John began to consider the possibility that the two fibrinogens might show different biological behavior. They were always on the lookout for clues—or approaches that might reveal clues—to functional differences between the two fibrinogens. One evening, while prowling in the NIH library, John came across a series of just-published articles by Ariel Loewy. They dealt with a plasma protein that, like many proteins of the blood clotting system, had many names. To these, Loewy had added yet another: 'Fibrinase.' Whatever its name, this protein seemed to act *after* clotting had occurred and somehow made the clot more stable. Thinking that this might be the long-awaited clue, John flipped through these articles. Essentially, he concluded that (1) these articles were very long and somewhat complex, (2) Loewy was convinced that this protein acted as a catalyst, as opposed to a building-block, and (3) John's own reading time was limited, so he had better move on to other articles. Nonetheless, the next morning he mentioned these papers to Mike, fully expecting Mike to have the same reaction.

Mike, however, was full of surprises. He soon read all the papers in Loewy's series and concluded, "We can set up his assay." As usual, the "we" turned out to be Mike; John simply continued to provide chromatographic fractions. Whatever the division of labor, the results were truly remarkable. Having, as promised, set up the assay, Mike found that Fibrinase (soon to become known to blood clotters as Factor XIII of the blood coagulation system) was concentrated in peak 2. Moreover, much of peak 1 was free of this factor, making it an ideal substrate for assaying the clot-stabilizing activity of Factor XIII.

Poor Ariel Loewy had labored intensely to prepare "Fibrinase-free" fibrinogen and had obtained it with approximately a 2% yield. In a single chromatographic step, we had achieved the same thing, with a yield that was 20 or 30 times higher. These findings continued to be important long after Mike had left NIH. Some five years later, factor-free fibrinogen was used by John and his NIH colleague, John Pisano (as well as independently, and essentially simultaneously, by Loewy), to demonstrate exactly what the biochemical action of Factor XIII really is. Much later, Kevin Siebenlist and Mike showed that peak 2 fibrinogen binds tightly to Factor XIII, whereas peak 1 fibrinogen and Factor XIII hardly bind to each other at all.

Emboldened by this discovery, Mike and John (well, mostly Mike) began to look for other biologically active proteins that might ride along with fibrinogen during chromatography. They found that if plasminogen had not been removed from the fibrinogen preparation before the latter was chromatographed, the plasminogen emerged from the column at the same time as peak 2.

Remember, now, that Mike's original idea was to study the action of plasmin (the active form of plasminogen) on fibrinogen. This meshed nicely with the search for different biological behaviors of different fibrinogens. Therefore, Mike began to study the rate at which various chromatographic fractions of fibrinogen underwent hydrolysis (digestion) when treated with plasmin. Of course, Mike didn't do things by halves. He made these measurements not only on the fibrinogen itself, but also on the fibrin made by clotting the chromatographic fractions. Furthermore, he didn't limit the study to plasmin treatment. He carried out the same kinds of experiments with trypsin, a well-known enzyme that is secreted by the pancreas and has many characteristics in common with plasmin.

The results of this work were striking. Fibrinogen that came off the column early was hydrolyzed relatively rapidly; so was that which came off late. However, the fibrinogen that appeared in the mid-part of the chromatographic pattern was digested much more slowly. This was true regardless of which enzyme was used and whether fibrinogen or fibrin was studied. Thus, an inhibitor of plasmin and trypsin was present even in highly purified preparations of fibrinogen, and it emerged from DEAE cellulose columns on the descending side of peak 1. ("Ascending peak 1," as it came to be known, was inhibitor-free, and was a convenient substrate for investigating this heretofore unknown inhibitor.)

Needless to say (which people always say before going ahead and saying it anyway), all this activity had generated an enormous amount of data, so some of the next important steps were involved with reporting it to the scientific community. One of these was the presentation of papers at a congress of the International Society of Hematology in Mexico City. Mike, John, and Dave each presented a paper. It was the first international meeting for Mike and John. Mike presented the work dealing with the various biological activities and their distribution during chromatography. John reported the details of the chromatographic separation and the heterogeneity.

For John, it was almost instant replay. The session in which he spoke was chaired by Dr. Benjamin Alexander. He was famous in the blood clotting world for having discovered coagulation Factor VII. Moreover, he was the scientific advisor for the Coagulation Section (albeit he usually obtained more advice—and free samples of purified proteins—than he gave). Hoping to keep the meeting on schedule, he announced that there would be no discussion or question-and-answer exchange after each individual paper. All the discussion would take place at the end of the session.

John, as he had been taught in graduate school, tried to eliminate all extraneous words. Consequently, his presentation style was (as described by Barbara Alving about 15 years later) "highly distilled." As a result, he finished his ten-minute talk in eight minutes. Thus, the session was in danger of proceeding *ahead* of schedule and thus frustrating listeners who might arrive in mid-session to hear a particular paper. Ben, of course, could not say something as simple as "We have a couple of extra minutes, so we can take a few questions." Instead, he said, "Because of the unusual nature of these results, I am going to rescind my previous announcement and open this fascinating paper for discussion." ("Fascinating," along with "kinetics," was the favorite word in Ben's lexicon.) Nonetheless, his invitation, "Are there any questions?" was followed by two minutes of absolute silence. Mike and John had struck again.

Not to be discouraged, they decided to accept the invitation to describe their research at the meeting of the Protein Foundation later that year. By this time, the method for preparing plasminogen-free fibrinogen was old news. This year's paper would focus on the chromatographic behavior of fibrinogen, as well as the various biological activities found in the chromatographic fractions. Whereas the previous talk in Boston had clearly been Mike's bailiwick, this time around the issue of who was the "senior" author was less certain. What to do? The answer was what American boys always do—flip a coin. Whoever won the toss would be first author; whoever lost would present the paper. The outcome was truly fortunate. John became first author; Mike would present.

Why fortunate? The day before the meeting, John caught a terrible cold. By the time the paper came up on the program, he had full-blown laryngitis. The only unfortunate aspect was that Mike did such an excellent job with the talk that, afterward, people converged on John wanting to know the experimental details. With something between a whisper and a croak, he tried to give intelligible answers. Giving talks is good, but publishing papers establishes a permanent record of one's work. Thus, even before departing for Mexico City, the intrepid authors had to decide on an appropriate journal for reporting the heterogeneity. The American Chemical Society, of which John was a member, had just established a new journal. It was called simply "Biochemistry." Because the Society wished to proceed cautiously, it was published only bimonthly. It seemed like the right place to tell the story.

The good news was that the paper was accepted and published. The less good news was that it did not make it into Volume 1. Mike and John had missed that chance at history by 42 pages. Nevertheless, 1963 brought forth a bumper crop. Two more papers (now focusing on the biological activities) were published. And the second presentation at the Protein Foundation continued to have fallout.

Somewhere along the line Mike had "discovered" that, lodged deep in the lab refrigerator, there were some bottles of crude, commercially prepared, animal fibrinogens. Who had ordered them (or why) was unknown, but they were intriguing. Mike had put them through an additional purification step, and John had put them on his column. Most of them showed some degree of heterogeneity, albeit generally less striking than that of human fibrinogen. When the experiment with the fibrinogen of a particular species was repeated with protein freshly prepared from animal plasma, the results agreed closely with those obtained by using the cleaned-up commercial material. This provided some assurance that the findings were "real." Furthermore, it seemed that they might be of general interest, in view of the fact that many workers used bovine fibrinogen in their research.

Therefore, the chromatography of animal fibrinogens was mentioned in the Protein Foundation talk. As it turned out, Dr. Jessica Lewis (*University of Pittsburgh*) was in the audience. Lewis's interest in blood coagulation was wide-ranging. Among other things, it included comparative studies of the clotting systems of various animals—some rather exotic. She offered to send plasma from all kinds of creatures. Thus, before long, Mike and John had data about the chromatographic behavior of fibrinogen from alligators, armadillos, green sea turtles, loggerhead turtles, etc.

Mike's time in Bethesda was running short; he would be heading for St. Louis to complete his medical training at Washington University with Dr. Sol Sherry. *(Sherry along with his associates Tony Fletcher and Norma Alkjaersig were widely known experts on basic and clinical fibrinolysis at that time.)* John hurried to prepare a short manuscript on animal fibrinogens. Literally, as they were preparing to mail it to a journal, Dr. Lewis telephoned. Wouldn't we like to examine some other species? Thank you, but no thank you. But couldn't we look at just a few more kinds of fibrinogen? Unfortunately, no. At least harbor seal fibrinogen? According to a popular song of the day, there must be 50 ways to leave your lover, but it wasn't easy to leave this project.

Nonetheless, what was done was done. In St. Louis, Mike began exploring other aspects of fibrinogen. Eventually the little paper on chromatography of animal fibrinogens was published, and John turned (or returned) to other subjects—albumin, plasminogen, and mouse and rat urinary proteins, *inter alia*. However, as anyone who has ever worked with fibrinogen knows, it's sticky. Once you've touched it, it's hard to let go.

Among the many visitors to Mike's and John's lab had been Professor J. P. Soulier, one of the towering figures of French hematology. (In the field of medicine, once you have a disease named after you, you become immortal, and he had been immortalized in the 'Bernard-Soulier Syndrome'.) He had been intrigued with their chromatographic separation methods and wanted one of his younger colleagues to learn the technique. Mike and John were happy to oblige. They gave him a copy of a manuscript before publication and even sent him a bottle of DEAE cellulose to help launch the project.

About two years later, his young colleague, Dr. Doris Ménaché (now written without the accents because, as she said, "everyone knows where they belong") arrived at NIH. She was going to work in the lab of two famous scientists, Drs. Koloman Laki and Jules Gladner. The problem was that, as far as she could discern, they were not doing any work. Therefore, she called up John and asked if she could spend some time in his lab.

So, John and Doris embarked on a little project. Naturally, it was about fibrinogen. The chromatographic part was relatively straightforward. (In reality, as any researcher will verify, nothing is ever straightforward; the expression simply means that the mechanical difficulties could be overcome.) But then Doris said, "Now, how do you do the clottability measurements?" John had never done them. Not even one. In fact, he had never even touched thrombin to fibrinogen. Nevertheless, after a quick cramming session, which consisted of John reading his own paper, he was able to set up the procedure and "teach" Doris how it was done.

After a few weeks, that project ran its course, and Doris migrated across the hall to Dave's lab. There, she undertook a project that lasted a little longer. Over the next three years, they published two papers together. And about a decade later they were married. Meanwhile, John again set fibrinogen aside—but not for long. Soon, he decided to see how fibrinogen would behave if the chromatography were performed on a different kind of column, namely, hydroxylapatite.

Hydroxylapatite is an interesting mineral. It is made up of calcium, phosphorus, hydrogen, and oxygen. It is the stuff of which our bones are constructed, and it can exist in many different forms, all of which delight mineralogists, inorganic chemists, and their ilk. In the presence of the right salt solutions, it also proved to be a very good substrate for growing mold, especially *Aspergillus niger*. Moreover, the enzymes from the mold were very adept at digesting fibrinogen.

Some years later, another group of workers made similar observations and immediately turned this problem to their advantage. They discovered that, unlike intact fibrinogen, the partially digested protein was relatively easy to crystallize. John simply wanted to circumvent the problem, which he did by flushing the column with liberal doses of a fungicide. Eventually, he found that chromatography on hydroxylapatite could separate fibrinogen into two peaks. These were somewhat similar to, but not identical with, those obtained by DEAE cellulose chromatography.

When Mike heard John describe this work at the congress of the International Society of Hematology in New York, his only comment was, "I see what you mean, Guy." John took that to mean that they were both equally baffled by the results. In retrospect, it may have stirred in Mike some uneasiness about that nagging question, "What is the difference between peak 1 and peak 2 fibrinogen?" After another year had passed (Mike had been away from Bethesda for about six years by now), he had decided that the question should be answered or, at least, actively pursued.

And thus the Mike-and-John collaboration entered its next phase. By the time of the next congress, which took place in Munich, Mike had separated the individual polypeptide chains of fibrinogen, and John had obtained their peptide maps (so-called "fingerprints") after digesting them with trypsin. It was already clear that two of the three kinds of chains showed no difference. The difference between peak 1 and peak 2, whatever its exact nature, appeared to lie in the third kind of chain, designated the γ chain. When John presented this work in Munich, the response was nothing short of astounding. It was not that the audience was particularly impressed by the studies of the individual polypeptide chains. On the contrary, it seemed that people had finally grasped the concept that there were two major kinds of fibrinogen that differed in electrical charge.

All the questions that should have been asked in Boston, or at least in Mexico City, came pouring forth. It was obvious that our finding was (finally!) of mainstream interest and had to be followed up as quickly as possible. Looking at the individual chains by means of tryptic peptide mapping proved to be very useful. It was applicable not only to the study of the peak 1/peak 2 heterogeneity but also to the investigation of a second kind of heterogeneity that Mike had discovered while he was in St. Louis. There was, however, a small geographic problem. Mike was separating the chains in Brooklyn. John was mapping them in Bethesda. How could they be transported, quickly and reliably, between the two labs?

The answer, of course, was Aronson Airlines. Dave, serving as pilot and crew, would fly up to New York in his own airplane and bring back the chains. Days were saved, and, as the saying goes, we never lost a sample. Less than 18 months after the Munich meeting, John and Mike submitted three manuscripts to the Journal of Biological Chemistry. They showed that (1) the basis of the heterogeneity that Mike had discovered was that various portions of one kind of polypeptide chain (the α chain) had been digested away; (2) the kind of fibrinogen that was missing these portions (i.e., high-solubility fibrinogen) could not form as many cross-links as could more intact fibrinogen; and, (3) the basis for the chromatographic heterogeneity was that peak 2 fibrinogen had two different kinds of γ chains, initially designated γ and γ', and the latter was more highly charged. (As you might expect, the second paper was carried out in collaboration with John Pisano and his group. He and John had continued to work together on the biochemical action of Factor XIII and the effects of its absence.)

The simultaneous publication of three papers in the Journal of Biological Chemistry was, for Mike and John, unprecedented. At the end of the third, there appeared a small acknowledgement to Dr. David Aronson for "his air transport services." Mike and John had decided that the august Journal might not take kindly to "Captain David Aronson of Aronson Airlines," and had modified the draft acknowledgement accordingly.

Afterward, Mike and John continued to collaborate. It wasn't as if John had exhausted his interest in fibrinogen. When Harvey Gralnick from the NIH Clinical Pathology Department had sought his help in studying a family with congenitally abnormal fibrinogen, John had pitched in. Together, they developed a strategy that, for a number of years, was the prototype for working up cases of abnormal fibrinogen. Meanwhile Mike had, in a sense, returned to his roots. His original objective in Bethesda had been to study the action of plasmin on fibrinogen. Now, he was again looking at that action, albeit from new perspectives.

One of these focused on the comparison of naturally occurring fibrinogen derivatives ("metabolites," i.e., those highly soluble fibrinogens that were missing parts of their α chains) with products created by treating purified fibrinogen with plasmin. Just how well did these two kinds of derivatives match each other? The answer was "fairly closely, but not exactly."

The other was even more global. The idea was to analyze the "pieces" that resulted from breaking up fibrinogen by digesting it with plasmin and thereby to obtain a detailed picture of what fibrinogen looked like in the first place. It was truly (to borrow the title from a review that Mike and John wrote) "the search for the structure of fibrinogen." Well, they didn't find that either, but, like the Princes of Serendip, they made some interesting and useful observations along the way. More importantly, as Elemer Mihalyi pointed out, Mike's provocative questions and interpretations revitalized a field that had been in the doldrums.

Throughout this time, some significant changes had taken place. While Mike had migrated from Bethesda to St. Louis to Brooklyn to Milwaukee, John had undergone major life alterations without ever leaving one building. The first of these was that, on July 1, 1972, the Division of Biologics Standards was swept out of NIH. "Under new management," i.e., with a new director, a new deputy director, and a new administrative assistant, it became the Bureau of Biologics of the Food and Drug Administration (FDA).

There was no physical migration, only administrative. The building was the same, the working personnel were the same, the problems were the same. But the culture began to shift, slowly but surely.

A little over three years later, John was given an ultimatum. He was to leave the Coagulation Section (now called the Coagulation Branch in FDA terminology) and become the Director of the Plasma Derivatives Branch. It wasn't that this was a new scientific area; he had worked on virtually all the proteins that fell within the purview of that Branch. It was just that he would now have to become a manager, and his days as a laboratory worker were numbered.

Nevertheless, both before and after this life-altering event, John's interest and primary allegiance remained with the lab, and the clotting system continued to haunt his days. For example, although he and Dave had worked cheek-by-jowl for a decade and a half, they had never published a paper together. This changed when Dave decided to set up a rabbit assay to assess the "thrombogenicity" of various commercial therapeutic protein preparations. That is to say, he wanted to see which of these, if any, would promote clotting "not wisely, but too well."

This assay involved some simple surgery on rabbits. The idea was to determine whether a particular preparation caused a clot to form in the animal's jugular vein and, if so, how long that took. John offered to serve as scrub nurse for surgeon Dave—shaving the rabbit's neck and performing related clinical chores. The assay proved to be quite useful, clots did form under some circumstances (sometimes very rapidly, suggesting that the preparation might be hazardous in the clinic), and all-in-all it was a successful endeavor.

Then Dave suggested that John might be able to learn something from the clots that did form. As an extension of his work with John Pisano, John decided to look at cross-linking in those clots. He learned how to dissect the fibrin clot away from the entrapped blood cells and to bring the biochemical processes (including clotting and cross-linking) to a halt—all within about two minutes. The remarkable finding was that, as soon as one could get one's hands on a clot, the γ chains were already completely cross-linked.

Among the implications of this finding was that although it was convenient to think of clotting as taking place in distinct stages (and, in fact, to slow down the process in the lab so as to study these stages individually), in real life these stages occurred in an overlapping fashion. This seemed a worthwhile subject for a scientific paper and, indeed, it was John's and Dave's first joint publication.

The first, but not the last. Over the next several years, they managed to co-author a few research papers, a review article, a chapter in a book, etc. One of the research papers involved a mutual co-author—a very bright, very persistent, and extremely dour biochemist named John Fenton. (Why were so many of John's collaborators named John?) John had met Fenton at a conference. The latter had worked out a way to prepare highly purified human thrombin in large quantities and wanted to examine as many of its properties as possible. Upon learning of the capabilities of the Bethesda folks, he asked John (Finlayson, that is) if he would be willing to do a couple of analyses. Those were the days when the usual response to such a request could be characterized as "Just say yes." (About 15 years later, scientists began to sign contractual agreements with each other, thus ushering in a new, but not necessarily better, era.)

This "couple" of analyses stretched into numerous replicate runs, under different conditions and with various controls. It was followed by analyses performed by other methods, each with its own variants. And then came a crusade to find the precise molecular weight of this so-called α-thrombin. Meanwhile, Dave had been enlisted to look at its catalytic properties. By the time this was published, some four years after John Fenton had come into our lives, the paper had accrued six authors—three from Bethesda and three from John Fenton's lab in Albany.

Among the findings was a precise molecular weight, 36 600 (or 36 500, if one wished to acknowledge the limits of said precision). Whichever was chosen, Dave delighted in noting that, after all this labor, the value differed by less than 5% from the one that he and Buster Preiss had reported 15 years previously from target-volume irradiation data. Nonetheless, sometimes earnest effort and sheer persistence pay off in unexpected ways.

After this paper was published, John and John Fenton (and oodles of co-authors) wrote a couple of extensive reviews about thrombin. In the course of this collaboration, the latter gave Dave several large batches of highly purified human thrombin. A mixture of these, after suitable filling into ampoules and calibration in a study involving many laboratories, became the new U.S. Standard Thrombin, against which manufacturers of therapeutic thrombin preparations compared the potency of their products. Of course, virtually nothing the government does escapes at least some degree of suspicion, and this was no exception. To distinguish it from the previous Standard, the supply of which had been exhausted, this material was designated "Lot J." This came about simply because the previous "candidate" preparation, which proved to be insufficiently uniform to meet requirements for a U.S. Standard, was Lot H, and a capital I is indistinguishable from the Roman numeral I. Still, there were those who wondered if the two Johns might have named it after themselves.

Through all of this, John's life continued in a somewhat schizophrenic fashion. Much of it was consumed by regulatory tasks such as reading and editing package inserts for biological drugs, managerial functions such as (as John put it at the time) arbitrating disputes between two so-called adults fighting over two square feet of cold-room space, and other equally exciting ventures. Occasionally, however, there could be an exhilarating burst of science.

One of the most notable of these occurred thanks to a colleague of John and Dave— Sadaaki Iwanaga of Osaka University. He invited John to spend a mini-sabbatical in the University's Protein Research Institute. Needless to say, John was happy to accept. More remarkably, both the Bureau of Biologics and John's wife agreed to let him "disappear" for a little over three months.

One can't accomplish a great deal in three months, but one can certainly learn a lot. John learned to speak a little Japanese and, taught by Takashi ("Tak") Takagi, who was also a visiting scientist at the Institute, to determine the amino acid sequence of proteins. He worked on chicken fibrinogen and on the clotting protein from the Japanese horseshoe crab. In his time away from the lab bench (other than the time in which Tak was showing him more temples and shrines than he ever knew existed), he was going over a manuscript of which Dave had generously made him a coauthor.

In this study, Dave wanted to learn what was really the first "piece" of prothrombin that came off when prothrombin was converted to the active enzyme, thrombin. Numerous elegant studies had been reported by other workers, but these were performed in purified systems. Dave's quest was to learn what happens when unpurified plasma (or, even better, whole blood) clots. It turned out that, unlike the situation in purified systems, about half of the prothrombin molecule comes off in one piece. Furthermore, when clotting occurs, essentially all the prothrombin undergoes this cleavage, even though only a small percentage of it shows up as thrombin at any one time. The reason for this is that, as thrombin is created, it is inactivated by the inhibitors in the plasma.

After John returned to Bethesda, this became another of Dave and John's joint publications. Following the apparently requisite fits and starts, it eventually came out in print. However, this was not the only spin-off of John's stay in Japan. It seems that a number of investigators were working on the clotting protein of the horseshoe crab. Among these was Mike. Still another was Dr. T.-Y. ("Darrell") Liu, who worked in the same building as John and Dave. Despite the similarity of their studies, these workers were drawing different conclusions.

Now this is not a particularly new phenomenon in science. In fact, it may be the rule rather than the exception, especially when the area of investigation is relatively new. Sometimes there is a simple explanation. For example, were there different proteins in the Japanese and American horseshoe crabs, even though both had the same functional property, namely, forming a clot? This is the sort of thing that is usually worked out sooner or later (occasionally much later) through mutual exchange of correspondence, samples, draft manuscripts, etc.

The problem in this case was that there seemed to be a great deal of mistrust. To put it briefly (probably too briefly to accommodate all the nuances of the situation), Mike wasn't sure what Iwanaga was up to; Tak, who had worked with Russ Doolittle, didn't trust Mike; and Darrell didn't seem to trust anybody. On the other hand, everyone trusted John, probably for a number of reasons, including the fact that he was too busy to be doing much research. As a result, all three groups gave John some of their protein. John and his technician put all the samples, side-by-side, in the same experiment and looked at their migration in an electrical field. There was no detectable difference among them. Thus, one couldn't blame the differences on the protein (or, by extension, on the crabs). It had to be a matter of differences in experimental design, experimental conditions, or the individual workers' interpretations.

In every good western there is a scene or a paragraph that begins, "Meanwhile, back at the ranch…" The time has arrived to inject it into this story. Nearly a year earlier, while John was still in the Coagulation Branch, he had received a visit from an enthusiastic young physician/hematologist named Barbara Alving. She was a fellow at Johns Hopkins University, working in the laboratory of Dr. William Bell on the biosynthesis of fibrinogen. (Just to close the ring, we note that Bill had taken John's course in biochemistry while he was working at NIH.) Barbara was going to come to the FDA as a commissioned officer in the Public Health Service. She particularly wanted to work in the Coagulation Branch with John because of their mutual background in fibrinogen research.

It was a nice visit. All the arrangements were made to the satisfaction of the administrators, the scientists, and all other participants. Now fast-forward for a year but recall that the medical world moves on the first of July. Barbara arrived on July 1. Irony point 1: about ten months previously, John had left the Coagulation Branch and migrated to Plasma Derivatives. Irony point 2: on June 30, John had left Bethesda, bound for Osaka.

Not to worry. Barbara was (and no doubt still is) the quintessential self-starter. She stepped right into the Plasma Derivatives Branch; ordered, requisitioned, begged, and borrowed the necessary equipment; and began the next phase of her study on the biosynthesis of fibrinogen. Little did she suspect that it would be more than six years before a paper describing this work would ever be published. This huge delay was not due to any lack of effort or to poor experimental design, or even to the possibility that, as John used to say, "the rabbits didn't understand the experiment." In the old days, one might have said that somebody threw a monkey wrench in the works.

By the time John returned from Japan, much progress had been made, and Barbara laid out the experiments and results in her characteristically clear, enthusiastic fashion. After suitable treatment of the bunnies, she had injected them with a radioactive compound that was an analogue of the amino acid, methionine. Then, at various time intervals, she had taken blood samples and measured the radioactivity of the fibrinogen in each sample.

John listened intently, but without any particular insight, inasmuch as he had never worked on the biosynthesis of fibrinogen. Nonetheless, he managed to toss in monkey wrench number one. More in the spirit of making conversation than as the wise mentor bestowing sage advice, he asked, "Which chains of fibrinogen become labeled?" "What?" "I mean, which of the polypeptide chains of the fibrinogen molecule end up being radioactive?" "I never did that kind of experiment. How would you do it?"

Recall, now, that the fibrinogen molecule consists of six chains of amino acids— two of each of three different kinds of chains. John was simply wondering if the methionine analogue that was being incorporated into each polypeptide chain of the newly-synthesized fibrinogen was all starting out with the same radioactivity, or if it might have undergone different degrees of dilution in the rabbit's body. In the language of biochemistry, did it all come from the same metabolic "pool"?

John suggested a simple approach to learning where (within the fibrinogen molecule) the radioactivity went, as well as how much of it ended up there. Barbara went one step further. Because she had been used to taking blood samples at timed intervals, she continued this practice, but analyzed the individual polypeptide chains at those intervals. Her results indicated that, at the end of the experiment, the methionine in all the chains had the same level of radioactivity. (In more technical terms, they all reached the same "specific activity," i.e., radioactivity per milligram.) Along the way, however, there were differences between the individual chains, even though the specific activity increased at the same rate in each chain.

By the end of the year, Barbara had accumulated enough information to prepare an abstract for the meeting of the International Society on Thrombosis and Haemostasis that would take place the following summer. After learning that it had been accepted for presentation, she continued working on the project in an attempt to refine the data and, more importantly, to figure out the basis for the differences. Then, that spring, the second monkey wrench landed. And it was a big one.

To take advantage of Barbara's medical training, the Division Director had put her in charge of reviewing adverse reactions to products for which the Division was responsible. This is a major function of the FDA, that is, to receive and evaluate reports from people (physicians, pharmacists, patients, and others) when something seems not to be right. These reports can involve anything from an apparent product defect (for example, a product that should be clear looks discolored or cloudy) to a catastrophic side-reaction in a patient.

In the case of an adverse patient reaction, the FDA's job includes deciding whether it was really caused by the product, determining how severe and how wide-spread it is, learning (if possible) the reason for it and, finally, figuring out what the manufacturer and the FDA need to do about it. All of this is often easier said than done. It usually involves two main endeavors: (1) trying to get as much information as possible, and (2) trying to understand the real basis of the problem.

In the case of this particular monkey wrench, Barbara had been receiving reports about patients who were given intravenous infusions of a particular plasma derivative (often, but not always, when they were having surgery). These patients were showing large decreases in their blood pressure. This was especially disturbing because the usual way of monitoring whether the product was working was to observe whether the patient's blood pressure was being maintained or increased. When it dropped, the attending medical person (usually a nurse or an anesthesiologist) would infuse more of the product at a greater flow rate. The result would be an even larger fall in the blood pressure.

Barbara's inquiries to follow up these reports revealed that almost all of them involved a product from a single company. And sometimes, when she talked directly to the medical personnel at the hospital, she learned that there were still more cases that had never been reported. By May, the reports had become so numerous that the manufacturer was told to stop distributing the product and to recall any product that was still on the market.

Then came the problem of figuring out what caused all of this. Clearly, it was a crisis—so much so that it had escalated to the office of the Bureau Director. His response was exactly the same as it usually was when any kind of crisis (except those involving infectious diseases) arose in the blood world. He told John to "get on an airplane," go to the manufacturing plant, and "find out what's going on."

John, as usual, did as he was told. Before leaving, however, he spoke with his longtime collaborator, John Pisano, who for years had been working on peptides and proteins that affect blood pressure. The latter's response was to give John a copy of a large (some 600 pages) book containing the papers presented at a conference about three years earlier. John (Pisano) was the senior editor.

So John (Finlayson), book in hand, got on an airplane. By the time he arrived at the plant to meet with the manufacturer's scientists, he had read most of it. By the end of a day of data presentations and discussion, he was saturated with knowledge, but "what was going on" was beginning to emerge. Clearly, the FDA, the Plasma Derivatives Branch, and the various layers in between all had their work cut out for them.

When an exciting story unfolds and a problem is solved, there is a natural desire to tell the whole story, detail by detail. This desire seems to be particularly strong in fishermen, hunters, and scientists. The saga of the hypotensive episodes readily falls into this category; however, an abbreviated and somewhat global summary will suffice. It is illustrative of two well-known phenomena: the lurking possibility of unintended consequences and the consummate power of cooperation.

For years scientists, research physicians, and manufacturers had been aware that this kind of episode could occur sporadically. There were even a few strong clues about the cause, but it seemed that the adverse clinical events were few and far between. Therefore, there was not a strong driving force to pursue any long-term investigation of them. Then, in February 1975, FDA and NIH held a workshop on albumin. It was wide-ranging and well attended, covering virtually all aspects of this abundant (and abundantly studied) plasma protein: its history, biochemistry, physiology, clinical use—and misuse—and even adverse clinical reactions to it.

Scientists from one of the companies whose representatives had attended this workshop returned to their home base convinced that they knew what was responsible for these precipitous drops in blood pressure. It had to be a small peptide (or "oligopeptide," in the language of biochemistry) with big pharmacological activity. Its name is bradykinin, and it is only nine amino acids long. This means that it is less than two percent of the size of albumin, which itself is not a particularly large protein. It is, however, very potent in its ability to cause blood vessels to dilate. If you can imagine water flowing through a pipe at a constant pressure, and then the pipe suddenly having a much larger diameter, you can see that the water pressure will fall equally suddenly.

Substitute "blood vessel" for "pipe" and "blood pressure" for "water pressure," and the strategy (at least, according to this company's scientists) became obvious: get rid of the bradykinin. Before too long, the company had modified its manufacturing method so as to produce a product that was virtually bradykinin-free. The approach was as follows: allow as much bradykinin as possible to be generated (from its naturally occurring plasma precursor) during the production process and then, at the end, perform an ultrafiltration step to remove it. Because of its small size, this removal was very efficient.

The approach was ingenious, but the failure to tell FDA about a change in the manufacturing method was not. And the consequences were disastrous. The problem arose because, in the course of generating bradykinin, other pharmacologically active substances were produced. These were not small enough to be removed by the ultrafiltration step and, consequently, remained in the final product.

One of these substances was an active enzyme (let's call it "activator") that was created from a piece of a clotting factor (not one of the clotting factors that we have spoken of previously). It could hardly have been a more devilish contaminant. When the product was infused into the patient's vein, the activator acted on a protein in the bloodstream to produce a second active enzyme. This second enzyme then catalyzed a pair of reactions that released bradykinin from its precursor. All of this took place in the patient, so that the bradykinin was being formed exactly where it could do the most harm. Moreover, at each of these steps there was a "multiplier" effect, so that one molecule of activator could potentially generate thousands of molecules of bradykinin.

The job of the Plasma Derivatives Branch was straightforward. "All" it had to do was to, (1) learn how to measure the amount of activator in a product; (2) prove that the enzyme activity measured actually was due to this activator molecule; (3) demonstrate that the severity of the adverse clinical reactions correlated with the amount of activator in the product; (4) test other companies' products—not only the same product that set off all this concern, but closely related products as well—to see if some of them contained the activator; (5) inform all the other manufacturers of this problem and the results of our investigation; (6) teach them how to perform the test; and, (7) establish a standard reference preparation that could be tested side-by-side with the products so that every lab's test results could be compared. And, did we mention, do this in a hurry.

In retrospect, it is difficult to believe that all this was accomplished. It was certainly not accomplished by anyone's singular effort alone. John Pisano was absolutely unstinting with his time and effort, but this was only the beginning. He also 'gave' Barbara and John his top postdoctoral fellow, Yoshio Hojima, on what today would probably be called "indefinite loan"—in other words "for as long as it takes." (In reality, one has to wonder if such generosity would ever be experienced today.)

Yoshio was a brilliant, imaginative, utterly indefatigable, and infinitely patient worker. His laboratory skill was remarkable, and his ability to teach laboratory techniques was without parallel. But even this was not the extent of the collaboration. Despite the obvious tension that exists between FDA and regulated industries (multiplied many-fold when the FDA says that millions of dollars' worth of product must be taken off the market), the company whose product was in jeopardy offered full cooperation. (Perhaps this had something to do with the fact that John and the company's director of chemical and biological research had known each other since their graduate school days.) Anesthesiologists with whom Barbara had been in contact (and, sometimes, their clinical assistants as well) provided additional case reports. The other companies, perhaps relieved that their products were not the ones to launch this furious endeavor, enthusiastically attended "activator" workshops in Bethesda, learned to perform the test, shared their results, and offered suggestions for improving the test.

There were several results from all this effort. One (one hopes) was improved safety for patients who might be recipients of the product. Another was that the research program of the Plasma Derivatives Branch took a new turn (definitely away from the biosynthesis of fibrinogen). A third was a direct result of John's visit to the company. Although he had met most of the company's scientists previously, there were a few new faces in the crowd. One of these belonged to Donald Tankersley. Don came to visit (and to work in) Barbara's and John's lab during the Christmas holidays. He evidently found it to his liking because by the following September he had joined the Plasma Derivatives Branch, and he remained with the organization for 17 years.

One might imagine that, from the company's point of view, this would have been adding insult to injury—first demanding a recall of a huge quantity of product and then stealing one of its valued employees. In reality, the response of John's old grad school buddy (Milt Mozen) was extraordinarily gracious. When it became apparent that Don's decision to leave the company and join FDA was irreversible, he telephoned John to congratulate him. His exact words were, "Don is one of the most brilliant, if not *the* most brilliant, employee the company has ever had." This was no exaggeration. Even though Barbara left two years later, Don became the nucleus of a research group that made a host of both fundamental and practical discoveries. After eight years at FDA, he replaced John as head of Plasma Derivatives, and eventually he was made Deputy Division Director.

As expected, the new direction of research in Plasma Derivatives generated a great deal of excitement. It also permitted the recruiting of additional scientists. Diligent searching revealed that "activator" and its fellow-traveling proteins could be contaminants of plasma products that, at first glance, seemed to be unrelated to the one whose problems set off the whole endeavor. Furthermore, these proteins not only contributed to adverse clinical reactions but also affected the stability (and therefore the shelf life) of these products.

In the midst of all this, John's work on fibrinogen sank to a minimum, but remarkably, it did not sink to zero. He and his technician managed to continue the collaboration with Doris Menache's group that had begun even before they had migrated from Coagulation to Plasma Derivatives. Both of the projects in this collaboration involved congenitally abnormal fibrinogens. Most of the methods used in studying these proteins had already been developed, especially during John's work with Harvey Gralnick. By contrast, some of the most challenging problems involved simply getting the patients' frozen plasma from Paris to Bethesda (and through Customs) without melting or other damage. Unfortunately, Aronson Airlines did not fly the trans-Atlantic route.

Nonetheless, the challenges were met; the experiments were done (although often with long lapses of time between them); and papers reporting the results were published. The last of these, fittingly enough, was the last paper that John and Mike Mosesson coauthored. It was a short communication about the abnormal fibrinogen that Doris had discovered some 17 years previously. And, to complete the ring of nostalgia, the editor who accepted it for publication was Mike's and John's longstanding colleague, Peter Harpel.

This is not to say that all contact between Mike and John, or even the part that one could call FDA-centered contact, ceased at that point. On the contrary, the latter included such things as Mike's serving as a member of FDA's Blood Products Advisory Committee. (Presumably, this would make him a sort of spiritual descendant of Ben Alexander, but neither Mike nor John would put too much credence in that metaphor.)

Another of their many path-crossings came about four or five years after John had left Plasma Derivatives. The Division of Blood and Blood Products had become so large (in terms of the number of employees) that it was unwieldly. Upper management had decided to split it into two new divisions, namely, the Division of Transfusion Science and the Division of Hematology. The director of the existing Division would assume directorship of the former; management would have to recruit a director for the latter.

To facilitate the split, however, and to fill the gap until the recruitment was completed, there had to be an Acting Director. John, who had been offered the permanent directorship (and who wanted no part of it, having been supersaturated with 15 years of management trivia) agreed to serve as Acting Director for ten weeks. This soon became one of the standing jokes throughout the Center, inasmuch as two full recruitment cycles, consuming 25 months, were needed before a permanent director was chosen.

In the first of these cycles, Mike was one of the candidates. In fact, he was far and away the top candidate. Of course, John, as "The Acting," had to interview all candidates and provide his evaluation. So, conflict of interest notwithstanding, John interviewed Mike. Usually, during such an interview, the interviewer stops asking questions and says something like, "Is there anything you would like to ask me?" Mike was so well informed about the job that he had only one question for John: "Are you *sure* you don't want the job?"

John was "sure" on two counts. He was sure he didn't want the job for himself, and he was sure that he wanted Mike to fill it. With this established, both of them were really excited by the prospect. Then came the crushing fact that the FDA couldn't pay enough to make the position attractive enough to induce Mike to leave his current position. (It went without saying that it couldn't pay him what he was worth, but that is the nature of government.)

So, for the moment, both Mike and John stayed put. Eventually, a permanent director was ensconced, and then an even more extensive reorganization took place. This allowed John to escape into a non-supervisory position, which he held for the next 11 years, i.e., until his retirement. But he never did column chromatography of fibrinogen again.

Part 5

Two Guys Named Bob

Bob Fletcher

It was early in the summer of 1961, and something was bothering Dr. Tripp (not an unusual situation). Apparently, pressure was coming from on high at NIH. It was one of those gentle bureaucratic requests that cannot, under any circumstances, be refused. Someone would have to provide summer employment for a nephew of Jack Masur (after whom the auditorium of the NIH Clinical Center was named). As the request trickled down, the Laboratory of Blood and Blood Products became the favored locus. Therefore Dr. Tripp, the Lab Chief, passed the favor on to John. John would be said nephew's boss for the summer.

Let it be said at the outset that, despite all the social baggage (relatives in high places, nobility of birth, fine New England university, etc.) with which he arrived, Bob Fletcher proved to be an outstanding find. John's collaborations with Mike were in full swing, so there was much to be done. Chromatographic columns had to be packed, the ultraviolet absorption of the fractions collected during the course of chromatography had to be measured in a spectrophotometer, and, at the end of each chromatographic run, the DEAE cellulose had to be removed from the column and washed with the appropriate series of reagents so that the process could begin again.

All these procedures were new to Bob, but he learned them almost immediately. And, as might be expected, some required less concentration than others. These were the ones that provided an opportunity for conversation. Among the topics were sports. It turned out that Bob had been quite an athlete. He had experience both as a hurdler and a pole vaulter, and he was currently on Wesleyan University's soccer team. In this connection he mentioned that he would like to do "something to stay in shape."

John had just the answer, or, to be specific, the "something." When John was in high school, he had caught what some refer to as "the running bug." Although he was nowhere near fast enough to compete in high school track meets, and his college had dropped track during World War II and never re-instituted it, John continued to run by himself. (In fact, he continued to do so until he was past the age of 60.)

Now, because the situation in the U.S. was so different from that existing today, some societal background should be provided. In those days, in virtually any locus other than Boston, distance running by an adult male had a level of social acceptability somewhere between that of bank robbing and child molesting. (Distance running on the part of adult females was essentially nonexistent.) Unlike golf, tennis, swimming, or a host of other informal sport activities, it was viewed with huge suspicion. At the very least, it had to be justified—for, example, running as part of a conditioning program for boxing, mountain climbing, etc. was considered appropriate (or at least not totally insane), whereas running for the sheer exhilaration of running most definitely was not.

This attitude underwent an abrupt change when the American runner, Frank Shorter, won the marathon at the 1972 Olympics. At that point, distance running became not only socially acceptable, but *de rigueur*. Over the period between his departure from high school and this salient event, however, John plodded on—not exactly alone, but certainly in very limited company.

The summer in question, though, was a minor exception. It was enhanced not only by Bob's arrival, but by another factor that also demands some historical attention. In those days there were many fewer buildings at NIH than there are today, and the grounds were filled with abundant swaths of green. In fact, a golf course had existed on those grounds, albeit it had recently ceased operation. The entire aspect of NIH was very much like that of a college campus. However, woe betide anyone who had the temerity to call it a campus. That one would be told, in no uncertain terms, that this was *not* a campus— it was a government *reservation*!

Some 30 or 40 years later, when the proliferation of buildings had created an aura reminiscent of Manhattan (and, even more so, post-9/11, when it took on the aspect of a military base), it became common practice to refer to "the NIH campus." This delightful irony, however, was far in the future, as were the not-so-delightful alterations of the geography.

John had usually run each day, either before or after work. When he suggested that Bob accompany him, Bob proposed that they run at noon. This seemed to be a good idea, even though the noonday heat, when compounded with Bethesda's legendary humidity and NIH's hilly terrain, made the run extremely challenging. Soon it became a daily activity for Bob and John, and they invited others to join them. Remarkably, many accepted, at least briefly or sporadically. One of the few persistent members of the hardy little band was Mike. (*Dave Aronson used to light his cigarette, run with us for about 100 yards, and then wish us good tidings! 'mm'*)

The summer passed quickly, and Bob returned for his senior year at Wesleyan University. He wrote to John fairly regularly. In one of his early letters he noted that, at soccer practice, he was so "bouncy and peppy" that his teammates all hated him. He finished his undergraduate studies and entered Harvard Medical School. John saw him in Boston on a few occasions, at the time of the Protein Foundation meetings. Bob had married a fellow medical student, Sue. They had some interesting adventures together. For example, one summer they had worked in Nigeria.

Despite Bob's diligent labor in John's lab, they never coauthored a scientific paper. The closest approach was an acknowledgement in the Biochemistry paper that John and Mike published. However, many years later, when searching in the NIH library for a suitable reference text, John found that Bob and Sue had become authors in their own right. They had written a very successful textbook of clinical epidemiology. It is now in its fourth edition.

Bob Morton

This story begins about two years before John ever met Morton. His mentor, Dr. James Hampton of the University of Oklahoma Medical Center, drove into the parking lot behind John's building at NIH (a feat that was possible in those days), parked, and walked into John's building (also possible). After a few brief inquiries, he found John's lab, which was quite easy, inasmuch as it was on the ground floor, just down the hall from the director's office.

In his pocket he had a bottle of dried fibrinogen. He had discovered a family in Oklahoma that had some kind of bleeding problem. Initially, two brothers came to his attention. As he had said, they did not bleed spontaneously (as a severe hemophiliac would), but they did bleed from trauma. In view of the fact that one of them was a construction worker, always subject to bumps and scrapes, and sometimes to worse, this was a significant problem. The fibrinogen had been purified from the plasma of that brother.

Initially, Jim Hampton and his coworkers believed that this was a family that was deficient in Factor XIII. The blood of such people clots at a normal rate, but the clots tend to be unstable. After 24 to 48 hours, they can begin to come apart. A scenario like this would be consistent with the "bleeding from trauma" observation. However, as more experiments were performed, some inconsistencies arose. Jim began to suspect that the problem might not be deficiency of Factor XIII (which, in its activated form, would promote the cross-linking—and therefore the stability—of the fibrin clot) but might lie in the fibrinogen itself.

Such so-called "congenital dysfibrinogenemias" (i.e., inborn abnormalities of fibrinogen) had been reported in the medical research literature, albeit rarely. Doris Menache had described the first one that was really proved to be a fibrinogen abnormality. Because it was discovered in Paris, she called it "Fibrinogen Paris." (Later, as other cases were discovered in the same locale, it was designated Fibrinogen Paris I.) Mike had worked on characterizing another, which was called Fibrinogen Baltimore. Jim had decided that the abnormality in this family should be "re-characterized." He had now tentatively called it Fibrinogen Oklahoma.

John agreed to analyze this sample of fibrinogen and asked Jim to send him some of the patient's plasma. Thus, began a collaboration that ultimately lasted more than a decade. (No, in case you're wondering, Jim did not drive all the way from Oklahoma City to Bethesda just to deliver one small bottle of fibrinogen—he had other business at NIH.)

When presented with a sample for analysis, a scientist's usual tendency (all other things being equal), is to perform the analysis with which he or she is most familiar. In John's case, this was chromatography. Immediately, John and his technician dissolved the fibrinogen, prepared it for chromatography, and put it on the column. The results were striking. In fact, they looked too good to be true. Such experiments were not common, but usually they revealed either no difference between normal fibrinogen and that of the patient or, at most, a very subtle difference.

In this case, the shape of the elution pattern was the same as that for normal fibrinogen, but "Fibrinogen Oklahoma" came off the column much later than expected. Such a finding, if confirmed, would indicate a great difference in the electrical charge carried by the protein molecule and would imply that its composition was vastly abnormal. To avoid prolonging the suspense, let us say simply that it *wasn't* confirmed, and it *was* too good to be true.

It seems that, as luck would have it, John's lab was almost out of a reagent needed to make a salt solution for the chromatography. Accordingly, John's technician, very sensibly, had weighed out only half the usual amount. Unfortunately, she neglected to use only half the usual quantity of water to dissolve it. When dissolved in the usual volume of water, it yielded a solution of only half the usual strength, meaning that about twice as much of it would have to be pumped through the column before the conditions for washing off the fibrinogen were reached.

As might be expected, it took some detective work to figure this part out. Then, when a new supply of the reagent was available, the "wrong" experiment had to be repeated with normal fibrinogen to see if the exciting (read "spurious") result could be reproduced. And, finally, the "right" experiment had to be done with another sample of the putative abnormal fibrinogen (that's what happens when you can't verify the conditions of an experiment—one goes on and on because you simply cannot let it go!)

Eventually, chromatographic patterns of fibrinogen from each of the brothers were obtained. They looked exactly like that of normal fibrinogen. Furthermore, when the second peak of each was tested to see if it contained Factor XIII, those results were also normal. Meanwhile, Jim had sent some of the patients' frozen plasma. John and John Pisano found that, upon clotting, the plasma yielded a fibrin clot with the normal number of cross-links.

Thus the fibrinogen seemed to be normal, and there was no hint of Factor XIII deficiency. To be sure of this, John used some of the other methods he had worked out during his collaboration with Harvey Gralnick on another congenitally abnormal fibrinogen (Fibrinogen Bethesda, later designated Fibrinogen Bethesda I). Again, the fibrinogen from the brothers behaved completely normally. Nonetheless, the fact remained that some members of this family had a bleeding problem. Now that it appeared certain that neither fibrinogen nor Factor XIII was the culprit, the problem for John and Jim was to find the real underlying cause.

Although these experiments and results have been described in an embarrassingly few sentences, they took a considerable amount of time to perform. The passage of this time made it possible for Jim to suggest the next step in the quest. He had a student who would soon be coming to NIH to spend a month in a hematology lab in the Clinical Center. Perhaps, if funding could be arranged, the student could work in John's lab for a month.

As you can guess, funding was arranged (otherwise there would be no story of the second Bob), and Jim informed John that Bob Morton would be arriving soon. Before coming to John's lab, he would attend a meeting in Atlantic City and give a talk, and he would send John a copy of the talk. Upon arrival in Bethesda, Bob would begin work in John's lab. He would spend a month there and then work for a month in the Clinical Center before returning to Oklahoma City in preparation for his last year of medical school.

By the time Bob arrived, John had received, read, and re-read the text of Bob's talk. So, intending to put him at ease by letting him discuss things he obviously knew very well, John asked Bob a few questions about the laboratory methods he had used to obtain the data presented in the talk. The result was just the opposite of what John had anticipated. Bob was unable to describe any of the methods or procedures and was clearly embarrassed by his inability to do so.

It seems that Bob had learned how to do research from his mentor, Jim, and had adopted his modus operandi. That is, as Bob described it later, "You would arrive at the office, straighten your cufflinks, and pick up the telephone." In other words, all the experiments had been performed by technicians, who were given essentially full responsibility for the experimental details. Jim had been the director of the operation, and Bob had become the deputy director.

Thus, before Bob had touched even one item in John's lab, his worldview underwent a major shift. A scientist could carry out his own experiments. And even if a particular experiment was done by a technician, the scientist should know all the details of the methods, their strong points, their weak points, and their interpretation. So profound was this shift that Bob immediately adopted a new approach to research. He wanted to learn all the experimental details, learn to perform the experiments himself, and develop an understanding of just how far one could (and couldn't) go in interpreting the results.

To accommodate Bob's new outlook, as well as to be realistic about what could be accomplished in a month, John decided that Bob should begin by learning one particular technique and should apply it to the plasma samples from the family with the bleeding problem. First, though, he should perform it with plasma from a normal person.

The technique was one that John and his technician had used for some time. It was the same one that Barbara Alving later used to great advantage to examine the individual peptide chains of fibrinogen. John had developed a simple procedure for "harvesting" clots. As diluted plasma clotted in a test tube, one just wound the clot up on a glass rod. When clotting was complete, all one had to do was to pull the rod (with clot firmly attached) out of the tube and put it into a beaker of salt solution to wash off the clot. After a suitable amount of washing, one could dissolve the clot in an appropriate reagent and proceed to the next step, i.e., separation of the peptide chains.

John had determined the time of washing, the volume of wash solution, and the number of washes needed. Depending on the analysis to be performed, washing had to be extensive or could be minimal. He thought that for Bob's purposes, they might be able to eliminate the washing step altogether. So, now all that was necessary was to find this normal person, obtain a sample of his or her plasma, and try out the idea. And who could be more normal than John himself?

Therefore, with John showing each step and Bob carefully following along, the intrepid team diluted a sample of John's plasma, clotted it, wound up the clot, and after a suitable period of time to be sure that no more clotting would occur, harvested the clot. After dissolving it (a step that was allowed to occur overnight), they separated the peptide chains and examined the resulting pattern. During the various times that required waiting, e.g., for clotting, dissolving, and/or separating, John explained to Bob what the expected results would be.

The solution used for diluting the plasma contained a number of reagents that would promote cross-linking but none that would prevent it. Therefore, the clot would be completely cross-linked. When the experiment was finished, this would be evident from the pattern given by the clot. That is, certain peptide chains (seen as bands in the pattern) typical of fibrinogen would disappear, whereas others, i.e., the cross-linked chains, would be seen.

The actual results, however, were not those detailed in John's explanations. One of the peptide bands that was supposed to disappear (viz., that corresponding to the γ chain) cooperated very nicely and did so. Moreover, the corresponding band indicating cross-linking of that peptide appeared exactly where it should have. However, the other band (the one corresponding to the α chain) not only failed to disappear—it sat there at least as strong, broad, and bold as in non-cross-linked fibrin. Obviously, or at least apparently, it had failed to cross-link.

What could this mean? Well, the quick interpretation was that John was partially deficient in Factor XIII. What should he do? Call for help, of course. (John never wore cufflinks, but now it was his turn to pick up the telephone.) He phoned John Pisano. "What would you think if I told you I am Factor XIII-deficient," he asked after describing the experiment and the outcome. "Nah," was (the other) John's reply, "you've been the 'control' in too many other experiments; it must be some contaminant."

In a sense, that wise counsel was reassuring. But now, John and Bob had two thorny problems confronting them. Why did the family members bleed? And what was this mysterious contaminant? It seemed that it would be better to attack the latter one first. If it could be solved, they could be sure that (1) John was not XIII-deficient and thus could continue to serve as a control when needed, and (2) the method (possibly with some modification) could be trusted.

Therefore, if one were to express it by compounding the current clichés, the epicenter of the problem had undergone a sea change. The overriding question was how to mount this vaunted attack. John Pisano had already provided his input. Bob did not yet have enough background to offer any suggestions. Hence, the responsibility fell to John. He could, of course, design some experiments, but without a guiding hypothesis they would be nothing but random activity. So his only recourse was to think. And to worry.

What is the appropriate length of time for worrying before one either gives up or reaches a breakthrough? In this case it was about a day and a half. John kept asking himself, "If it is a contaminant, what is the most likely suspect?" He must have asked it out loud more than once because Bob, taking his cue and focusing on the other problem, began to chant, "The brothers bleed."

One must not disparage the power of positive worry. Although the intervening steps have disappeared from John's memory, at some point he must have made the subtle conversion from asking, "What is the most likely suspect [contaminant]?" to "What is the most abundant potential contaminant in plasma?" When couched in these terms, the problem seems almost trivial. The answer, however, arrived with a jolt. "Of course," John thought, "it's the most abundant protein in plasma!" Albumin. It had literally been staring him in the face.

John was so excited that he could hardly wait to tell John Pisano about his "breakthrough"—or to begin the experiments that would either confirm or refute his conclusion. Bob sensed this excitement and dove into the action. In short, albumin proved to be the contaminant. It is, by far, the most abundant protein in human plasma. It has a molecular weight very similar to that of an α chain (hence it appeared as a band in the position of a non-cross-linked α chain). It can be washed off of the clot by a very brief period of stirring in saline solution. However, the difference between brief washing and none at all had a huge impact on the results.

Because others might use this technique to assess Factor XIII deficiency, John and Bob decided to write a little paper describing their experience. In such a paper, definite proof of the identity of the contaminant would have to be provided. To accomplish this, they performed the experiment again. This time, several replicate clots were prepared. Some were washed extensively, some were washed briefly, and some were not washed at all. Furthermore, the washings were concentrated and examined. Concentrated washings were also added back to a washed clot.

The overall picture that emerged was as follows. The band patterns of briefly washed and extensively washed clots were virtually the same. The confounding band appeared in both the pattern given by the unwashed clot and that of the washed clot to which concentrated washings had been added and, furthermore, appeared at the same position. The same pattern could be created by adding purified albumin to the washed clot. The major band in the pattern given by the washings appeared in the same position as that of purified albumin. (Bands other than this major band were very faint.) Finally, the major protein of the washings was shown to be immunologically identical to albumin.

It was exciting for Bob to have participated "hands-on" in both the performance of the experiments and their interpretation. The little paper, which was published early the following year, was a sort of bonus. Now they could return to the business of trying to discover why the family had the bleeding problem.

Bob still had the commitment to work in the NIH Clinical Center. He fulfilled that commitment and found the experience to be instructive and enriching. In addition, he proved to be very persuasive. He not only convinced Jim Hampton to let him spend another month in John's lab; he also talked the dean of the medical school into letting him begin his senior year a month late. Thus, his one month in John's lab grew into three.

During this time, Bob learned additional lab techniques, but he also participated in various other activities, two of which spring to mind. One was running. Ever since the summer of Bob Fletcher's sojourn in his lab, John had become a committed noon runner. Bob Morton, unlike Bob Fletcher, did not have a background of participation in team sports. However, being from the Southwest, he was adept at calf- and steer-roping. He had even tried bull riding. And, to complete the picture, he had a lean, cowboy build.

So, for that summer, the second Bob became a daily runner. He seemed to enjoy it and to like the idea that he was improving his physical condition as well as his grasp of science. The second "activity," if it can be called that, stemmed from the fact that Jim Hampton was quite keen to learn what his prize student was up to. He telephoned John every week to inquire about progress on the joint project.

John would dutifully answer the telephone (with Bob standing by, absorbing every word) and describe the previous week's observations. In reality, numerous observations were made, but no salient conclusions emerged. Nevertheless, each week Jim became more eager to publish the results that had accumulated. Consequently, each week John had to stand more firmly, insisting that there could be no meaningful publication until there was a story to be told. In doing so, he had to walk a fine line. On the one hand, he was very appreciative of Jim's willingness to send additional plasma samples. On the other, he felt that with two previous misdiagnoses of this bleeding condition, no one would be served by rushing into print.

Bob came to describe John's verbal resistance to Jim's eagerness as "Horatio at the bridge," a reference to the Roman hero of Macaulay's poem, "Horatius at the Bridge." (In that poem there is a line about "facing fearful odds.") It was the source of considerable amusement for him. At the same time, it reinforced his understanding of the contrast between the two research styles that he had encountered in his short career.

Eventually, fall came, and Bob returned to finish medical school. He then went to Massachusetts General Hospital for a residency and subsequently migrated to the NIH Clinical Center for additional training. During the latter stint, he and John were able to get together on several occasions. Afterward, Bob returned to the South. Exquisitely trained and credentialed, he became a full-time clinician.

John continued to spend part of his time wrestling with the business of Jim's bleeding patients. And Jim continued to be willing and able to send him plasma samples. Among the techniques that John used was that simple one that he had taught to Bob years previously, namely, clotting diluted plasma and winding up the clot. When cross-linking was prevented, the peptide chains of the patients' fibrin sometimes resembled those of the high-solubility fibrinogen or the plasmin-digested fibrinogen that Mike and John had studied.

This gave John the idea that maybe something *was* missing from the patient's fibrinogen after all. However, the true situation became clear after a few simple experiments. (Almost all experiments are simple—after you know the answer.) If the clots were wound up and allowed to incubate in their own serum, they underwent digestion. They continued to undergo digestion if the incubation was prolonged. By contrast, if both the cross-linking and the digestion were prevented by the use of appropriate inhibitors, the fibrin clots were stable, and the peptide chains looked perfectly normal. In other words, there was (just as all the previous experiments had indicated) nothing abnormal about the fibrinogen. The apparent abnormality was being *created* during the incubation.

This suggested two things. Either there was too much of the digesting enzyme (plasmin) or its precursor (plasminogen), or there was not enough of a plasmin inhibitor. The first possibility was ruled out by some straightforward assays. The latter required outside help. Peter Harpel, who had spent much of his career making elegant measurements of one particular plasmin inhibitor, graciously analyzed some patient samples. Sadly (for revealing the nature of the problem, not for the patients), the concentration of the inhibitor in their plasma was normal.

At about this time Jack Folk had a senior postdoctoral fellow, Franco Carmassi, working in his lab. Franco was setting up an immunological analysis for another plasmin inhibitor and agreed to run some samples for John. As the results accumulated, the situation became somewhat like that in the old days when stock market quotations were received on tickertape. One felt the excitement rising but tried not to become too excited by the news. But, in this case, the news was genuinely exciting.

Finally, some 11 years after Bob had arrived in John's lab, it was possible for John to report (in a conference co-organized and co-chaired by Mike, of all things) that this long-studied "Fibrinogen Oklahoma" family had a partial deficiency of the inhibitor that Franco was studying. This meant that the blood of the afflicted family members clotted in normal fashion but that the clots were being digested away before they had completed their job, that is, not only to stop bleeding but also to prevent its recurrence.

Remarkably, we now know, thanks to much additional work carried out in Mike's lab, that this inhibitor was exactly the same one that Mike and John had discovered in the course of investigating normal fibrinogen 20 years earlier ($\alpha 2$ antiplasmin). Bob Morton would have been so pleased (and, probably, more than a little excited). By this time, however, he had moved far beyond the ivory tower of research and was busy saving lives.

~ *January 23, 2014*

ANNOTATED BIBLIOGRAPHY

1. **THE PREPARATION OF HUMAN FIBRINOGEN FREE OF PLASMINOGEN.** MW Mosesson. *Biochim Biophys Acta* 57:204-213, 1962. *My first publication! JSF helped me with the writing. The method works and many still use it for preparing plasminogen-free fibrinogen.*

2. **THE PREPARATION AND CERTAIN PROPERTIES OF PLASMINOGEN FREE HUMAN FIBRINOGEN.** MW Mosesson, JS Finlayson. *Vox Sang* 7:99, 1962. *My debut presentation at the Protein Foundation.*

3. **MOLECULAR WEIGHTS OF FACTOR VIII AND FACTOR IX BY ELECTRON IRRADIATION.** DL Aronson, JS Preiss, MW Mosesson. *Thromb Diath Haemorr* 8:270-275, 1962. *Molecular weight values for factor VIII by this technique were accurate and preceded more classical estimations of its molecular weight. The work has not been cited much. This was mainly DLA's experimental idea and was carried out by John Preiss, who deserves credit for its development-I prepared the FVIII-rich fibrinogen for this analysis. See John Finlayson's essays about the origins of FDA.*

4. **CERTAIN BIOLOGICAL ACTIVITIES ASSOCIATED WITH PLASMINOGEN FREE FIBRINOGEN PREPARATIONS.** MW Mosesson, JS Finlayson. *Proc IX Cong Int'l Soc Hematol* 2:283-289, 1962. *First met Tony Fletcher at these meetings in Mexico, and that encounter sure changed my life. I wound up going to St. Louis to finish Medical Residency training and beyond.*

5. **CHROMATOGRAPHIC BEHAVIOR OF HUMAN FIBRINOGEN.** JS Finlayson, MW Mosesson. *Proc IX Cong Int'l Soc Hematol* 2:205-210, 1962. *Oral presentation.*

6. **HETEROGENEITY OF HUMAN FIBRINOGEN.** JS Finlayson, MW Mosesson. *Biochemistry* 2:42-46, 1963. *The first 'peak 1'/'peak 2' fibrinogen paper.*

7. **CHROMATOGRAPHIC AND RELATED BIOCHEMICAL STUDIES OF FIBRINOGEN.** JS Finlayson, MW Mosesson. *Vox Sang* 8:108-109, 1963. *Once again, I presented at the Protein Foundation. I guess they liked what I had said the first time. But not many questions were posed.*

8. **BIOCHEMICAL AND CHROMATOGRAPHIC STUDIES OF CERTAIN ACTIVITIES ASSOCIATED WITH HUMAN FIBRINOGEN PREPARATIONS.** MW Mosesson, JS Finlayson. *J Clin Invest* 42:747-755, 1963. *The original observations leading to recognition forty or so years later that α2-antiplasmin was covalently bound to circulating fibrinogen*

9. **SUBFRACTIONS OF HUMAN FIBRINOGEN-PREPARATION AND ANALYSIS.** MW Mosesson, JS Finlayson. *J Lab Clin Med 62:663-674, 1963. This method is still used in its original format to prepare fibrinogen subfractions.*

10. **CHROMATOGRAPHIC HETEROGENEITY OF ANIMAL FIBRINOGENS.** JS Finlayson, MW Mosesson. *Biochim Biophys Acta 82:415-417, 1964. Jessica Lewis (Univ Pittsburgh) gave us most of the animal samples. Nowadays I'd have added her name on the paper, but regrettably I hadn't learned the rules of the game at that point.*

11. **THE PREPARATION AND PROPERTIES OF HUMAN FIBRINOGEN OF RELATIVELY HIGH SOLUBILITY.** MW Mosesson, S Sherry. *Biochemistry 5:2829-2835, 1966. This was the first description and characterization of plasma fibrinogens that were separable according to their solubilities, and soon led to the recognition that they represented fibrinogen catabolic processes. WE called them 'Catabolites'.*

12. **HÄMORRHAGISCHE DIATHESE MIT DOMINATEM ERBGANG, VERURSACHT DURCH EIN ANOMALES FIBRINOGEN (FIBRINOGEN BALTIMORE).** EA Beck, MW Mosesson, P Charache, DP Jackson. *Schweiz Med Wschr 96:2296-2299, 1966. Gene Beck was from Switzerland and was doing a fellowship with Dudley Jackson-he sent the 'fibrinogen Baltimore' plasma samples. This was one of the first dysfibrinogens that was clearly described.*

13. **HUMAN FIBRINOGEN OF RELATIVELY HIGH SOLUBILITY. COMPARATIVE BIOPHYSICAL, BIOCHEMICAL AND BIOLOGICAL STUDIES WITH FIBRINOGEN OF LOWER SOLUBILITY.** MW Mosesson, N Alkjaersig, B Sweet, S Sherry. *Biochemistry 6:3279-3287, 1967. Follow up on the 1966 paper. Bernie Sweet, my lifelong friend, was a fellow with Sol Sherry at the same time I was there. He returned to Australia after his fellowship and went into medical practice. I met up with him again 29 years later, and several more times after that.*

14. **CHRONIC INTRAVASCULAR COAGULATION SYNDROME-REPORT OF A CASE WITH SPECIAL STUDIES OF AN ASSOCIATED PLASMA CRYOPRECIPITATE ('CRYOFIBRINOGEN').** MW Mosesson, R Colman, S Sherry. *New Eng J Med 278:815-821, 1968. Mrs Alma Beene became my patient as described in one of the monographs. A lovely person with a great disposition and unfortunately a bad illness. This report described the discovery of a new plasma protein now known as Fibronectin. Franz Ingelfinger was the Journal editor and he made it a worthwhile experience for me. Larry Sherman did the clinical follow up on Mrs. Beene after I had departed to New York at SUNY Downstate- I forgot to include him as a co-author and that may account for him leaving my name off his paper on the in vivo transformation of intact.(low solubility) fibrinogen to α chain degraded (high solubility) fibrinogen, 'fibrinogen catabolites' (Chapter IV).*

15. **ISOLATION AND CHARACTERIZATION OF THE CLOTTABLE LOW MOLECULAR WEIGHT FIBRINOGEN DERIVED BY LIMITED PLASMIN HYDROLYSIS OF HUMAN FRACTION I-4.** LA Sherman, MW Mosesson, S Sherry. *Biochemistry 8:1515-1523, 1969. Larry Sherman was 'assigned' to me by Sol Sherry as a post-doctoral fellow in order that Tony Fletcher not use him in that same capacity. We showed that plasma fibrinogen could be transformed from 'low' to 'high' solubility forms by limited plasmin hydrolysis, and that these products were similar but not identical to the high solubility fibrinogens found in plasma.*

16. **CHROMATOGRAPHIC, ULTRACENTRIFUGAL AND RELATED STUDIES OF FIBRINOGEN 'BALTIMORE'.** MW Mosesson, EA Beck. *J Clin Invest 48:1656-1662, 1969. This was a follow through on my earlier studies on fibrinogen Baltimore.*

17. **STUDIES OF THE AMINO ACID COMPOSITION AND CONFORMATION OF HUMAN FIBRINOGEN-COMPARISON OF FRACTIONS I-4 AND I-8.** R Huseby RM, MW Mosesson, M Murray. *Physiol Chem Phys 2:374-384, 1970. Rolf Huseby was working in Marvin Murray's lab (Louisville, KY) at the time I met and collaborated with him. I also met Agnes Henschen who was in Louisville during that time. Rolf went on to a career in industry with Dade, and we stayed in close touch for several years-he used me as a Dade consultant for a few years, and then he disappeared.*

18. **THE COLD INSOLUBLE GLOBULIN OF HUMAN PLASMA I. PURIFICATION, PRIMARY CHARACTERIZATION AND RELATIONSHIP TO FIBRINOGEN AND OTHER COLD INSOLUBLE FRACTION COMPONENTS.** MW Mosesson, RA Umfleet. *J Biol Chem 245:5728-5736, 1970. This report that described the discovery and the essential features of Plasma Fibronectin (aka, CIg). It was a major follow up on an earlier NEJM paper characterizing Mrs Beene's cold-insoluble plasma protein precipitate that contained Fibrinogen and 'Cold-Insoluble Globulin' (CIg) (see ref 14). There never was a number 'II' in the series.*

19. **FIBRINOGEN BALTIMORE-PHYSICOCHEMICAL CHARACTERIZATION.** MW Mosesson. *Hemophilia and New Hemorrhagic States,* (KM Brinkhous, ed) University North Carolina Press, Chapel Hill 247-253, 1970. *A solicited review.*

20. **MOLECULAR HETEROGENEITY OF HUMAN FIBRINOGEN.** MW Mosesson. *Thromb Diath Haemor Suppl 39:63-70, 1970. A review.*

21. **HIGH SOLUBILITY FIBRINOGEN AND PLASMIN-MEDIATED DEGRADATION PRODUCTS.** MW Mosesson. *Thromb Diath Haemor Suppl 39:255-258, 1970. I had one of several 'dustups' with Victor Marder about these derivatives (also see below). He never did understand that the catabolic fibrinogen derivatives in plasma were qualitatively different from those he had described based upon plasmin digestion products.*

22. **CURRENT STATUS OF KNOWLEDGE OF THE EARLY PLASMIN-MEDIATED HUMAN FIBRINOGEN DEGRADATION PRODUCTS.** MW Mosesson. *Thromb Diath Haemor* Suppl 51:277-281, 1972. *A review.*

23. **HETEROGENEITIES OF HUMAN FIBRINOGEN I. STRUCTURAL AND RELATED STUDIES OF PLASMA FIBRINOGENS WHICH ARE HIGH SOLUBILITY CATABOLIC INTERMEDIATES.** MW Mosesson, JS Finlayson, RA Umfleet, D Galanakis. *J Biol Chem* 247:5210-5219, 1972. *Number 'I' of the 'Trilogy' was a highlight. John and I spent countless hours together composing these papers and I learned much from him about writing and composition.*

24. **HETEROGENEITIES OF HUMAN FIBRINOGEN II. CROSSLINKING CAPACITY OF HIGH SOLUBILITY CATABOLIC INTERMEDIATES.** JS Finlayson, MW Mosesson, TJ Bronzert, JJ Pisano *J Biol Chem* 247:5220-5222, 1972. *Number 'II' was John's baby. He masterminded the interpretation of our findings.*

25. **HETEROGENEITIES OF HUMAN FIBRINOGEN III. IDENTIFICATION OF γ CHAIN VARIANTS.** MW Mosesson, JS Finlayson, RA Umfleet. *J Biol Chem* 247:5223-5227, 1972. *Number 'III' in the series. A great collaboration between John and me. I went on from there to and capitalize on these findings.*

26. **PROPERTIES OF SOLUBLE FIBRIN POLYMERS ENCOUNTERED IN THROMBOTIC STATES.** NU Bang NU, MS Hansen, GF Smith, MW Mosesson. *Thromb Diath Haemor* Suppl 56:75-**90, 1973**. *A report written with Nils Bang that related to 'CIg' (aka Fibronectin). Nils was a good scientist who became submerged by his commercial duties with Eli Lilly. For several years he provided me with an unsolicited $5,000 a year grant from Lilly-much appreciated!*

27. **DEGRADATION OF HUMAN FIBRINOGEN BY PLASMA α_2-MACROGLOBULIN-ENZYME COMPLEXES.** PC Harpel, MW Mosesson. *J Clin Invest* 52:2175-2184, 1973. *Peter and I holed up in a dingy hotel (replete with would-be hookers knocking on the door) in Dallas for two fun days to write this report. We had been searching for an explanation for the differences between plasma fibrinogen derivatives and those formed by plasmin, and we showed that 'plasmin α_2-M' complexes could not account for their existence in circulation.*

28. **CROSSLINKING OF α CHAIN REMNANTS IN HUMAN FIBRIN.** JS Finlayson, MW Mosesson. *Thromb Res* 2:467-478, 1973. *Follow up on ref 24.*

29. **THE ESSENTIAL COVALENT STRUCTURE OF HUMAN FIBRINOGEN EVINCED BY ANALYSIS OF DERIVATIVES FORMED DURING PLASMIC HYDROLYSIS.** MW Mosesson, JS Finlayson, DK Galanakis. *J Biol Chem* 248:7913-7929, 1973. *Wish I had this one back! I made interpretive errors concerning the covalent structure of fibrinogen, and I heard about this in spades from several sources. Although I*

wanted to crawl into a hole and disappear, I never was able to. With trepidation I went back to the experimental drawing board trying to explain the basis for my flawed hypothesis. In the process I learned a lot-Rule 1: 'verify before publishing'. Rule 2: go back and read rule 1. This exercise in humility benefited me for the remainder of my career. To the best of my knowledge, I have not again violated rule 1. I did, in fact, eventually provide a reasonable explanation for my interpretive errors, and I retracted those errant conclusions (see ref. 74). John Finlayson picked the word 'evinced' for the title of this paper.

30. **COMPARISON OF HUMAN PLASMA FIBRINOGEN SUBFRACTIONS AND EARLY PLASMIC FIBRINOGEN DERIVATIVES.** MW Mosesson, DK Galanakis, JS Finlayson. *J Biol Chem* 249:4656-4664, 1974. *Reprising earlier conclusions.*

31. **THE FIBRINOGENOLYTIC PATHWAY OF FIBRINOGEN CATABOLISM: A REBUTTAL.** MW Mosesson MW, JS Finlayson. *Thromb Res* 4:895-900, 1974. *A review.*

32. **THE COLD INSOLUBLE GLOBULIN OF PLASMA AND ITS RELATIONSHIP TO FACTOR VIII.** HA Cooper, R Wagner, MW Mosesson. *J Lab Clin Med* 84:258-263, 1974. *Here I was again in a controversy, but this time it involved factor VIII and fibrinogen. This time I was right-and I partnered with the right collaborators.*

33. **STEROID EFFECTS ON FIBRINOGEN SYNTHESIS BY CULTURED EMBRYONIC CHICKEN HEPATOCYTES**. J Pindyck, MW Mosesson, MW Roomi, RD Levere *Biochem Med* 12:22-31, 1975. *Johanna Pindyck's crowning research achievement.*

34. **THE COLD INSOLUBLE GLOBULIN OF HUMAN PLASMA-STUDIES ON ITS ESSENTIAL STRUCTURAL FEATURES.** MW Mosesson, AB Chen, RM Huseby. *Biochim Biophys Acta* 386:509-524, 1975. *The covalent structure of fibronectin and a significant extension of earlier groundbreaking studies.*

35. **STUDIES ON THE STRUCTURE AND FUNCTION OF α_2-MACROGLOBULIN AND C1 INACTIVATOR.** PC Harpel, MW Mosesson, NR Cooper. *Proteases and Biological Control.* Cold Spring Harbor Laboratory 387-404, 1975. *A reprise.*

36. **CHARACTERISTICS OF PLATELET PROTRANSGLUTAMINASE (FACTOR XIII)-BINDING ACTIVITY IN HUMAN PLASMA.** D Bannerjee, MW Mosesson. *Thromb Res* 7:323-338, 1975. *These results were a 'non--mistake' and I wish I had not lost track of David Bannerjee in the way it occurred. He was a fine, self-effacing investigator from India. I believed that his findings were correct and reproducible. Nevertheless, Jan and Rick McDonagh who also worked on FXIII, had written a half-baked commentary stating that the complexes we had observed were some sort of artifact, I approached David about this issue and asked him whether we should repeat some of the studies. My approach was not as tactful as I thought it had been, and that was all it took for him to 'lose face'. He didn't show up at the lab the next day or ever again, never picked up his paycheck, and I never could*

locate him to discuss this issue. About two years later, having carried out confirmatory studies on my own, I was able to explain why his results were essentially correct-but it was too late for Bannerjee. Although I placed him as first author of reference 43, he never learned about that as far as I knew. I heard he had returned to India, but I couldn't confirm that. The findings in this paper predated by more than twenty years studies that were published in 1996, describing complexation of FXIII with fibrinogen (see ref 147).

37. **STUDIES OF THE STRUCTURAL ABNORMALITY OF FIBRINOGEN PARIS I.** MW Mosesson, DL Amrani, D Ménaché. *J Clin Invest* 57:782-790, 1976. *A detailed follow-up on the first clearly described dysfibrinogen.*

38. **FIBRINOGEN STRUCTURE AFTER SPRAYING ON MICA: ASSESSING THE ELECTRON MICROSCOPIC BASIS FOR A TRINODULAR MODEL.** MW Mosesson. *Thromb Res* 8:737-744, 1976. *This was part of my errant mission to disprove the trinodular model of fibrinogen. It was a clever experiment but framed incorrectly and I soon recognized that (best forgotten).*

39. **IDENTIFICATION OF THE COLD-INSOLUBLE GLOBULIN OF HUMAN PLASMA (CIg) IN AMNIOTIC FLUID.** AB Chen, MW Mosesson, GI Solish. *Amer J Obst Gyn* 125:958-961, 1976. *George Solish was an obstetrician who provided amniotic fluid samples for our study. Shortly after my father's death, George also helped Shirley to abort her fourth pregnancy against my wishes, the one that might have been the child I named after my father.*

40. **EVALUATION OF THE ROLE OF *IN VIVO* PROTEOLYSIS (FIBRINOGENOLYSIS) IN PROLONGING THE THROMBIN TIME OF HUMAN UMBILICAL CORD FIBRINOGEN.** DK Galanakis, MW Mosesson. *Blood* 48:109-118, 1976. *This was one of Denny's independently conducted studies. Good for him!*

41. **HYDROLYSIS OF FIBRINOGEN PARIS I BY PLASMIN.** MW Mosesson, MH Denninger, D Ménaché. *Thromb Res* 9:115-121, 1976. *OK, but so what? Not an earth-shaking study.*

42. **AN IMPROVED METHOD FOR PURIFICATION OF THE COLD-INSOLUBLE GLOBULIN OF HUMAN PLASMA (CIg).** AB Chen, MW Mosesson. *Anal Biochem* 79:144-151, 1977. *Tony Chen now lives in California, and he keeps in touch. This was an improved purification procedure.*

43. **REAPPRAISAL OF THE GEL SIEVING PROPERTIES OF PLASMA PROTRANSGLUTAMINASE (FACTOR XIII).** D Bannerjee, MW Mosesson. *Thromb Res* 10:183-184, 1977. *See ref. 36 commentary.*

44. **CONTROL OF PRODUCTION OF A MAJOR CELL SURFACE GLYCOPROTEIN BY EPIDERMAL GROWTH FACTOR.** LB Chen, RC Gudor, TT

Sun, AB Chen, MW Mosesson. *Science* 197:776-778, 1977. *The first author was Lan Bo Chen. I met him at a Cold Spring Harbor symposium on fibronectin (see also ref. 50).*

45. **THE STRUCTURAL CHARACTERISTICS OF CHICKEN FIBRINOGEN.** J Pindyck, MW Mosesson, D Bannerjee, DK Galanakis. *Biochim Biophys Acta* 492:377-386, 1977. *Johanna Pindyck was completing a Fellowship in my laboratory.*

46. **HETEROGENEITY OF THE COLD-INSOLUBLE GLOBULIN OF HUMAN PLASMA (CIg), A CIRCULATING CELL SURFACE PROTEIN.** AB Chen, DL Amrani, MW Mosesson. *Biochim Biophys Acta* 493:310-322, 1977. *Another study advancing what we knew about CIg.*

47. **PRIMARY STRUCTURE OF THE AMINO TERMINAL REGIONS OF CHICKEN FIBRIN CHAINS.** G Murano, D Walz, L Williams, J Pindyck, MW Mosesson. *Thromb Res.* 11:1-10, 1977. *(Gene: A great study carried out mainly by you!)*

48. **INTERACTIONS AMONG HEPARIN, COLD-INSOLUBLE GLOBULIN, AND FIBRINOGEN IN FORMATION OF THE HEPARIN PRECIPITABLE FRACTION OF PLASMA.** NE Stathakis, MW Mosesson. *J Clin Invest* 60:855-865, 1977. *In this study, spearheaded by Nick Stathakis, we explained how heparin interacts with fibronectin ('cold-insoluble globulin') in the cold to induce what had long been known as the 'heparin-precipitable fraction'. Fibrinogen comes along for the ride whenever it is available. In the next publication we carried out additional studies on the role that fibronectin plays in cold-induced precipitation of fibrin-fibrinogen complexes.*

49. **CRYOPRECIPITATION OF FIBRIN-FIBRINOGEN COMPLEXES INDUCED BY THE COLD-INSOLUBLE GLOBULIN OF PLASMA.** NE Stathakis, MW Mosesson, AB Chen, DK Galanakis. *Blood* 51:1211-1222, 1978. *This study was initiated because we wanted to find an explanation for the components of the 'cryofibrinogen' precipitate that we had observed in Mrs. Alma Beene's plasma cold-insoluble plasma precipitate (see ref. 14). We nailed the key role played by fibronectin in producing such precipitates.*

50. **DISTRIBUTION OF CELL SURFACE LETS PROTEIN IN COCULTURES OF NORMAL AND TRANSFORMED CELLS.** LB Chen, FG Moser, AB Chen, MW Mosesson. *Exptl Cell Res* 108:375-383, 1977. *Everyone was happy with this one.*

51. **STUDIES ON THE STRUCTURE OF HUMAN PLASMA COLD-INSOLUBLE GLOBULIN (CIg) AND THE MECHANISM OF ITS PRECIPITATION IN THE COLD WITH HEPARIN OR FIBRIN-FIBRINOGEN COMPLEXES.** MW Mosesson. *Ann NY Acad Sci* 312:11-30, 1978. *A review of previous work on fibronectin.*

52. **HUMAN FIBRINOGEN HETEROGENEITIES. DISTRIBUTION AND CHARGE CHARACTERISTICS OF CHAINS OF Aα ORIGIN.** DK Galanakis, MW Mosesson, NE Stathakis. *J Lab Clin Med* 92:376-386, 1978. *Denny Galanakis' magnum opus. I was proud of his growth as an experimentalist.*

53. **COMPARISON OF PLASMIC HYDROLYSIS OF NORMAL FIBRINOGEN AND FIBRINOGEN GIESSEN I.** MW Mosesson, PD Natale, DL Amrani, LA Sherman, JH Joist, WH Krause *Thromb Res* 12:693-696, 1978. *I don't remember the details of this study anymore, but they were not mind bending.*

54. **HUMAN FIBRINOGEN HETEROGENEITIES. PREPARATION AND CHARACTERIZATION OF γ AND γ' CHAINS.** NE Stathakis, MW Mosesson, DK Galanakis, D Ménaché. *Thromb Res* 13:467-475, 1978. *A simpler method for separating γ chain variants.*

55. **CHARACTERIZATION OF AMEBOCYTE COAGULOGEN FROM THE HORSESHOE CRAB (LIMULUS POLYPHEMUS).** MW Mosesson, C Wolfenstein-Todel, J Levin, O Bertrand. *Thromb Res* 14:765-779, 1979. *Worked with Jack Levin at Woods Hole, MA, for several summers on this subject. My initial interest was to determine whether this primitive creature's coagulation protein bore any resemblance to mammalian fibrinogen-it did not! But it was still a wonderful subject and a great way to spend summers together with my family at Woods Hole.*

56. **EVALUATION OF TWO NEW ASSAYS FOR DETERMINATION OF SERUM FIBRINOGEN/FIBRIN DEGRADATION PRODUCTS.** K Sumner, E Feller, DK Galanakis, MW Mosesson *Ann Clin Lab Sci* 9:362-367, 1979. *Minor stuff!*

57. **DELAYED-TYPE HYPERSENSITIVITY SKIN REACTIONS IN CONGENITAL AFIBRINOGENEMIA-LACK OF FIBRIN DEPOSITION AND INDURATION.** RB Colvin, MW Mosesson, HF Dvorak. *J Clin Invest* 63:1302-1306, 1979. *Bob Colvin later became chairman of the Department of Pathology at Massachusetts General. Together, we studied the delayed hypersensitivity reaction in two afibrinogenemic subjects-important results on the role played by fibrinogen in delayed hypersensitivity reactions.*

58. **PRODUCTION OF FIBRONECTIN (LETS PROTEIN) BY HUMAN EPITHELIAL CELLS IN CULTURE.** HS Smith, JR Riggs, MW Mosesson. *Cancer Res* 39:4138-4144, 1979. *I met Helene Smith at a Cold Springs Harbor Symposium and we cooked up this collaboration.*

59. **RELEASE OF PLATELET FIBRONECTIN (COLD-INSOLUBLE GLOBULIN) FROM ALPHA GRANULES INDUCED BY THROMBIN OR COLLAGEN, AND THE LACK OF REQUIREMENT FOR PLASMA FIBRONECTIN IN ADP-INDUCED PLATELET AGGREGATION.** MB Zucker, MW Mosesson, MJ Broekman, KL Kaplan. *Blood* 54:8-12, 1979. *Marge Zucker was a platelet 'maven' at NYU, a member of our 'New York Clot Club'. We collaborated in this interesting study.*

60. **STRUCTURAL STUDIES OF THE COAGULOGEN OF AMEBOCYTE LYSATE FROM LIMULUS POLYPHEMUS.** MW Mosesson, C Wolfenstein-Todel, J Levin,

O Bertrand. *Progress in Clinical and Biological Research* (E. Cohen, ed) Alan R. Liss, Inc., New York, Pub. 29:159-168, 1979. *A reprise.*

61. **THE Aα CHAIN COMPOSITION OF PLASMA FIBRINOGEN CATABOLITES.** DK Galanakis, MW Mosesson. *Thromb Res* 15:287-289, 1979. *Denny played a key role in writing up this work. I took pride in his growth as an investigator.*

62. **STUDIES OF PLATELET FIBRINOGEN FROM A SUBJECT WITH A CONGENITAL PLASMA FIBRINOGEN ABNORMALITY (FIBRINOGEN PARIS I).** M Jandrot-Perrus, MW Mosesson, M-H Denninger, D Ménaché. *Blood* 54:1109-1116, 1979. *Martine was a post-doc with Doris, and this was her project. Marie-Hélène helped us a lot and was a joy to work with. We all remained friends for a long time. Martine spent a few weeks in my SUNY laboratory as a follow-up to this study and she lived with us during her visit. Aimee eventually spent a few weeks in Paris living with Marie-Hélène's family, mainly to improve her French and met some new people.*

63. **APPLICATION OF ELECTROIMMUNOASSAY TO THE STUDY OF PLASMA PROTEIN SYNTHESIS IN CULTURED HEPATOCYTES.** G Grieninger, J Pindyck, KM Hertzberg, MW Mosesson. *Ann Clin Lab Sci* 9:511-517, 1979. *An okay study! I did not become heavily engaged in it.*

64. **CELL SURFACE FIBRINOGEN FIBRIN RECEPTORS ON CULTURED HUMAN FIBROBLASTS: ASSOCIATION WITH COLD-INSOLUBLE GLOBULIN (FIBRONECTIN) AND LOSS IN SV-40 TRANSFORMED CELLS.** RB Colvin, PI Gardner, RO Roblin, EL Verderberg, JM Lanigan, MW Mosesson. *Lab Invest* 41:464-473, 1979. *A good study. No further comment.*

65. **ELECTRON MICROSCOPY OF METAL-SHADOWED FIBRINOGEN MOLECULES DEPOSITED AT DIFFERENT CONCENTRATIONS.** MW Mosesson, J Escaig, G Feldmann. *Brit J Haematol* 43:469-477, 1979. *I did this study at Jacque Escaig's laboratory while I was on sabbatical in Paris. Jacque had an engineering background and was developing new freeze-drying equipment for preparing EM specimens. (see Chapter V) He did not know much about fibrinogen, but his equipment was superb (except for the artefacts that Gérard Feldmann and I misinterpreted). We talked a lot and had much fun together doing ordinary things like eating Croque Monsieurs with a glass of wine for lunch. I liked him and his family, and we remained in close touch until his death by drowning in a California riptide in 1986.*

66. **PROPERTIES OF EPITHELIAL CELLS CULTURED FROM HUMAN CARCINOMAS AND NON-MALIGNANT TISSUES.** HS Smith, AJ Hackett, JL Riggs, MW Mosesson, JR Walton, MR Stampfer. *J Supramol Str* 11:147-166, 1979. *I collaborated with Helene Smith whom I met at a Cold Spring Harbor conference.*

67. Ibid in **TUMOR CELL SURFACES AND MALIGNANCY. PROGRESS IN CLINICAL AND BIOLOGICAL RESEARCH.** (RO Hynes, F Fox, eds) Alan R Liss, Inc., Pub. 41:93-112, 1980.

68. **FIBRINOPEPTIDE RELEASE FROM FIBRINOGEN PARIS I.** JS Finlayson, LA Reamer, MW Mosesson, D Ménaché. *Thromb Res* 17:577-579, 1980. *Peptide release was the same as the normal control, as expected.*

69. **ELECTRON MICROSCOPY OF FIBRIN PARIS I.** MW Mosesson, G Feldmann, D Ménaché. *Blood* 56:80-83, 1980. *Interesting results but difficult to interpret at that time.*

70. **HUMAN PLASMA FIBRINOGEN HETEROGENEITY: EVIDENCE FOR AN EXTENDED CARBOXYL-TERMINAL SEQUENCE IN A NORMAL γ CHAIN VARIANT (γ').** C Wolfenstein-Todel, MW Mosesson. *Proc Natl Acad Sci (USA)* 77:5069-5073, 1980. *Carlotta was especially good at amino acid sequencing (also see ref. 75 and Chapter VII).*

71. **THYROID HORMONE STIMULATION OF PLASMA PROTEIN SYNTHESIS IN CULTURED HEPATOCYTES.** KM Hertzberg, J Pindyck, MW Mosesson, G Grieninger. *J Biol Chem* 256:563-566, 1981.

72. **RECEPTORS FOR COLD-INSOLUBLE GLOBULIN (PLASMA FIBRONECTIN) ON HUMAN MONOCYTES.** MP Bevilacqua, D Amrani, MW Mosesson, C Bianco. *J Exp Med* 153:42-60, 1981. *This was a productive collaboration between me and Celso Bianco who was the thesis advisor for Michael Bevilacqua. I especially enjoyed participating in this with Celso, we had many productive discussions together, and I was able to make many useful contributions.*

73. **DETECTION AND QUANTITATION OF FIBRONECTIN IN SYNOVIAL FLUID FROM PATIENTS WITH RHEUMATIC DISEASE.** S Carsons, MW Mosesson, HS Diamond. *Arthr Rheum* 24:1261-1267, 1981.

74. **IDENTIFICATION AND MASS ANALYSIS OF HUMAN FIBRINOGEN MOLECULES AND THEIR DOMAINS BY SCANNING TRANSMISSION ELECTRON MICROSCOPY (STEM).** MW Mosesson, J Hainfeld, RH Haschemeyer, J Wall. *J Mol Biol* 153:695-718, 1981. *This was a great study! In s single stroke I disproved my earlier hypothesis on the covalent structure of fibrinogen (1973) and made valuable new contributions. By the time I met Rudy Haschemeyer he was an alcoholic, but smart and coherent at most times. He came with me on my first trip to Brookhaven to help me interpret the experiments. He had been married to Audrey Haschemeyer who started out as his graduate student and who I subsequently met at Woods Hole. She was an excellent singer, but I don't think she ended up very well. She was living in Paris last I heard.*

75. **CARBOXY-TERMINAL AMINO ACID SEQUENCE OF A HUMAN FIBRINOGEN γ CHAIN VARIANT (γ').** C Wolfenstein-Todel, MW Mosesson. *Biochemistry* 20:6146-6149, 1981. *(see ref. 70)*

76. **DISTRIBUTION OF PLASMA FIBRONECTIN (COLD-INSOLUBLE GLOBULIN) AND COMPONENTS OF THE FACTOR VIII COMPLEX AFTER HEPARIN-INDUCED PRECIPITATION OF PLASMA.** DL Amrani, MW Mosesson, L Hoyer. *Blood* 59:657-663, 1982. *A nice piece of work by David.*

77. **SYNOVIAL FLUID FIBRONECTIN.** S Carsons, BB Lavietes, HS Diamond, MW Mosesson. *Eur J Clin Invest* 12:8, 1982 (Letter-to-the-editor).

78. **EVIDENCE FOR CIRCULATING FIBRIN IN FAMILIAL MEDITERRANEAN FEVER.** MW Mosesson, JL Wautier, DL Amrani, M Dervichian, D Cattan. *J Lab Clin Med* 99:559-567, 1982. *This was a really interesting study. I do not understand completely why high levels of circulating soluble fibrin are so often found in FMF plasmas. The study is not cited very often, if at all, but someday it may have audience.*

79. **EVIDENCE FOR TWO CLASSES OF RAT PLASMA FIBRINOGEN γ CHAINS DIFFERING BY THEIR COOH-TERMINAL AMINO ACID SEQUENCES.** CD Legrele CD, C Wolfenstein-Todel, Y Hurbourg, MW Mosesson. *Biochem Biophys Res Comm* 105:521-529, 1982. *Between 1980 and 1981 Claude Legrele (The University of Reims), visited my laboratory for several weeks while I was still at SUNY, Downstate Medical Center, and we studied the fibrinogen of his favorite rodent, the rat. We had met while I was on sabbatical in Paris. Not only did we become close friends, but we showed that rat fibrinogen contained substantial quantities of the γ' chain variant. Years later I realized that the rat γ' chain was nearly identical to that of its cousin the mouse, and that neither rodent's fibrinogen possessed thrombin binding potential! That knowledge contributed to creation of the hu-γ' mouse (Chapter VIII).*

80. **NEAR ULTRAVIOLET CIRCULAR DICHROISM SPECTROSCOPY OF PLASMA FIBRONECTIN AND FIBRONECTIN FRAGMENTS.** NM Tooney, DL Amrani, GA Homandberg, JA McDonald, MW Mosesson. *Biochem Biophys Res Comm* 108:1085-1091, 1982. *Nancy was from Pace College in Brooklyn. She had been a post-doc with Carolyn Cohen, the 'Jewish Princess' from Brandeis University. I recruited Nancy to Milwaukee to enhance my biophysical section, but she turned out to be incapable of doing this. She wasn't 'focused' (my pun on electron microscopy), she didn't know or learn much about fibrinogen, and she was extremely rigid. I believe she moved to Milwaukee with me to have a well-paid leave-of-absence from Pace University. She stayed in Milwaukee for two years before returning to NYC to well-deserved obscurity. On balance, she was a bust!*

81. **STRUCTURAL ANALYSIS OF FIBRINOGEN SYNTHESIS BY CULTURED CHICKEN HEPATOCYTES IN THE PRESENCE OR ABSENCE OF**

DEXAMETHASONE. DL Amrani, PW Plant, J Pindyck, MW Mosesson, G Grieninger. *Biochim Biophys Acta* 743:394-400, 1983.

82. **FIBRINOGEN HETEROGENEITIES: DETERMINATION OF THE MAJOR Aα CHAIN DERIVATIVES IN BLOOD.** DK Galanakis, MW Mosesson. *Thromb Res* 31:403-413, 1983. *Good job, Denny!*

83. **PLASMA FIBRONECTIN-Clq COMPLEX FORMATION AND ITS EFFECT ON COLLAGEN-INDUCED PLATELET AGGREGATION.** JL Wautier, MP Wautier, H Kadeva, MW Mosesson. *Thromb Res* 32:283-290, 1983. *Shirley and I had several pleasant personal meetings with Jean-Luc and Marie-Paul Wautier during my sabbatical year in Paris.*

84. **HORMONAL REGULATION OF FIBRINOGEN SYNTHESIS IN CULTURED HEPATOCYTES.** G Grieninger, PW Plant, TJ Liang, RG Kalb, DL Amrani, MW Mosesson, KM Hertzberg, J Pindyck. *Ann NY Acad Sci* 408:97-113, 1983. *A reprise.*

85. **ANALYSIS OF HUMAN FIBRINOGEN BY SCANNING TRANSMISSION ELECTRON MICROSCOPY.** J Wall, J Hainfeld, RH Haschemeyer, MW Mosesson. *Ann NY Acad Sci* 408:164-179, 1983. *This was a reprise of our study published in The Journal of Molecular Biology (ref. 74).*

86. **SOLUTION AND SURFACE EFFECTS ON PLASMA FIBRONECTIN STRUCTURE.** NM Tooney, MW Mosesson, DL Amrani, JF Hainfeld, JS Wall. *J Cell Biol* 97:1686-1692, 1983. *Still trying to figure this one out.*

87. **SEPARATION AND ANALYSIS OF THE MAJOR FORMS OF PLASMA FIBRONECTIN.** DL Amrani, GA Homandberg, NM Tooney, C Wolfenstein-Todel, MW Mosesson. *Biochim Biophys Acta* 748:308-320, 1983. *This was the main piece of work for David's PhD thesis.*

88. **EVIDENCE THAT THE γ CHAIN POPULATION OF HUMAN PLATELET FIBRINOGEN LACKS THE γ' VARIANT THAT IS PRESENT IN PLASMA FIBRINOGEN.** Mosesson MW, GA Homandberg, DL Amrani. In *Fibrinogen and Its Degradation Products - Structure and Function* (Henschen A, ed) W de Gruyter, Pub 3:133-145, 1983. *A reprise.*

89. **HUMAN PLATELET FIBRINOGEN GAMMA CHAIN STRUCTURE.** MW Mosesson, GA Homandberg, DL Amrani *Blood* 63:990-995, 1984. *We had expected these results.*

90. **CLEAVAGE OF FIBRINOGEN BY HUMAN PLATELET CALCIUM-ACTIVATED PROTEASE.** TJ Kunicki, MW Mosesson, D Pidard. *Thromb Res* 35:169-182, 1984.

91. **FIBRONECTIN DEPOSITION IN DELAYED-TYPE HYPERSENSITIVITY. REACTIONS OF NORMALS AND A PATIENT WITH AFIBRINOGENEMIA.** RAF Clark, CR Horsburgh, AA Hoffman, HF Dvorak, MW Mosesson, RB Colvin. *J Clin Invest* 74:1011-1016, 1984. *Richard Clark became chairman of the Department of Dermatology at SUNY-Stony Brook. An extension of Colvin's and my study of Afibrinogenemic subjects (see ref. 57).*

92. **STUDIES ON THE STRUCTURE OF BOVINE FACTOR V BY SCANNING TRANSMISSION ELECTRON MICROSCOPY (STEM).** MW Mosesson, ME Nesheim, J DiOrio, JF Hainfeld, JS Wall, KG Mann. *Blood* 65:1158-1162, 1985... *Mike Nesheim had some interesting times at Brookhaven imaging factor V molecules.*

93. **EVIDENCE THAT RAT PLATELET FIBRINOGEN MOLECULES LACK THE γ' CHAIN VARIANT FOUND IN PLASMA FIBRINOGEN MOLECULES.** GA Homandberg, JE Williams, DB Evans, MW Mosesson. *Thromb Res* 38:203-209, 1985.

94. **PREPARATION OF FUNCTIONALLY INTACT MONOMERS BY LIMITED DISULFIDE REDUCTION OF HUMAN PLASMA FIBRONECTIN DIMERS.** GA Homandberg, DL Amrani, DB Evans, CM Kane, E Ankel, MW Mosesson. *Arch Biochem Biophys* 238:652-663, 1985...*Interesting project but then I also had to deal with Gene Homandberg.*

95. **STUDIES OF FIBRONECTIN SYNTHESIZED BY CULTURED CHICK HEPATOCYTES.** DL Amrani, MJ Falk, MW Mosesson. *Exp Cell Res* 160:171-183, 1985.

96. **HUMAN PLATELET FIBRINOGEN: PURIFICATION AND HEMOSTATIC PROPERTIES.** TJ Kunicki, PJ Newman, DL Amrani, MW Mosesson. *Blood* 66:808-815, 1985.

97. **AMINO ACID SEQUENCE OF COOH-TERMINAL REGIONS OF RAT PLASMA FIBRINOGEN γA AND γ' CHAINS.** GA Homandberg, D Evans, C Kane, MW Mosesson. *Thromb Res* 39:263-269, 1985

98. **EVIDENCE THAT PRODUCTION OF PLATELET FIBRINOGEN IS SYNCHRONOUS WITH PLATELET PRODUCTION IN THE TURPENTINE-INDUCED ACUTE PHASE RESPONSE.** JE Williams, JJ Cypher, MW Mosesson. *J Lab Clin Med* 106:343-348, 1985. *Jim Willams was an excellent anatomical pathologist who wanted to learn basic research. I picked this topic for him since it was a hot subject at the time and of well-circumscribed scope. Jim had a wonderful operatic singing voice and Jeff Cypher was a good technologist who carried out most of the bench analyses.*

99. **EVIDENCE THAT CHICKEN ANTITHROMBIN III IS A DEVELOPMENTALLY REGULATED HEPATOCYTE GLYCOPROTEIN.** DL Amrani, MW Mosesson, T Koide. *Biochim Biophys Acta* 847:324-334, 1985. *So it is!*

100. **EFFECT OF HEPATOCYTE STIMULATING FACTOR AND GLUCOCORTICOIDS ON PLASMA FIBRONECTIN LEVELS.** DL Amrani, D Mauzy-Melitz, MW Mosesson. *Biochem J* 238:365-371, 1986. *Debbie Mauzy-Melitz worked at my laboratory for a few years and finally earned her PhD at Marquette University.*

101. **EVIDENCE THAT PROXIMAL NH$_2$-TERMINAL PORTIONS OF FIBRINOGEN METZ (Aα16 Arg→Cys) Aα CHAINS ARE ORIENTED IN THE SAME DIRECTION.** MW Mosesson, KR Siebenlist, JP DiOrio, JF Hainfeld, JS Wall, J Soria, C Soria, M Samama. *Fibrinogen and Its Derivatives* (Müller-Berghaus G, U Scheefers-Borchel, E Selmayr, A Henschen, eds). Elsevier Science Pub, NY, 3-15, 1986. *This was a really cool study, most of it devised by Kevin. It never got much attention but turned out to be correct.*

102. **STUDIES ON THE ULTRASTRUCTURE OF FIBRIN LACKING FIBRINOPEPTIDE B (β-FIBRIN).** MW Mosesson, JP DiOrio, MF Müller, JR Shainoff, KR Siebenlist, DL Amrani, GA Homandberg, J Soria, C Soria, M Samama. *Blood* 69:1073-1081, 1987. *Nice study. Jim DiOrio was a key investigator.*

103. **EVALUATION OF FACTOR VIII-RICH CRYOPRECIPITATE AND THE PLASMA FIBRONECTIN-RICH HEPARIN-PRECIPITABLE FRACTION PREPARED FROM SINGLE DONOR UNITS.** JE Menitove, DL Amrani, D Meh, M Frenzke, MW Mosesson. *Transfusion* 27:491-494, 1987.

104. **ADP-INDUCED PLATELET AGGREGATION DEPENDS UPON THE CONFORMATION OR AVAILABILITY OF THE TERMINAL GAMMA CHAIN SEQUENCE OF FIBRINOGEN. STUDY OF THE REACTIVITY OF FIBRINOGEN PARIS I.** MH Denninger, M Jandrot-Perrus, J Elion, O Bertrand, GA Homandberg, MW Mosesson, M-C Guillin. *Blood* 70:558-563, 1987.

105. **FIBRINOGEN BIRMINGHAM: A NEW HETERODIMERIC DYSFIBRINOGENEMIA WITH DEFECTIVE FIBRINOPEPTIDE A RELEASE (Aα Arg 16→His).** KR Siebenlist KR, JT Prchal, MW Mosesson. *Fibrinogen 2. Biochemistry, Physiology, and Clinical Relevance* (Lowe GDO, JT Douglas, CD Forbes, A Henschen, eds) Elsevier Science Pub, NY, 63-66, 1987.

106. **THE ROLE OF FIBRINOGEN Aα CHAINS IN ADP-INDUCED PLATELET AGGREGATION IN THE PRESENCE OF FIBRINOGEN MOLECULES CONTAINING γ' CHAINS.** DL Amrani, PJ Newman, MW Mosesson. *Fibrinogen 2. Biochemistry, Physiology, and Clinical Relevance* (Lowe GDO, JT Douglas, CD Forbes, A Henschen, eds). Elsevier Science Pub, NY, 136-142, 1987.

107. **ESSENTIAL THROMBOCYTHEMIA IN PREGNANCY.** EC Jones, MW Mosesson, JL Thomason, TC Jackson. *Obst Gyn* 71:501-513, 1988. *This clinical project was my idea. Jones was a practicing obstetrician.*

108. **FIBRINOGEN BIRMINGHAM: A HETEROZYGOUS DYSFIBRINOGENEMIA (Aα16 ARG→HIS) CONTAINING HETERODIMERIC MOLECULES.** KR Siebenlist, JT Prchal, MW Mosesson. *Blood* 71:613-618, 1988.

109. **THE ROLE OF FIBRINOGEN Aα CHAINS IN ADP-INDUCED PLATELET AGGREGATION IN THE PRESENCE OF FIBRINOGEN MOLECULES CONTAINING γ' CHAINS.** DL Amrani, PJ Newman, D Meh, MW Mosesson. *Blood* 72:919-924, 1988.

110. **EVIDENCE THAT BINDING TO THE CARBOXYL-TERMINAL HEPARIN BINDING DOMAIN ('HEP II') DOMINATES THE INTERACTION BETWEEN PLASMA FIBRONECTIN AND HEPARIN.** MJ Benecky, CG Kolvenbach, DL Amrani, MW Mosesson. *Biochemistry* 27:7565-7571, 1988. *Mike Benecky was a Dweeb.*

111. **EVIDENCE FOR THE EXISTENCE OF TRIMERIC AND TETRAMERIC PLASMIC D FRAGMENTS DERIVED FROM FIBRIL JUNCTIONS OR TRIFUNCTIONAL BRANCH POINTS IN THE CROSSLINKED FIBRIN MATRIX.** MW Mosesson, KR Siebenlist, DL Amrani, JP DiOrio. *Fibrinogen 3. Biochemistry, Biological Functions, Gene Regulation and Expression.* (Mosesson MW, DL Amrani, JP DiOrio, KR Siebenlist, eds) Elsevier Science Pub, NY, 99-104, 1988. (*see ref. 114*).

112. **STUDIES ON THE POLYMERIZATION OF FIBRIN HAIFA (γ275 ARG→HIS).** KR Siebenlist, MW Mosesson, JP DiOrio, S Tavori, I Tatarsky, & A Rimon. *Fibrinogen 3. Biochemistry, Biological Functions, Gene Regulation and Expression* (MW Mosesson, DL Amrani, JP DiOrio, KR Siebenlist, eds) Elsevier Science Pub, NY, 271-274, 1988.

113. **THE ULTRASTRUCTURE OF FIBRIN PREPARED FROM FIBRINOGEN HAIFA (γ275 ARG→HIS).** KR Siebenlist, MW Mosesson, JP DiOrio, S Tavori, I Tatarsky, A Rimon. Proc. 46 Ann Mtg Electron Microscope Society of America (EMSA), 248-249, 1988.

114. **IDENTIFICATION OF COVALENTLY LINKED TRIMERIC AND TETRAMERIC D DOMAINS IN CROSSLINKED FIBRIN.** MW Mosesson, KR Siebenlist, DL Amrani, JP DiOrio. *Proc Natl Acad Sci (USA)* 86:1113-1117, 1989. (see Chapters VI and VII). *An important study bearing on fibrin branch junctions and transverse γ chain 'cross-linking'.*

115. **FATAL SMALL BOWEL NECROSIS AND PULMONARY HYPERTENSION IN SICKLE CELL DISEASE.** TE Hammond, MW Mosesson. *Arch Int Med* 149:447-448, 1989. *I engineered this publication as a teacher/student exercise with Tim Hammond, a*

promising clinician/investigator. I enjoyed doing this and even presented a 'Grand Rounds' on this subject.

116. **TERMINOLOGY FOR FIBRINOGEN γ–CHAINS DIFFERING IN CARBOXYL TERMINAL AMINO ACID SEQUENCE.** CW Francis, MW Mosesson. *Thromb Haemostas* 62:813-814, 1989.

117. **THE POLYMERIZATION OF FIBRIN PREPARED FROM FIBRINOGEN HAIFA (γ275 ARG→HIS).** KR Siebenlist, MW Mosesson, JP DiOrio, S Tavori, I Tatarsky, & A Rimon. *Thromb Haemostas* 62:875-879, 1989.

118. **STUDIES ON THE CONVERSION OF DES Bβ 1-42 FIBRINOGEN TO FIBRIN AND THE THROMBIN BINDING PROPERTIES OF DES Bβ 1-42 FIBRIN.** MW Mosesson, KR Siebenlist, JP DiOrio, AZ Budzinski. *Fibrinogen 4. Current Basic and Clinical Aspects* (M Matsuda, S. Iwanaga, A Takada, A Henschen, eds) Elsevier Science Pub, NY 13-20, 1990. *Presented at the Kyoto Fibrinogen Workshop in 1989.*

119. **HUMAN PLASMA FIBRONECTIN STRUCTURE PROBED BY STEADY-STATE FLUORESCENCE POLARIZATION: EVIDENCE FOR A RIGID OBLATE STRUCTURE.** MJ Benecky, CG Kolvenbach, RW Wine, JP DiOrio, MW Mosesson. *Biochemistry* 29:3082-3091, 1990 *I'm still not sure whether this was a verifiable conclusion.*

120. **STRUCTURAL MODEL OF FACTORS V AND Va BASED ON SCANNING TRANSMISSION ELECTRON MICROSCOPE IMAGES AND MASS ANALYSIS.** MW Mosesson, WR Church, JP DiOrio, S Krishnaswamy, KG Mann, JF Hainfeld, JS Wall. *J Biol Chem* 265:8863-8868, 1990. *Beautiful STEM images of Factor V and Va molecules, permitting a structural model to be presented.*

121. **STRUCTURAL MODEL OF FACTORS VIII AND VIIIa BASED ON SCANNING TRANSMISSION ELECTRON MICROSCOPE (STEM) IMAGES AND STEM MASS ANALYSIS.** MW Mosesson MW, DN Fass, P Lollar, JP DiOrio, CG Parker, GJ Knutson, JF Hainfeld, JS Wall. *J Clin Invest* 85:1983-1990, 1990 *This was a good study, providing the first high resolution STEM images of factor VIII. Pete Lollar was a key collaborator. He and I went to BNL several times to carry out these experiments together. Our extra-curricular activities included seeing 'Les Miserables' on Broadway and watching the Atlanta Braves get beaten that year.*

122. **THE POLYMERIZATION AND THROMBIN BINDING PROPERTIES OF DES-(Bβ 1-42)-FIBRIN.** KR Siebenlist, JP DiOrio, AZ Budzynski, MW Mosesson. *J Biol Chem* 265:18650-18655, 1990 *A study that provided new and still relevant information on Des-(Bβ 1-42)-Fibrin.*

123. **THE ACCELERATORY EFFECT OF THROMBIN ON FIBRIN CLOT ASSEMBLY.** MW Mosesson, M Kaminski. *Blood Coagulation & Fibrinolysis* 1:475-478, 1990. *What a story this turned out to be....'The Kamiski effect'! (see Chapter VIII).*

124. **EVIDENCE FOR THROMBIN ENHANCEMENT OF FIBRIN POLYMERIZATION THAT IS INDEPENDENT OF ITS CATALYTIC ACTIVITY.** M Kaminski, KR Siebenlist, MW Mosesson. *J Lab Clin Med* 117:218-225, 1991. *We called this 'The Kaminski Effect', and it turned into a rather big deal. Marek was a bust both experimentally and clinically, but I appreciated that he had some good ideas and therefore pursued this subject.*

125. **IONIC STRENGTH-AND pH-DEPENDENT CONFORMATIONAL STATES OF HUMAN PLASMA FIBRONECTIN.** MJ Benecky, RW Wine, CG Kolvenbach, MW Mosesson. *Biochemistry* 30:4298-4306, 1991...*Rich Wine was ideal for working in industry and while he was with me, he was also an excellent technologist, especially at biophysical techniques. He was a favorite of Jim DiOrio's and Kevin's. He married Robin Yamashita who also worked in my lab-the neatest handwriting, data-recording, color-coding technologist I have ever known. We still use some of the fibrinogen samples she prepared as 'gold standards.'*

126. **HEMOSTATIC EVALUATION OF SARNS/3M-VAD IMPLANTATION IN CALVES.** DL Amrani, C Christensen, L Hauerwas, M Rieder, MW Mosesson, D Schmidt, R Flemma, GA Prophet, W Pierce. *Trans Amer Soc Artif Intern Organs* 37:M308-M310, 1991 *A report on a part of the 'Milwaukee Heart Project' at the Winter Research Institute (1986-1999). I was one of three Directors, along with Robert Flemma and Donald Schmidt. Unfortunately, we failed to develop a transplantable, battery-driven, mechanical VAD for use in humans (mainly for lack of funding), but we did get close with a VAD that was successfully implanted in calves for more than two months.*

127. **FACTORS AFFECTING γ CHAIN MULTIMER FORMATION IN CROSS-LINKED FIBRIN.** KR Siebenlist, MW Mosesson. *Biochemistry* 31:936-941, 1992 *Kevin's work.*

128. **CHARACTERIZATION OF THE γ CHAIN PLATELET BINDING SITE ON FIBRINOGEN FRAGMENT D.** NE Kirschbaum, MW Mosesson, DL Amrani. *Blood* 79:2643-2648, 1992 *Nancy the Nebish couldn't take instruction and didn't want any. She was a dud!*

129. **THE ULTRASTRUCTURE OF FIBRIN PREPARED FROM FIBRINOGEN ASAHI (γ310 Met→Thr) AND FIBRINOGEN MORIOKA (γ275 Arg→Cys).** JP DiOrio, KR Siebenlist, S Terukina, K Yamazumi, M Matsuda, MW Mosesson. 50th Ann Mtg Electron Microscope Society of America (EMSA) 1090-91, 1992 *Jim DiOrio liked to present a poster at each EMSA meeting.*

130. **MOLECULAR BASIS OF FIBRINOGEN DUSART (Aα Arg 554→Cys) AND ITS ASSOCIATION WITH ABNORMAL FIBRIN POLYMERIZATION AND THROMBOPHILIA.** J Koopman, F Haverkate, J Grimbergen, ST Lord, MW Mosesson, JP DiOrio, KR Siebenlist, C Legrand, J Soria, C Soria, JP Caen. *J Clin Invest* 91:1637-43, 1993.

131. **PARIS I DYSFIBRINOGENEMIA: A POINT MUTATION IN INTRON 8 RESULTS IN INSERTION OF A 15 AMINO ACID SEQUENCE IN THE FIBRINOGEN γ CHAIN.** JB Rosenberg, PJ Newman, MW Mosesson, M-C Guillin, DL Amrani. *Thromb Haemost* 69:217-20, 1993 *Jonathan Rosenberg worked for DLA and moved to the BRI with me for a while. I don't remember how Peter Newman got his name on this publication unless it was because Jonathan had previously worked for him.*

132. **THE CLEAVAGE SEQUENCE OF FIBRINOPEPTIDE A FROM FIBRINOGEN FRAGMENT E BY THROMBIN, ATROXIN, OR BATROXOBIN.** DA Meh, KR Siebenlist, G Bergtrom, MW Mosesson. *Blood Coag Fibrinolysis* 4:107-112, 1993.

133. **THE POLYMERIZATION OF FIBRINOGEN DUSART (Aα 554 ARG→CYS) AFTER REMOVAL OF CARBOXY TERMINAL REGIONS OF THE Aα CHAIN.** KR Siebenlist, MW Mosesson, JP DiOrio, J Soria, C Soria, JP Caen. *Blood Coag Fibrinolysis* 4:61-65, 1993

134. **FACTORS AFFECTING FACTOR XIIIa-CATALYZED γ-CHAIN CROSSLINKING IN FIBRIN.** KR Siebenlist, MW Mosesson. *Factor XIII (Second Int'l Conf., Marburg) (McDonagh J, R Seitz, R Egbring, Eds) Schattauer, Stuttgart,* 46-51, 1993 *A good conference!*

135. **COMPARISON OF THE SEQUENCE OF FIBRINOPEPTIDE A CLEAVAGE FROM FIBRINOGEN FRAGMENT E BY THROMBIN, ATROXIN AND BATROXOBIN.** DA Meh, KR Siebenlist, G Bergtrom, MW Mosesson. *Thromb Res* 70:437-449, 1993.

136. **EVIDENCE FOR A SECOND TYPE OF FIBRIL BRANCH POINT IN FIBRIN POLYMER NETWORKS, THE TRIMOLECULAR JUNCTION.** MW Mosesson, JP DiOrio, KR Siebenlist, JS Wall, JF Hainfeld. *Blood* 82:1517-1521, 1993 *Kevin drew his idea of the scheme for trimolecular junction formation for me, and that was what I needed to complete this report.*

137. **PROGRESSIVE CROSSLINKING OF FIBRIN γ CHAINS INCREASES RESISTANCE TO FIBRINOLYSIS.** KR Siebenlist, MW Mosesson. *J Biol Chem* 269:28414-28419, 1994, *Kevin's project.*

138. **THE SEQUENCE OF RELEASE OF FIBRINOPEPTIDE A FROM FIBRINOGEN MOLECULES BY THROMBIN OR ATROXIN.** DA Meh, KR Siebenlist, G Bergtrom, MW Mosesson. *J Lab Clin Med* 125:384-391, 1995.

139. **THE DIMERIC Aα CHAIN COMPOSITION OF DYSFIBRINOGENEMIC MOLECULES WITH MUTATIONS AT Aα 16.** DA Meh, KR Siebenlist, DK Galanakis, G Bergtrom, MW Mosesson. *Thromb Res* 78:531-539, 1995.

140. **TERMINOLOGY FOR MACROMOLECULAR DERIVATIVES OF CROSSLINKED FIBRIN.** MW Mosesson. *Thromb Haemostas* 73(4):725-726, 1995.

141. **THE COVALENT STRUCTURE OF FACTOR XIIIa-CROSSLINKED FIBRINOGEN FIBRILS.** MW Mosesson, KR Siebenlist, JF Hainfeld, JS Wall. *J Structural Biol* 115:88-101,1995. *This was a dynamite paper, but it never got the attention it deserved. The first time that anyone had imaged the gamma chain 'transverse' cross-links. It was rejected by the Journal of Molecular Biology. I saved all the correspondence-it's good reading for those who want to experience denial statements by non-believers.*

142. **DEVELOPMENT OF A WHOLE PLATELET ELISA TO DETECT CIRCULATING ACTIVATED PLATELETS.** DL Amrani, L Stojanovic, **MN Mosesson**, Y Shalev, **MW Mosesson**. *J Lab Clin Med* 126:603-611, 1995 *Matt was working in my lab under David Amrani and he did a good job developing the assay. At that time he was thinking of a career in engineering research or medical school, or both, but unfortunately, he met Amber Jost and that changed everything for the worse. This was Matt's only research publication, and I was pleased to share authorship with him.*

143. **THE ROLE OF FIBRINOGEN D DOMAIN INTERMOLECULAR ASSOCIATION SITES IN THE POLYMERIZATION OF FIBRIN AND FIBRINOGEN TOKYO II (γ275 ARG→CYS).** MW Mosesson, KR Siebenlist, JP DiOrio, M Matsuda, JF Hainfeld, JS Wall. *J Clin Invest* 96:1053-1058, 1995 *A good idea!*

144. **ORIENTATION OF THE CARBOXY-TERMINAL REGIONS OF FIBRIN γ CHAIN DIMERS DETERMINED FROM THE CROSSLINKED PRODUCTS FORMED IN MIXTURES OF FIBRIN, FRAGMENT D, AND FACTOR XIIIa.** KR Siebenlist, DA Meh, JS Wall, JF Hainfeld, MW Mosesson. *Thromb Haemostas* 74:1113-1119, 1995. *Another successful set of experiments supporting a 'Transverse' cross-linking arrangement (see Chapter VI).*

145. **THE RELATIONSHIP BETWEEN THE FIBRINOGEN D DOMAIN SELF-ASSOCIATION/CROSSLINKING SITE (γXL) AND THE FIBRINOGEN DUSART ABNORMALITY (Aα R554C-ALBUMIN) – CLUES TO THROMBOPHILIA IN THE 'DUSART SYNDROME'.** MW Mosesson, KR Siebenlist, JF Hainfeld, JS Wall, J Soria, C Soria, JP Caen. *J Clin Invest* 97:2342-2350, 1996 *A creative idea that offered a rationale for the 'Dusart' Syndrome.*

146. **EVIDENCE FOR INTRAMOLECULAR CROSSLINKED Aα·γ CHAIN HETERODIMERS IN PLASMA FIBRINOGEN.** KR Siebenlist, MW Mosesson. *Biochemistry 35:5817-5821, 1996. We're still not sure how these cross-linked chains arise in the circulation, but they surely exist. My guess is: the intrinsic cross-linking activity of circulating Factor XIII.*

147. **PLASMA FACTOR XIII BINDS SPECIFICALLY TO FIBRINOGEN MOLECULES CONTAINING γ' CHAINS.** KR Siebenlist, DA Meh, MW Mosesson. *Biochemistry 35:10448-10453, 1996. This was an important discovery and with our subsequent interest in Antithrombin I, was often cited for its methodology and its concepts.*

148. **THE BASIS FOR FIBRINOGEN CEDAR RAPIDS (γ R275C) FIBRIN NETWORK STRUCTURE.** JP DiOrio, MW Mosesson, KR Siebenlist, JD Olson, JF Hainfeld, JS Wall. *Proc Microscopy Microanalysis 1:928-929, 1996. Part of our workup on Cedar Rapids fibrinogen.*

149. **IDENTIFICATION AND CHARACTERIZATION OF THE THROMBIN BINDING SITES ON FIBRIN.** DA Meh, KR Siebenlist, MW Mosesson. *J Biol Chem 271:23121-23125, 1996. An exposition of previous observations on the two classes of binding sites in fibrin.*

150. **EVALUATION OF THE FACTORS CONTRIBUTING TO FIBRIN-DEPENDENT PLASMINOGEN ACTIVATION.** MW Mosesson, KR Siebenlist, M Voskuilen, W Nieuwenhuizen. *Thromb Haemostas 79: 796-801, 1998.*

151. **HUMAN FIBROBLASTS BIND DIRECTLY TO FIBRINOGEN AT RGD SITES THROUGH INTEGRIN αvβ3.** J Gailit, C Clarke, D Newman, MG Tonneson, MW Mosesson, RAF Clark. *Exptl Cell Res 232:118-126, 1997.*

152. **THE ROLE OF PUTATIVE FIBRINOGEN Aα, Bβ and γA-CHAIN INTEGRIN BINDING SITES IN ENDOTHELIAL CELL MEDIATED CLOT RETRACTION.** RA Smith, MW Mosesson, MM Rooney, ST Lord, AU Daniels, TK Gartner. *J Biol Chem 272:22080-22085, 1997.*

153. **ENDOTHELIAL CELLS OF DIFFERING ORIGIN AND THEIR ADHESION TO THE FIBRINOGEN GAMMA CHAIN.** RA Smith, MM Rooney, ST Lord, MW Mosesson, AU Daniels, TK Gartner. *J Biol Chem, 1997.*

154. **FIBRINOGEN KURASHIKI (γ G268E) FIBRIN NETWORK STRUCTURE.** JP DiOrio, MW Mosesson, M Matsuda. *Microscopy Microanalysis* Suppl 2:1160-1161, 1998.

155. **THE LOCATION OF THE CARBOXY-TERMINAL REGION OF γ CHAINS IN FIBRINOGEN AND FIBRIN D DOMAINS.** MW Mosesson, KR Siebenlist, DA Meh, JS Wall, JF Hainfeld. *Proc Natl Acad Sci (USA)* 95:10511-10516, 1998 *One of my best in terms of insightful analyses of STEM mages. Should become an EM classic!*

156. **FIBRINOGEN MARBURG FIBRIN NETWORK STRUCTURE.** JP DiOrio, MW Mosesson, I Hernandez, T Sugo, M Matsuda. *Microscopy Microanalysis* Suppl 2:1119-1120, 1999.

157. **FIBRINOGEN NIIGATA WITH IMPAIRED FIBRINOGEN ASSEMBLY: AN INHERITED DYSFIBRINOGEN WITH A Bβ ASN-160 TO SER SUBSTITUTION ASSOCIATED WITH EXTRA GLYCOSYLATION AT Bβ ASN-158.** T Sugo, Nakamikawa, H Takano, J Mimuro, S-I Yamaguchi, MW Mosesson, DA Meh, JP DiOrio, N Takahashi, H Takahashi, K Nagai, M Matsuda. *Blood* 94:3806-3813, 1999.

158. **EVIDENCE FOR NEW ENDOTHELIAL CELL BINDING SITES ON FIBRINOGEN.** RA Smith, MM Rooney, ST Lord, MW Mosesson, TK Gartner. *Thromb Haemostas* 84:819-825, 2000.

159. **COEXISTING DYSFIBRINOGENEMIA (γR275C) AND FACTOR V LEIDEN DEFICIENCY ASSOCIATED WITH THROMBOEMBOLIC DISEASE (FIBRINOGEN CEDAR RAPIDS).** KR Siebenlist, MW Mosesson, DA Meh, JP DiOrio, RM Albrecht, JD Olson. *Blood Coag & Fibrinol* 11:293-304, 2000. *This study took some time to complete, and the answers we found were not readily explained, but it was worth the struggle. Among the ancillary findings was that α2-antiplasmin was tightly bound to fibrinogen.*

160. **POSITION OF γ CHAIN CARBOXY-TERMINAL REGIONS IN FIBRINOGEN:FIBRIN CROSSLINKING MIXTURES.** KR Siebenlist, DA Meh, MW Mosesson. *Biochemistry* 39:14171-14175, 2000. *We exploited the size differences between γ and γ' chains to prove that these two chains are transversely oriented between fibril strands when they become inter-molecularly cross-linked. One of several definitive experiments to examine this issue. Another nail in the 'D-D long' coffin.*

161. **CROSS-LINKING OF PLASMINOGEN ACTIVATOR INHIBITOR 2 AND α2-ANTIPLASMIN TO FIBRIN(OGEN).** H Ritchie, LC Lawrie, PW Crombie, MW Mosesson, NA Booth. *J Biol Chem* 275:24915-24920, 2000. *A collaboration originating at an International Fibrinogen Workshop Conference.*

162. **ADHESION OF MICROVASCULAR ENDOTHELIAL CELLS TO METALLIC IMPLANT SURFACES.** RA Smith, MW Mosesson, AV Daniels, TK Gartner. *J Mater Sci: Materials in Medicine* 11:279-285, 2000.

163. **THE AMINO ACID SEQUENCE IN FIBRIN RESPONSIBLE FOR HIGH AFFINITY THROMBIN BINDING.** DA Meh, KR Siebenlist, SO Brennan, T Holyst, MW Mosesson. *Thromb Haemostas 85:470-474, 2001 A key publication demonstrating the sequence in γ'chains that accounts for high affinity thrombin binding. It led to several more publications on this subject and remains a beacon for workers in this field.*

164. **PROTRANSGLUTAMINASE (FACTOR XIII) MEDIATED CROSSLINKING OF FIBRINOGEN AND FIBRIN.** Siebenlist KR, DA Meh, MW Mosesson. *Thromb Haemostas 86:1221-1228, 2001 Introducing a new concept concerning the fact that factor XIII is not a zymogen (an enzyme precursor) but rather an active enzyme. Kevin carried out these experiments. To this day, there are investigators who avoid coming to grips with these observations and conclusions. Among other things, this activity likely accounts for α2-antiplasmin that is covalently bound to circulating fibrinogen.*

165. **FOCUS ON HEMATOLOGY: FIBRINOGEN AS A DETERMINANT OF THE METASTATIC POTENTIAL OF TUMOR CELLS.** MW Mosesson. *Blood 96:330, 2000. An interpretive editorial.*

166. **FIBRINOGEN NAPLES I (Bβ A68T) NON- SUBSTRATE THROMBIN BINDING CAPACITIES.** DA Meh, MW Mosesson, KR Siebenlist, PJ Simpson-Haidaris, SO Brennan, JP DiOrio, K Thompson, G Di Minno. *Thromb Res 102:1-11, 2001 A middle author, Kevin Thompson, worked for me as a technologist for a year or two. He was shy and self-effacing person, yet I was nevertheless aware of him and his contributions to the study. He rewarded me with a clever diorama presenting several unused remnants from our laboratory at the time. The Naples paper itself was an outstanding piece of work that introduced a logical explanation for the pathophysiology of the Naples' affliction. A precursor project leading to the Thrombotic Microangiopathy study was reported a few years later (see ref. 187)*

167. **FIBRINOGEN AND FIBRIN ARE ANTI-ADHESIVE FOR KERATINOCYTES: A MECHANISM FOR FIBRIN ESCHAR SLOUGH DURING WOUND REPAIR.** M Kubo, L Van De Water, LC Plantefaber, MW Mosesson, M Simon, MG Tonnesen, L Taichman, RAF Clark. *J Invest Dermatol 117:1369-1381, 2001 I provided some key materials for this collaborative study with Richard Clark, then Chairman of the Dermatology Department at Stony Brook Medical Center.*

168. **CHARACTERIZATION OF A MOUSE MODEL FOR THROMBOMODULIN DEFICIENCY.** H Weiler, V Lindner, B Kerlin, B Isermann, SB Hendrickson, BC Cooley, DA Meh, MW Mosesson, NW Shworak, MJ Post, EM Conway. JH Ulfman, UH von Abdrian, JI Weitz. *Arterioscl Thromb Vasc Biol 21:1531-1537, 2001 Hardy Weiler liked to include everyone possible on his publications, including me (I'm somewhere in the middle of this one) and probably the BRI janitor as well. Problem was he didn't bring people like me aboard as intellectual partners. I would just as soon have been excluded from authorship.*

169. **DISINTEGRATION AND REORGANIZATION OF FIBRIN NETWORKS DURING tPA-INDUCED CLOT LYSIS.** DA Meh, MW Mosesson, JP Diorio, KR Siebenlist, I Hernandez, DL Amrani, L Stojanovic. *Blood Coag Fibrinol 12:627-637, 2001 A nice piece of work that has not to my knowledge, received the notoriety that it deserves. I surreptitiously included one of the EM images of 'disintegrating fibrin' as the picture on the cover page of Willem Nieuwenhuizen's and my New York Academy of Sciences 'Fibrinogen' book. Most people who commented upon that cover picture told me it was the most beautiful image of a fibrin clot they had ever seen-until I brought them back to reality by pointing out that the cover page 'clot' was an image of a dissolving clot that no longer had structural integrity.*

170. **FIBRINOGEN ASSEMBLY AND CROSSLINKING ON A FIBRIN FRAGMENT E TEMPLATE.** MW Mosesson, KR Siebenlist, I Hernandez, JS Wall, JF Hainfeld. *Thromb Haemostas 87:651-658, 2002 This was an outstanding investigation, largely supported by STEM images recorded at the Brookhaven Laboratory. This study further put to rest any credibility of John Weisel's arguments for a longitudinal cross-linking arrangement, or so I strongly believed. The analyses and my arguments were sharply honed to drive a dagger into Weisel's previous report. The results concerned as they were with the subject of γ chain cross-linking, were prominently featured in the written formal debate with John Weisel (see refs 175 and 176). With clearly outlined experiments such as these, I thought I would or at least, should, win the debate about the positioning of fibrin γ-chain cross-links. Weisel never capitulated and neither did Russ Doolittle (if anything Russ made it a political issue rather than one based upon scientific merit). I don't think Russ clearly understood the power of well-designed and conducted experiments. He remained fixated on the crystal structures of fragment D-dimers that really had little to do with a structured fibrin clot. Nothing I ever said to him, or wrote to him, made a lasting impression, nor did it change his personna. Let history and future events settle this issue. (Reminds me of Daniel Moynihan's aphorism: "Everyone can have his own set of own opinions, but not his own set of facts.")*

171. **THE INHIBITORY EFFECT OF FIBRINOGEN IN PLASMA ON THROMBIN GENERATION. ANTITHROMBIN I (FIBRIN).** NB De Bosch, MW Mosesson, A Ruiz-Sáez, M Echenagucia, A Rodriguez-Lemoin. *Thromb Haemostas* 88:253-258, 2002. *This was a memorable presentation recalling Walter Seegers' timely statement about 'Antithrombin I' ("It's in the right place at the right time").*

172. **CAUSE-EFFECT RELATION BETWEEN HYPERFIBRINOGENEMIA AND VASCULAR DISEASE.** B Kerlin, BC Cooley, BH Isermann, C Hartwig, DA Meh, M Zogg, SB Hendrickson, MW Mosesson, S Lord, H Weiler. *Blood* 103:1728-1734, 2004. *The many co-authors once again reflected Hardy Weiler's sense of 'democracy' and justice for all authors.*

173. **CRYSTAL STRUCTURE OF THE COMPLEX BETWEEN THROMBIN AND THE CENTRAL 'E' REGION OF FIBRIN.** I Pechik, J Madrazo, MW Mosesson, I Hernandez, GL:Gilliland, L Medved. *Proc Natl Acad Sci (USA)* 101:2718-2723, 2004. *It was a pleasure to be included as an author on this seminal work. I provided the hementin E fragments for the study.*

174. **REGULATION OF TRANSGLUTAMINASE ACTIVITY IN ARTICULAR CHONDROCYTES THROUGH THROMBIN RECEPTOR-MEDIATED FACTOR XIII SYNTHESIS.** AK Rosenthal, MW Mosesson, CM Gohr, I Masuda, D Heinkel, KR Siebenlist KR. *Thromb Haemostas* 91:558-568, 2004. *Ann Rosenthal was a rheumatologist at MCOW who was having great difficulties characterizing the transglutaminase (cross-linking) activity derived via articular chondrocyte production of factor XIII. She consulted us because her submitted work had been rejected by several rheumatology-style journals. Kevin and I discussed her problems at length, and we helped her clarify the situation. Into the bargain we all learned a great deal. The paper was finally accepted by TH.*

175. **CROSS-LINKED γ CHAINS IN FIBRIN FIBRILS BRIDGE 'TRANSVERSELY' BETWEEN STRANDS: YES.** MW Mosesson. *J Thromb Haemostas* 2:388-393, 2004. *This is a subject to which I devoted an entire chapter in these memoirs (see Chapter VI).*

176. **CROSS-LINKED CHAINS IN FIBRIN FIBRILS BRIDGE 'TRANSVERSELY' BETWEEN STRANDS.** (Forum) MW Mosesson. *J Thromb Haemostas* 2:1469-1471, 2004.

177. **EVIDENCE THAT CATALYTICALLY-INACTIVATED THROMBIN FORMS NON-COVALENTLY LINKED DIMERS THAT BRIDGE BETWEEN FIBRIN/FIBRINOGEN FIBERS AND ENHANCE FIBRIN POLYMERIZATION.** MW Mosesson, I Hernandez, KR Siebenlist. *Biophysical Chemistry* 110:93-100, 2004. *This article started out as what we call 'The Kaminski Effect' (Marek 'The Great' Kaminski that is). See ref 123 and Chapter VIII.*

178. **THE ULTRASTRUCTURE OF FIBRINOGEN-420 AND THE FIBRIN-420 CLOT.** MW Mosesson, JP DiOrio, I Hernandez, JF Hainfeld, JS Wall, G Grieninger. *Biophysical Chemistry* 112:209-214, 2004. *This was published in the 'Festschrift' I edited in honor of John Ferry. Gerd Grieninger had discovered fibrinogen-420, and I took advantage of the Festschrift issue to report on the remarkable ultrastructural features we had found.*

179. **JOHN FERRY AND THE MECHANICAL PROPERTIES OF CROSS-LINKED FIBRIN.** MW Mosesson. *Biophysical Chemistry* 112:215-218, 2004. *Another article I wrote for the Ferry Festschrift.*

180. **JOHN D FERRY'S PATENTS.** JL Schrag, MW Mosesson. *Biophysical Chemistry* 112:95-101, 2004. *In the Ferry Festschrift.*

181. **STUDIES ON THE BASIS FOR THE PROPERTIES OF FIBRIN PRODUCED FROM FIBRINOGEN CONTAINING γ' CHAINS.** KR Siebenlist, MW Mosesson, I Hernandez, LA Bush, E Di Cera, JR Shainoff, JP DiOrio, L Stojanovic. *Blood* 106:2730-2736, 2005. *Another article relating to γ' chains. Worth a read. By the way, Laura Bush was a computer programmer at St Luke's who helped us immensely in converting our data from BNL to a readable form. One day I questioned some of her procedures and asked, "Why are you insisting on doing it this way?" Her reply, "Because I'm the Mother!" I never forgot her comment and I never interrupted her again.*

182. **FIBRINOGEN SAINT-GERMAIN II: HYPOFIBRINOGENEMIA DUE TO HETEROZYGOUS γ N345S MUTATION.** E De Raucort, P de Mazancourt, GJ Maghzal, SO Brennan, MW Mosesson. *Thromb Haemostas* 94:965-968, 2005. *In August 2010 we visited Paris on a 'reunion' journey. Marie-Helene Denninger arranged for us to meet Emmanuele in person at a Bistro-a pleasure!*

183. **HYPOFIBRINOGENEMIA RESULTING FROM NOVEL SINGLE NUCLEOTIDE DELETION AT CODON Bβ58 (3404del A) ASSOCIATED WITH THROMBOTIC STROKE IN INFANCY.** SO Brennan, MW Mosesson, R Lowen, KR Siebenlist, A Matsunaga. *Thromb Haemostas* 95:738-739, 2006. *Ask Steve Brennan about this one.*

184. **STRUCTURAL BASIS FOR SEQUENTIAL CLEAVAGE OF FIBRINOPEPTIDES UPON FIBRIN ASSEMBLY.** I Pechik, S Yakovlev, MW Mosesson, GL Gilliland, L Medved. *Biochemistry* 45:3588-3597, 2006. *A rewarding collaboration with Leonid.*

185. **DYSFIBRINOGENEMIA (FIBRINOGEN WILMINGTON) DUE TO A NOVEL Aα CHAIN TRUNCATION CAUSING DECREASED EXPRESSION AND IMPAIRED FIBRIN POLYMERIZATION.** SO Brennan, MW Mosesson, R Lowen, C Frantz. *Thromb Haemostas* 96:88-89, 2006. *Another thorough job by Steve.*

186. **CRYSTAL STRUCTURE OF THROMBIN IN COMPLEX WITH FIBRINOGEN γ′ PEPTIDE.** AO Pineda, Z-W Chen, F Marino, FS Mathews, MW Mosesson, E Di Cera. *Biophys Chem* 125:556-559, 2006. *This one was a rewarding collaboration with Enrico Di Cera and Gus Pineda.*

187. **PLASMA FIBRINOGEN γ′ CHAIN CONTENT IN THE THROMBOTIC MICROANGIOPATHY SYNDROME.** MW Mosesson, I Hernandez, TJ Raife, L Medved, S Yakovlev, PJ Simpson-Haidaris, S Uitte de Willige, RM Bertina. *J Thromb Haemostas* 5:62-69, 2006. *An important paper in developing the basis for γ′ function.*

188. **THE EFFECT OF A THROMBIN EXOSITE 2-BINDING DNA APTAMER (HD-22) ON NON-CATALYTIC THROMBIN-ENH-ANCED FIBRIN POLYMERIZATION.** MW Mosesson. *Thromb Haemostas* 97:327328, 2007. *I did this study on my own. Sink or swim! An addendum to the 'Kaminski effect'.*

189. **FIBRINOGEN COLUMBUS: A NOVEL γ GLY200VAL MUTATION CAUSING HYPOFIBRINOGENEMIA IN A FAMILY WITH ASSOCIATED THROMBOPHILIA.** RL Davis, MW Mosesson, B Kerlin, J Canner, Ruymann, SO Brennan. *Haematologia* 92:1151-52, 2007. *Another dysfibrinogen study.*

190. **CONGENITAL HYPODYSFIBRINOGENEMIA (FIBRINOGEN DES MOINES, γ320ASP DELETED) ASSOCIATED WITH SEVERE SPONTANEOOUS PERIPHERAL ARTERIAL THROMBOEMBOLISM.** SO Brennan, Davis RL, Mosesson MW, Hernandez I, Lowen R, Alexander SJ. *Thromb Haemostas* 98:467-469, 2007 *Another in the series of collaborative works on dysfibrinogenemia with Steve Brennan.*

191. **CHANGES IN FIBRINOGEN AND FIBRIN INDUCED BY A PEPTIDE ANALOG OF FIBRINOGEN γ365–380.** C-E Dempfle, N Bindeballe, M Münchbach, C Blume, M Borggreffe, MW Mosesson. *J Thromb Haemostas* 5:1707-1714, 2007.

192. **CAVEOLIN-1 DEPENDENT APOPTOSIS INDUCED BY FIBRIN DEGRADATION PRODUCTS.** Y-H Guo, I Hernandez I, B Isermann B, T-B Kang, L Medved, R Sood, EJ Kerschen, T Holyst, MW Mosesson, H Weiler. *Blood* 113:4431-4439, 2009 *There were many problems in writing this paper. Even though I was next-to-last author I played a major role that I later regretted having played. To effect the changes that I had insisted were necessary, I refused to put my name on the paper (or Irene's or Leonid's) unless changes were made in the text. In the end the changes were made. Hardy Weiler further revealed his Teutonic and closed-minded nature. Read the related account of this work that can be found in my notes on this paper and in these memoirs.*

193. **NANOSCALE PROBING REVEALS THAT REDUCED STIFFNESS OF CLOTS FROM FIBRINOGEN LACKING 42 N-TERMINAL BBETA-CHAIN RESIDUES IS DUE TO THE FORMATION OF ABNORMAL OLIGOMERS.** RH Abou-Saleh, SD Connell, R Harrand, RA Ajjan, MW Mosesson, DA Smith, PJ. Grant, RA Ariens. *Biophys J* 18:2415-2427, 2009. *An idea that I planted with Robert a few years ago based upon my interpretation of images that he showed to me while he was visiting the BloodCenter as a lecturer.*

194. **EVIDENCE THAT α2-ANTIPLASMIN BECOMES COVALENTLY LIGATED TO PLASMA FIBRINOGEN IN THE CIRCULATION: A NEW ROLE FOR PLASMA FACTOR XIII IN FIBRINOLYSIS REGULATION.** MW Mosesson, KR Siebenlist, I Hernandez, KN Lee, VJ Christiansen, PA McKee. *J Thromb Haemostas* 6:1565-1570, 2008. *This study was an ongoing project with the Diagnostics lab at the BloodCenter. We were trying to develop an ELISA for plasma fibrinogen-bound α2-AP in partnership. The hard part was creating a calibration standard (see Chapter IX).*

195. **THROMBOSIS RISK MODIFICATION IN TRANSGENIC MICE CONTAINING THE HUMAN FIBRINOGEN THROMBIN-BINDING GAMMA' CHAIN SEQUENCE.** MW Mosesson, BC Cooley, I Hernandez, JP DiOrio, HW Weiler. *J Thromb Haemostas* 7:102-110, 2009. *I had to argue at length with hardy Weiler about preserving the original organization and focus of this work. Glad that I did! I've kept some of the dialogue that took place with Hardy Weiler.*

196. **SHORT BY ONE MECHANISM: A REBUTTAL*** (Letter-To-The-Editor) MW Mosesson. *J Thromb Haemostas* 8: 2089-2090, 2010. *No new information of any value to the cross-linking issue had appeared since the formal debate between Weisel and me in 2004. In 2010 Martin Guthold uncritically joined the Doolittle/Weisel 'DD-long' camp. Guthold is a biophysicist who carried out atomic force microscopy experiments on stretching and breaking of noncross-linked and cross-linked fibrin fibers. That report stimulated my 'Letter-to-the-Editor'. They had posited three mechanisms that could account for their observations, but they did not consider the most likely one, 'transverse cross-linking'-not one mention! (see Chapter VI).*

*Without my knowledge or permission the editors added "A REBUTTAL" to my Letter in order to accommodate a response by Guthold and Carlisle (p. 2090-91) entitled: "REPLY TO A REBUTTAL".

197. **EVIDENCE FOR COVALENT LINKAGE BETWEEN SOME PLASMA α2-ANTIPLASMIN MOLECULES AND Aα CHAINS OF CIRCULATING FIBRINOGEN** (Letter-To-The Editor). MW Mosesson, T Holyst, J Hernandez, KR Siebenlist. *J Thromb Haemostas* 11:995-8, 2013. *My earlier observations and reports demonstrated tight binding between α2-AP and fibrinogen, but the nature of the bond was unknown. Evidence that the bond was covalent (i.e., a presumed factor XIII–catalyzed 'cross-link') had been lacking. I carried out these studies using Western Blotting. Took me over two years to complete the experiments and interpret them!*

BOOKS, MONOGRAPHS, CHAPTERS, EDITORIALS, MEMORIALS, REVIEWS

1. **THE FIBRINOGENOLYTIC PATHWAY OF FIBRINOGEN CATABOLISM.** MW Mosesson. *Thromb Res* 2:182-300, 1973 *A review emphasizing circulating fibrinogen catabolites.*

2. **FIBRINOGEN CATABOLIC PATHWAYS-DETERMINATIONS FROM ANALYSIS OF THE STRUCTURAL FEATURES OF CIRCULATING FIBRINOGEN AND OF DERIVATIVES PRODUCED IN VITRO BY THE ACTION OF PLASMIN OR THROMBIN.** MW Mosesson. *Semin Thromb Hemost* 1:63-84, 1974. *A Review.*

3. **INTRODUCTION.** (HJ Day, MW Mosesson, R Colman, eds) *Thromb Diath Haemor* 33:405, 1975. NATIONAL CONFERENCE ON THROMBOSIS AND HEMOSTASIS, Dallas Texas, 20-22 November 1974. *Conference proceedings.*

4. **THE SEARCH FOR THE STRUCTURE OF FIBRINOGEN.** MW Mosesson, JS Finlayson *Prog Hemostas Thromb* (TH Spaet, ed) 3:61-107, 1976 (chapter). *A detailed review of knowledge at the time. One important hypothesis about fibrinogen structure was not correct, and I corrected my mistake in later studies (see Chapter V).*

5. **COLD INSOLUBLE GLOBULIN (CIg), A CIRCULATING CELL SURFACE PROTEIN.** MW Mosesson. *Thromb Haemost* 38:742-750, 1977. *A Review.*

6. **THE STRUCTURE AND BIOLOGICAL ACTIVITIES OF PLASMA FIBRONECTIN.** MW Mosesson, DL Amrani. *Blood* 56:145-158, 1980. *A Review.*

7. **THE POTENTIAL OF HEPARIN AS AN AGENT FOR PRECIPITATION OF PLASMA FIBRONECTIN (CIg) AND CERTAIN COMPONENTS OF THE PLASMA FACTOR VIII COMPLEX.** MW Mosesson, DL Amrani. *The Chemistry*

and Biology of Heparin (Brown WV, KG Mann, HR Roberts, RL Lundblad, eds) Elsevier North-Holland, NY, Pub. 105-111, 1981. *A Review.*

8. **THE ROLE OF PLASMA FIBRONECTIN IN MONOCYTE/MACROPHAGE FUNCTION.** MW Mosesson. *Verhand Deutsche Gesell Inn Med* 88:1277-1288, 1982. *A Review,*

10. **MOLECULAR BIOLOGY OF FIBRINOGEN AND FIBRIN.** (MW Mosesson, RF Doolittle, eds) *Annals of the New York Academy of Sciences* 408:1-672, 1983 (book). *This was a timely conference that convened most of the key players in the field and led to what was referred to for a long time as the 'Fibrinogen Bible'.*

9. **FIBRINOGEN HETEROGENEITY.** MW Mosesson. *Ann NY Acad Sci* 408:97-113, 1983. *A Review.*

11. **PLASMA FIBRONECTIN: ROLES IN HEMOSTASIS, MACROPHAGE FUNCTION, AND RELATED PROCESSES.** DF Mosher, MW Mosesson. *Hematology (vol. 2): Haemostasis and Thrombosis,* Butterworth and Co., Pub, 173-196, 1985. *A Book Chapter. Deane Mosher did most of the writing for this review, but he wanted me to co-author something with him and I gladly agreed.*

12. **INTERACTIONS BETWEEN GLYCOSAMINOGLYCANS AND FIBRONECTIN.** MW Mosesson, DL Amrani, *Plasma Fibronectin. Structure and Function.* (McDonagh J, ed) Marcel Dekker, NY, Pub, 77-97, 1985. *A Book Chapter.*

13. **ORGANIZATION AND STRUCTURE OF THE FIBRINOGEN GENES.** MW Mosesson. *Fibrinogen and Its Derivatives 2. Biochemistry, Physiology and Clinical Relevance* (Lowe GDO, JT Douglas, CD Forbes, A Henschen, eds) Elsevier Science Pub, NY, 3-8, 1987. *A review. Patrick Gaffney talked me into presenting a summary of the fibrinogen genes. A good learning experience for me and I hope for those who listened to my presentation.*

14. **FIBRINOGEN 3. BIOCHEMISTRY, BIOLOGICAL FUNCTIONS, GENE REGULATION AND EXPRESSION.** (MW Mosesson, DL Amrani, JP DiOrio, KR Siebenlist, eds) Elsevier Science Pub, NY., 1-361, 1988. *Book. This meeting of the International Fibrinogen Workshop Fibrinogen Research Society was held in Milwaukee at the Marc Plaza. A great success! (see Chapter XI).*

15. **D-DIMER, AN AMBIGUOUS MARKER OF THROMBOLYSIS.** MW Mosesson. *J Lab Clin Med* 113:662, 1989. *Editorial commentary.*

16. **FIBRIN POLYMERIZATION AND ITS REGULATORY ROLE IN HEMOSTASIS.** MW Mosesson. *J Lab Clin Med* 116:8-17, 1990. *A Review.*

17. **FIBRIN POLYMERIZATION AND ITS ROLE IN REGULATING HEMOSTASIS.** MW Mosesson. In New Trends in Haemostasis (Harenberg J, Heene DL, Stehle G, Schettler G, eds.) Springer-Verlag, Berlin 27-43, 1990. *A Book Chapter.*

18. **COLLAGEN AND THE DEVELOPMENT OF RESISTANCE TO FIBRIN CLOT LYSIS.** MW Mosesson. *J Lab Clin Med* 117:265, 1991. *An Editorial.*

19. **FIBRONECTINS.** MW Mosesson. *Cell* 64:1054-55, 1991. *A Book Review.*

20. **THE ROLES OF FIBRINOGEN AND FIBRIN IN HEMOSTASIS AND THROMBOSIS.** MW Mosesson. *Seminars in Hematology* 29:177-188, 1992. *A Review.*

21. **THE ASSEMBLY AND STRUCTURE OF THE FIBRIN CLOT.** MW Mosesson. *Nouv Rev Fr Hematol* 34:11-16, 1992. *A Review.*

22. **THROMBIN INTERACTIONS WITH FIBRINOGEN AND FIBRIN.** MW Mosesson. *Sem Thromb Hemostas* 19:361-367, 1993. *A Review.*

23. **A MEMORIAL TO SOL SHERRY, M.D. (1916-1993).** MW Mosesson. *Thromb Res* 72:91-98, 1993. *A Memorial. Sol Sherry was like a father to me and I admired him for his wisdom and his perspectives.*

24. **FIBRINOGEN AND FIBRIN POLYMERIZATION: APPRAISAL OF THE BINDING EVENTS THAT ACCOMPANY FIBRIN GENERATION AND FIBRIN CLOT ASSEMBLY.** MW Mosesson. *Blood Coag Fibrinolysis* 8:257-267, 1997. *A Review.*

25. **FIBRINOGEN STRUCTURE AND FIBRIN ASSEMBLY.** MW Mosesson. *Sem Thromb Hemostas* 24;169-174, 1998. *A Review.*

26. **FIBRIN(OGEN) STRUCTURE AND THE MULTIPLE EVENTS THAT ACCOMPANY FIBRIN CLOT ASSEMBLY. MW** Mosesson *International Symposium on Clot Formation and Lysis* (Hamamatsu, Japan, March 1997) *in:* Recent Progress in Blood Coagulation and Fibrinolysis (A Takada, D Collen, PJ Gaffney, eds) Elsevier Science, Amsterdam, The Netherlands, 1997. *A Book Chapter. I attended and participated in this meeting in Hamamatsu. The only problem I had subsequently, was that Aki Takada forgot to include my manuscript in the final publication. There were some memorable pictures that were published in the book. Among them is one of me with my head bowed at a dinner held on the first day. You guessed it; I was asleep.*

27. **DYSFIBRINOGENEMIA AND THROMBOSIS.** MW Mosesson. *in:* Seminars in Thrombosis and Hemostasis (Bick RL, ed) 25:311-319, 1999. *A Review.*

28. **FIBRINOGEN UND FIBRIN.** MW Mosesson. *in:* Hämostaseologie (G Müller-Berghaus, B Pötzsch, eds) Springer-Verlag, Berlin, pp 285-290, 1999. *A Book Chapter (translated into German by Gert Müller-Berghaus' wife, Rotraut.)*

29. **FIBRINOGEN AND FIBRIN POLYMERIZATION AND FUNCTIONS.** MW Mosesson. *Blood Coag Fibrinolysis* 10 (suppl 1):45-48, 1999. *A Review.*

30. **FIBRINOGEN FUNCTIONS AND FIBRIN ASSEMBLY.** MW Mosesson. *Fibrinol Proteol* 14:182-186, 2000. *A Review.*

31. **HEREDITARY DISORDERS OF FIBRINOGEN.** MW Mosesson. *in: Williams' Hematology, 6th edition* (E Beutler, MA Lichtman, BS Coller, TJ Kipps, U Seligsohn, eds) McGraw-Hill, New York, pp 1659-1671, 2001. *A Textbook Chapter. This was the best organized and comprehensive review of hereditary fibrinogen disorders written up to that time.*

32. **FIBRINOGEN.** W Nieuwenhuizen, MW Mosesson, M De Maat, eds. *The New York Academy of Sciences*, vol 936: 1-643, 2001. *A Book. This meeting was sponsored by the NY Academy of Sciences and held in Leiden, The Netherlands. It was the successor to the 'Fibrinogen Bible' (1983).*

33. **THE STRUCTURE AND BIOLOGICAL FEATURES OF FIBRINOGEN OF FIBRINOGEN AND FIBRIN.** MW Mosesson, KR Siebenlist, DA Meh. *in* **Fibrinogen** (W Nieuwenhuizen, MW Mosesson, M De Maat., eds). *The New York Academy of Sciences* 936:11-30, 2001. *A Chapter.*

34. **CHARACTERIZATION OF CROSSLINKING SITES IN FIBRINOGEN FOR PLASMINOGEN ACTIVATOR INHIBITOR 2 (PAI-2).** H Ritchie, LC Lawrie, MW Mosesson, NA Booth. *in* Fibrinogen (W Nieuwenhuizen, MW Mosesson, M De Maat., eds). *The New York Academy of Sciences*, vol 936: pp 215-218, 2001. *A Review Article.*

35. **FIBRINOGEN γ CHAIN FUNCTIONS. MW Mosesson.** *J Thromb Haemostas.* 1:231-238, 2003. *A Review Article.*

36. **ANTITHROMBIN I. INHIBITION OF THROMBIN GENERATION IN PLASMA BY FIBRIN FORMATION.** MW Mosesson. *Thromb Haemostas.*89:9-12, 2003 (review article)

37. **STEWART ANTHONY CEDERHOLM-WILLIAMS, PhD (1947-2002).** L Medved, MW Mosesson, I Sandys, N Lukinova, M MacPhee. *Thromb Haemostas.* 89 (2):XII, 2003. *A Memorial.*

38. **JOHN DOUGLASS FERRY (1912-2002)-A MEMORIAL TRIBUTE.** MW Mosesson. *Biophysical Chemistry* 104:1-4, 2003. *In the Festschrift honoring John Ferry.*

39. **THEME ISSUE: FIBRINOGEN AND FIBRIN–STRUCTURE, FUNCTION, INTERACTIONS AND CLINICAL APPLICATIONS.** C-E Dempfle, MW Mosesson. *Thromb Haemostas* 89:599-600, 2003. *An Editorial.*

40. **AFIBRINOGENEMIA IN A COMPOUND HETEROZYGOTE-MAKING SENSE OUT OF MISSENSE.** MW Mosesson. *Blood* 102:4247-4248, 2003. *Inside Blood-Editorial.*

41. **FIBRINOGEN CONTRIBUTIONS TO ARTERIAL THROMBUS FORMATION-VESSEL SIZE COUNTS.** MW Mosesson. *Blood* 103:1977-1978, 2004. *Inside Blood Editorial.*

42. **FIBRINOLYSIS.** MW Mosesson. *Clin Lab Haem* 26 (suppl 1): 1-4, 2004. *A Review.*

43. **JOHN D FERRY-SPECIAL ISSUE.** (MW Mosesson, E Di Cera, eds). *Biophysical Chemistry* 112 (2/3):89-302, 2004. *A Festschrift to honor John Ferry.*

44. **JOHN D FERRY-SPECIAL ISSUE.** (MW Mosesson, E Di Cera, eds). **EDITORIAL.** MW Mosesson, E Di Cera. *Biophysical Chemistry* 112 (2/3):89-90, 2004. *An Editorial.*

45. **JOHN D FERRY-SPECIAL ISSUE.** (MW Mosesson, E Di Cera, eds). **JOHN DOUGLASS FERRY (1912-2002)-A MEMORIAL TRIBUTE.** MW Mosesson. *Biophysical Chemistry* 112 (2/3):91-93, 2004. *A Memorial Reprised.*

46. **FIBRINOGEN AND FIBRIN STRUCTURE AND FUNCTIONS.** MW Mosesson. *J Thromb Haemostas* 3:1894-1904, 2005. *ISTH State-of-the-Art Lecture.*

47. **HEREDITARY FIBRINOGEN ABNORMALITIES.** MW Mosesson. *in: Williams' Hematology*, 7th edition (E Beutler, MA Lichtman, BS Coller, TJ Kipps, U Seligsohn U, eds) McGraw-Hill, New York, pp, 2005. *A Textbook Chapter. An update of my original chapter-twice was enough!*

48. **STRUCTURE AND FUNCTIONS OF FIBRINOGEN AND FIBRIN.** MW Mosesson. *in: Recent Advances in Thrombosis and Hemostasis* (K Tanaka, EW Davie, Y Ikeda, S Iwanaga, H Saito, K Sueishi, eds) Springer, Japan, pp3-26, 2008. *A Review.*

49. **UPDATE ON ANTITHROMBIN I (FIBRIN).** Mosesson MW. *Thromb Haemostas* 98:105-108, 2007. *A Review.*

50. **JOHN DOUGLASS FERRY (1912-2002). A BIOGRAPHICAL MEMOIR.** Landel RF, MW Mosesson, JL Schrag. *Proc Nat'l Acad Sci (USA)* 2008. *The 'official' Memorial for John Ferry who was a member of the National Academy of Sciences. Robert Landel asked me to contribute part of this article.*

January 23, 2014

THE AUTHOR

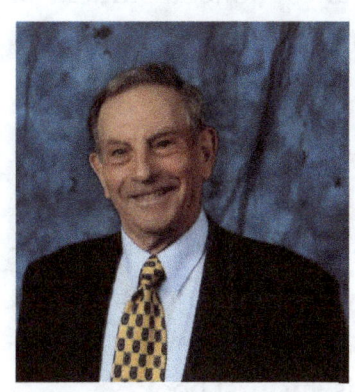

Dr. Michael Mosesson, the author.

Born in New York City and raised in Brooklyn, Michael Mosesson's formal education was entirely local: PS 134, Montauk Jr. High School, Erasmus Hall High School, Brooklyn College [BS], State University of New York, Downstate Medical Center (SUNY) [MD]. Medical School graduation led him to post-graduation clinical training at Boston City Hospital's Harvard Medical Service and subsequently at Barnes Hospital's Ward Medical Service in St Louis, Missouri. Between clinical training periods, he spent three years in the US Public Health Service (USPHS) stationed at The Division of Biologics Standards (DBS) on the National Institutes of Health (NIH) campus. During USPHS service he completed courses in Biophysics, Differential Equations, Protein Chemistry, and Enzyme Kinetics, and applied this knowledge at DBS (which evolved to become an FDA subsidiary) to initiate research projects on protein purification, blood coagulation, and fibrinolysis, and to conduct oversight of Blood Banks and licensing of Biological Reagents.

Mosesson spent 36 years as an academic Faculty Member, Teacher, Research Investigator, and Clinician at Washington University-Barnes Hospital, at SUNY-Downstate Medical Center, and at The University of Wisconsin Medical School's Milwaukee Clinical Campus [Research Division Director]. During that period he became a member of several prestigious societies that included The American Society for Clinical Investigation (ASCI) and The Association of American Physicians (AAP), and he attained the academic ranks of Professor of Medicine and Professor of Biochemistry. Following these experiences, he relocated to The Blood Research Institute of the BloodCenter of Wisconsin where he continued to pursue his research interests for 15 additional years.

His research focus was on Hemostasis, Thrombosis, and Fibrinolysis with emphasis on blood clotting proteins Fibrinogen and Fibrin, Factor VIII (Hemophilia Factor A}, and Factor XIII (Plasma Protransglutaminase), the fibrinolytic proenzyme Plasminogen, and the fibrinolytic agents Streptokinase and Urokinase. These productive adventures were supplemented by several summer detours at The Marine Biological Laboratory to investigate the clotting system of the Horseshoe Crab (*Limulus Polyphemus*).

Over a career spanning more than fifty years he authored more than 250 scientific papers, books, and review articles. He founded The International Fibrinogen Research

Society (IFRS) in 1990 and served as its President for more than thirteen years. In addition to his academic and scientific achievements, Mosesson is a Francophone, a student of Classical Music, and was an active pilot for more than fifty years.

One special interest was Electron Microscopy which he first studied during a sabbatical year at Hôpital Beaujon in Paris, France, and then vastly expanded that knowledge at The Scanning Transmission Electron Microscopy (STEM) facility at the Brookhaven National Laboratory. He successfully applied STEM to elucidate ultra-structural, quantitative, and functional aspects of proteins such as Fibrinogen, Fibrin, Factor V, Factor VIII, and Fibronectin. He remains actively engaged in publishing non-technical accounts of his previously published work, such as this, his first book.